Lower Extremity Nerve Entrapments

Marcelo J. S. Magalhães

Lower Extremity Nerve Entrapments

Clinical Diagnosis and Treatment

Springer

Marcelo J. S. Magalhães
Department of Neurosurgery
Hospital Aroldo Tourinho
Montes Claros, Minas Gerais, Brazil

ISBN 978-3-031-90057-0 ISBN 978-3-031-90058-7 (eBook)
https://doi.org/10.1007/978-3-031-90058-7

The original submitted manuscript has been translated into English. The translation was done using artificial intelligence. A subsequent revision was performed by the author(s) to further refine the work and to ensure that the translation is appropriate concerning content and scientific correctness. It may, however, read stylistically different from a conventional translation.

This Springer imprint is published by the registered company Springer Nature Switzerland AG
The registered company address is: Gewerbestrasse 11, 6330 Cham, Switzerland

Prologue

Compressive pathology of peripheral nerves is a prevalent entity, which in many communities exceeds the incidence of traumatic and compressive pathology. In the world literature, compressive neuropathies of the upper limbs have traditionally attracted the attention of clinicians, researchers, and surgeons, so compressions of the lower limbs have been relegated to the background. This book, which I am sure will become a must-read for neurosurgeons, traumatologists, and plastic surgeons, provides an updated look at a constellation of compressive syndromes that are often forgotten. Those who are beginning their journey in the exciting world of peripheral nerve surgery and those who have experience in the subject will be seduced by its content. Inside, the reader will find a complete development of the most frequent neuropathies, such as peroneal nerve compression or meralgia paresthetica, but will also have the opportunity to update and deepen their anatomical and clinical knowledge of other much less frequent or controversial entities, such as piriformis syndrome.

Likewise, its modern content includes considerations regarding classic neurophysiological studies and ultrasound and resonance, among others. Tendon transfers for Stepagge have also been carefully addressed.

The indications for surgery in compressions are not exempt from discussion and controversy. Conservative treatment is imposed as the initial approach in sensitive cases but should not be delayed when there is motor involvement. Indeed, these considerations, pillars of management in compressive pathologies, are discussed in depth in this work.

In summary, I would like to congratulate Dr. Marcelo Magalhães, who has dedicated this work exclusively to exploring a topic not always looked at by the literature as it should be.

Mariano Socolovsky

Head of Neurosurgery, Hospital de Clínicas
University of Buenos Aires
Buenos Aires, Argentina

Professor of Neurosurgery, Faculty of Medicine
University of Buenos Aires
Buenos Aires, Argentina

Chairman, Peripheral Nerve Committee
World Federation of Neurosurgical Societies
(2013–2019 and 2023–2025)
Prague, Czech Republic

Preface

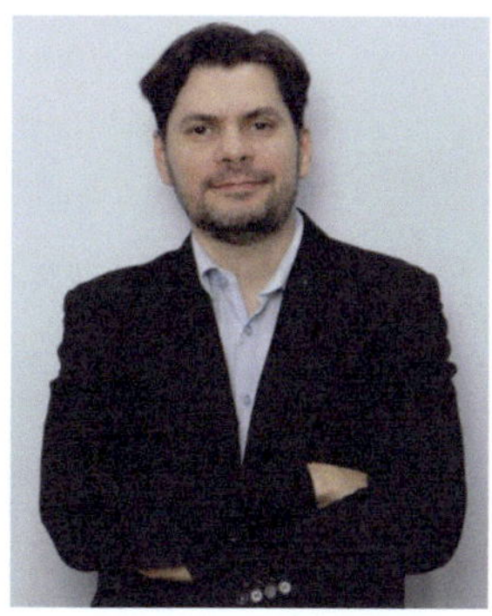

Peripheral nerve surgery is a broad field that has grown significantly in recent decades. Currently, we identify orthopedists, plastic surgeons, and neurosurgeons as professionals involved in the treatment of peripheral nerve diseases. This universe of diseases includes brachial plexus injuries, nerve tumors, traumatic injuries of peripheral and cranial nerves, as well as neuropathies of different etiologies. Compressive syndromes constitute a heterogeneous group of neuropathies, where much scientific activity has been developed, especially with regard to the different treatment modalities of the most prevalent neuropathies, such as those involving the fibular nerve. On the other hand, some of these syndromes still have significant gaps in knowledge, particularly the rare neuropathies that affect the lower limbs.

Thanks to the exchange between the different medical specialties that manage patients with compressive neuropathies of the lower limbs, a lot of new knowledge has been added in relation to differential diagnoses, imaging exams, and new techniques for pain control.

This book offers the surgeon a holistic view of the patient with compressive neuropathy in the lower limbs. Each chapter addresses epidemiological aspects, anatomical aspects, as well as those related to conservative and surgical management.

Greater emphasis is given to the surgical treatment of compressive neuropathies. Each chapter includes anatomical illustrations and photographs of surgical approaches that will assist in the management of your patients. Some videos address both the surgical aspects of neuropathies and other topics.

There is a chapter that deals with myotendinous transfer for the treatment of foot drop, a technique of great value for the management of neurological injuries that result in paresis of foot dorsiflexion.

I believe this work will be of great value to surgeons who wish to delve into peripheral nerve surgery, an area that, unlike others, provides the surgeon with a good quality of life.

I hope this work provides you with the necessary theoretical substrate for your clinical-surgical practice to promote patient well-being, which is the ultimate goal of all areas of medicine.

Buenos Aires, Argentina Marcelo J. S. Magalhães

Acknowledgments

First and foremost, I thank God for the opportunity to work in the field of nerve surgery and for the chance to share a bit of my experience with other surgeons who are passionate about this fascinating field.

To my wife, Aline, and my daughter, Clara, for their unwavering support, even during my absences throughout the process of writing this text and participating in conferences around the world.

To the Peripheral Nerve Surgery Group of the Brazilian Society of Neurosurgery, of which I have the honor to be a member. Without you, I would not have advanced or fallen in love with this field.

To my colleagues at Aroldo Tourinho Hospital and Vila da Serra Hospital in Brazil.

To my colleagues at Clínica Aliviar, Policlínica Bom Jesus, and Clínica Sempre Saúde, where I also have the privilege to practice.

To the medical schools at FUNORTE and UNIFIPMoc, where I have been teaching for over a decade.

To Dr. Mariano Socolovsky, for the opportunity to complete the Fellowship in Buenos Aires, Argentina.

To Dr. Lukas Rasulic, for the chance to participate in the Fellowship at the University Clinical Centre of Serbia.

To the team at Springer Nature, for believing in my work.

And finally, to my patients, who are the greatest inspiration for this book.

Contents

Chapter 1
Epidemiology of Lower Limb Nerve Entrapments

1.1 Introduction

Knowledge about the epidemiology of compressive neuropathies helps health professionals to direct their neurological examination and save financial resources during the diagnosis process of peripheral neuropathies. Also knowing the risk factors most associated with a certain compressive neuropathy increases the chances that the doctor makes the correct diagnosis. It is important to keep in mind that some of these risk factors are curable or controlled through appropriate clinical management, such as diabetes mellitus (DM), Hansen's disease, hypothyroidism, and deficiencies of B complex vitamins.

About 2.4% of the world population is affected by peripheral neuropathy (PN), so that in the elderly population, this prevalence reaches 8% [1].

The study by Trivedi et al. (2017), which involved a review of epidemiological studies between 1991 and 2004, showed that the prevalence of PN in the population of different parts of India varied between 5 and 2400 for every 10,000 inhabitants [2]. Gosh et al. (2006) in a study, also conducted in India, evaluated 225 patients with diagnoses of acute and chronic neuropathies. This study revealed that Guillain-Barré syndrome (GBS) was the most prevalent neuropathy, accounting for 24.8% of cases, diabetic polyneuropathy 11.1%, hereditary sensorimotor neuropathy 7.55%, Hansen's disease 4.8%, nutritional/alcoholic 3.55%, and compressive neuropathy 3.55% [3]. These authors also revealed that in 17.3% of cases it was not possible to identify the etiology associated with the patient's PN [3].

Regarding the epidemiology of neuropathies in North America, the study by Hicks et al. (2021) described that the prevalence of PN in the US population aged ≥40 years, defined by insensitivity to monofilament, was 13.5%, equivalent to 18.6 million inhabitants. These same authors also evaluated the population with DM that presented 28.4% (4.2 million inhabitants) of PN. It was observed that among

M. J. S. Magalhães, *Lower Extremity Nerve Entrapments*,
https://doi.org/10.1007/978-3-031-90058-7_1

individuals without DM the prevalence of PN was 11.8% (14.4 million inhabitants) [4]. This study also revealed that female individuals and those with a black phenotype had higher chances of developing PN. Other risk factors identified in this study were described: high body mass index (BMI), tall stature, low level of education, and peripheral arterial disease [4]. Some risk factors offered the patient a moderate relative risk for the development of PN such as systemic arterial hypertension (SAH), cardiovascular disease, and chronic kidney disease (CKD) [4].

It is noted that few articles on the epidemiology of compressive syndromes of the lower limbs are available in the medical literature. In a study conducted with the Egyptian population regarding neuropathies revealed that peroneal nerve neuropathy is the most prevalent among those identified, with an incidence around 19–40/100,000 inhabitants/year, totaling between 0.6% and 1.2% of all identified neuropathies [5, 6]. When disregarding the location of the neuropathy, carpal tunnel and cubital tunnel syndromes occupy the first two positions [5].

The objective of this chapter is to discuss the epidemiological data of the main compressive neuropathies of the lower limbs, as well as, comment on the risk factors most associated with these neuropathies.

1.2 Risk Factors for Peripheral Neuropathies

The process of investigating the risk factors/etiology of PN is often difficult and sometimes, no etiology is identified. The correct identification could allow the patient, suffering from a potentially serious underlying disease, to receive appropriate management. See Table 1.1 for identification of the most common clinical findings of risk factors/etiology of peripheral neuropathies.

Table 1.1 Etiology/risk factors of peripheral neuropathies and some complementary exams that can assist in the diagnosis

Name of neuropathy/ disease	Symptoms, signs, and laboratory findings	Complementary exams
Carpal tunnel syndrome [7]	Pain/paresthesia in the palmar region of the I, II, III digits of the hand and lateral face of the IV digit and thenar atrophy	Electroneuromyography of the upper limbs, wrist US
Cubital tunnel syndrome [7]	Pain/paresthesia in the palmar region on the medial face of the IV digit and V digit. Atrophy of the interosseous muscles.	Electroneuromyography of the upper limbs, elbow US
Common peroneal syndrome [7]	Pain/paresthesia in the region of the dorsum of the foot and lateral face of the leg. Paresis for dorsiflexion of the foot, eversion of the foot, and extension of the toes and hallux	Electroneuromyography of the lower limbs. Fibular tunnel US

(continued)

Table 1.1 (continued)

Name of neuropathy/ disease	Symptoms, signs, and laboratory findings	Complementary exams
Piriformis syndrome [7]	Pain in the gluteal region, ipsilateral sciatica	Electroneuromyography of the lower limbs, pelvis MRI
Posterior tarsal tunnel syndrome [7]	Pain in the medial region of the foot, plantar region pain	Electroneuromyography of the lower limbs, MRI of the foot, US of the foot
Anterior tarsal tunnel syndrome [7]	Pain in the region of the first interdigital space	Electroneuromyography of the lower limbs. Foot X-ray. Computed tomography of the foot. Foot MRI
Hypothyroidism [8]	Neuropathy, fatigue, alopecia, edema in lower limbs, mood changes, weight gain, trophic skin changes, hoarseness, speech slowing, facial changes, cold intolerance	TSH, Free T4. Electroneuromyography of the limbs. Ultrasound of the thyroid gland
Diabetes mellitus [8]	Increased thirst, hyperphagia, weight loss, polyuria, neuropathy in lower limbs. Pain and burning in the lower limbs	Fasting blood glucose, HBA1C, glucose tolerance test, electroneuromyography of the lower limbs
Sjögren's syndrome [9]	Xerostomia, dry eye, parotid enlargement	Anti-Ro, anti-La, electroneuromyography of the limbs. Schirmer's test
Vitamin B12 deficiency [10]	Peripheral polyneuropathy, degeneration of the posterior funiculus, cognitive changes, megaloblastic anemia	Serum vitamin B12 dosage, methylmalonic acid, homocysteine, upper digestive endoscopy, schilling test. Electroneuromyography of the limbs. MRI of the cervical and thoracic spine
HIV [11]	Weight loss, recurrent infections, chronic diarrhea, polyneuropathy, fatigue, night sweats, persistent fever, oral candidiasis, lymphadenopathies, herpes zoster, anemia, thrombocytopenia, leukopenia, anorexia, Kaposi's sarcoma, oral hairy leukoplakia	HIV serology Complete blood count (lymphocyte count)
Amyloidosis [12]	Neuropathy, heart failure, nephrotic syndrome, painless hepatomegaly, dyspnea, hoarseness, cerebral hemorrhage, gastric atony, malabsorption, goiter	Genetic test for transthyretin, biopsy, electroneuromyography of the limbs
Lyme disease [13]	Erythema migrans, fatigue, chills, fever, headache, neck stiffness, myalgias, arthralgias, arthritis, polymorphic erythema, atrioventricular blocks and rarely myopericarditis and cardiomegaly	Serology for *Borrelia* spp., electroneuromyography of the limbs

(continued)

Table 1.1 (continued)

Name of neuropathy/ disease	Symptoms, signs, and laboratory findings	Complementary exams
Cytomegalovirus [14]	Neuropathy, fever, flu-like symptoms	Serology for cytomegalovirus, electroneuromyography of the limbs
Zika virus [15]	Arthralgias, retroocular pain, polyneuropathy, fever, fatigue, maculopapular rash, conjunctivitis, headache	Serological test for the Zika virus, electroneuromyography of the limbs
COVID-19 [16]	Fever, cough, diffuse myalgia, peripheral neuropathies, anosmia, arthralgias	PCR for COVID-19, electroneuromyography of the limbs
Guillain-Barré syndrome [17]	Polyneuropathy, symmetric paresis, areflexia, and progressive, usually initiated in the lower limbs, paresthesias, in severe cases respiratory failure and ocular involvement	Lumbar puncture–cytoproteic dissociation, normal cellularity with elevated proteins, electroneuromyography of the limbs
Miller-Fisher syndrome [17]	Ataxia, ophthalmoplegia, areflexia, diplopia	Lumbar puncture—cytoproteic dissociation, normal cellularity with elevated proteins, electroneuromyography of the limbs
Charcot-Marie-Tooth disease [18]	Slow progressive paresis that starts in the lower limbs, “stork leg” deformity, thermal-painful and vibratory hypoesthesia in a glove and sock pattern, deep tendon reflexes are absent, foot deformity with hammertoes and high arches, hand paresis starts later	Genetic test for the *PMP22* gene, electroneuromyography of the limbs
Dejerine-Sottas disease [19]	Symptoms start in childhood, progressive paresis, hypoesthesia, and abolition of deep tendon reflexes, thickening of nerves	Search for mutation in the genes *PMP22*, *MPZ*, *EGR2*, electroneuromyography
Hereditary motor neuropathy with susceptibility to pressure palsy [20]	Development of multiple mononeuropathies after minor traumas, paresis, muscle hypotrophy, pain, and hypoesthesias	Search for mutation in the *PMP22* gene, electroneuromyography of the limbs
Sarcoidosis [21]	Dyspnea, cough, fatigue, weakness, weight loss, low fever, polyneuropathy, dacryocystitis, erythema nodosum, hypercalcemia, skin changes	Biopsy of the affected site: lymph nodes, dermatological lesions, conjunctiva, etc. Serum dosage of ACE (angiotensin converting enzyme), electroneuromyography of the limbs

(continued)

Table 1.1 (continued)

Name of neuropathy/ disease	Symptoms, signs, and laboratory findings	Complementary exams
Vitamin B1 deficiency [22]	Polyneuropathy predominantly in lower limbs, with burning pain, paresthesias, dysesthesias, cognitive changes, psychosis, cardiomyopathy, nystagmus, ataxia, ophthalmoplegia	Serum dosage of vitamin B1, electroneuromyography
Vitamin B6 intoxication [23]	Polyneuropathy compromising proprioceptive and vibratory sensitivity	Serum dosage of vitamin B6, electroneuromyography of the limbs
Hansen's disease [24–26]	Paucibacillary form—skin lesions, hypoesthetic macules, centrally hypopigmented, the lesions are not itchy, thickening of peripheral nerves. Lepromatous form—papules, nodules, skin plaques, polyneuropathy, loss of eyebrow and eyelashes. Complications: collapse of the nasal cartilage, plantar ulcers, erectile dysfunction, glaucoma, iritis, and corneal insensitivity	Skin biopsy, IgM serology for *M. leprae*, electroneuromyography of the limbs
(Chronic acquired demyelinating polyneuropathy; chronic recurrent polyneuropathy) CIDP [27]	Symptoms similar to Guillain-Barré syndrome, but with symptoms lasting longer than 2 months	Lumbar puncture—cytoproteic dissociation, normal cellularity with elevated proteins, electroneuromyography of the limbs
Lead poisoning [28]	Cognitive deficiency, neuropathies, chronic renal dysfunction, colic abdominal cramps, constipation, mood changes, encephalopathy, male infertility	Serum lead dosage, X-ray of long bones, electroneuromyography of the limbs
Paraneoplastic syndrome [29]	Polyneuropathy	Anti-Hu antibody, computed tomography of the chest to exclude lung cancer, electroneuromyography of the limbs
POEMS [7]	Polyneuropathy, organomegaly, endocrinopathy, monoclonal gammopathy and skin changes	Protein electrophoresis, serum levels of VEGF (vascular endothelial growth factor), complete blood count, immunoglobulin electrophoresis (immunofixation), electroneuromyography of the limbs

(continued)

Table 1.1 (continued)

Name of neuropathy/ disease	Symptoms, signs, and laboratory findings	Complementary exams
Cryoglobulinemia [30, 31]	Polyneuropathy, purpura, arthralgias, weakness	Serum cryoglobulin dosage, HIV, hepatitis C serology, rheumatoid factor, ANA, hepatitis B serology, electroneuromyography of the limbs
Systemic lupus erythematosus [32, 33]	Fever, weight loss, arthralgias, arthritis, skin lesions, photosensitivity, oral ulcers, anemia, optic neuritis, myelitis, psychiatric changes, headache, neuropathy, pleural effusion, nephritis, alopecia, pericarditis	ANA, anti-β2GP1 antibody, anti-dsDNA antibody, anti-Smith antibody, anticardiolipin antibody, complement C3, complement C4, electroneuromyography of the limbs
Rheumatoid arthritis [33]	Joint pain, morning joint stiffness, neuropathy, skin nodules, interstitial lung disease, associated Sjögren's syndrome	Rheumatoid factor, anti-Ro, anti-La, electroneuromyography of the limbs

1.2.1 Diabetes Mellitus

It is known that at least half of the patients with type 1 and 2 DM will develop diabetic neuropathy [6]. The estimated prevalence for the PN present in the adult population suffering from this metabolic disease revolves around 28% [34]. Young et al. (1993) published a study in the UK involving 6487 adult patients with DM. It was revealed that the prevalence of PN was 5% among participants aged 20–29 years and 44% among individuals aged 70–79 years [35]. On the other hand, the Spanish study by Cabezas-Cerato et al. (1998), which involved 2644 adult patients with DM, revealed that 30% of patients aged 70–74 years had PN [36].

1.2.2 Chronic Kidney Disease

Metabolic diseases such as chronic kidney disease (CKD) provide evidence that they can compromise the function of the central and peripheral nervous system. CKD can lead to PN, especially patients over 65 years old, with long-standing disease, male, and with creatinine clearance values <15 mL/min [37, 38]. In a study involving 74 patients with CKD, it was observed that 65% of the participants had PN [38].

1.2.3 Hansen's Disease

Hansen's disease is among the treatable causes of PN most commonly identified in different parts of the world [39]. In 2013, it was estimated that the global number of this bacterial infection reached the figure of 240,000 cases, with prevalence around 0.37 cases/10000 inhabitants [40]. In 2013, it was also estimated that 72% of the world's cases were concentrated in Southwest Asia, with 58.8% of cases in India [41]. In about 4–8% of all patients with this bacterial infection, the disease's involvement is restricted to the peripheral nerves [42, 43].

Trivedi et al. in a review of this disease revealed that the most common neurological picture is multiple mononeuritis, in which several peripheral nerves are compromised [2].

1.2.4 Long Stay in the Intensive Care Unit

Patients who stay for long periods in intensive care units (ICUs) can develop compressive neuropathies. Some prospective studies have revealed that the incidence of neuropathy of this nature revolves around 25–36% [44, 45].

Leijten et al. (1995) revealed that patients who stayed for more than 7 days in ICU presented in electroneuromyography, changes compatible with the diagnosis of myopathy and neuropathies in 52–57% of cases [46].

1.2.5 Collagen Diseases

Collagen disease or connective tissue disease is a group of diseases in which a persistent autoimmune inflammatory process is present. This group of diseases can include Sjögren's syndrome, systemic lupus erythematosus, systemic sclerosis, dermatopolymyositis, polymyositis, and undifferentiated connective tissue disease and mixed connective tissue disease [47].

The incidence of peripheral neuropathy in patients with Sjögren's syndrome is around 10–60%, and many patients develop PN as an initial symptom of the disease (40–93%) [47, 48].

Patients with systemic lupus erythematosus can develop NP in 25–50% of cases when based on electrodiagnostic studies, on the other hand, in only 5% of cases when based on clinical criteria [47, 49, 50].

The presence of NP in systemic sclerosis, mixed connective tissue disease, polymyositis, and dermatopolymyositis is rare [47, 48].

1.2.6 Vitamin B12 Deficiency

In a meta-analysis, there was statistical significance for the development of NP in the group of patients with low levels of vitamin B12, high levels of methylmalonic acid, and high levels of homocysteine [51].

1.3 Epidemiology of Meralgia Paresthetica

Meralgia paresthetica (MP) is a disease resulting from impairment of the lateral femoral cutaneous nerve (LFCN) that presents with symptoms of neuropathic pain, paresthesia, and dysesthesia in the lateral region of the thigh.

This syndrome was initially described in the 1880s independently, by two authors, Bernhardt and Roth. The term "meralgia" was first coined by Roth, whose words "meros" and "algos" mean in Greek, respectively, thigh and pain.

As for its epidemiological characteristics, MP can occur at any time in life; however, this syndrome is most commonly manifested in the fifth decade of life. It is a neuropathy that tends to occur more in males and be unilateral [52, 53].

It is estimated that the incidence of this disease is 4.3 cases per 10,000 per year in the general population and among the population with DM it is 24.7 cases per 10,000 [54, 55].

In a study conducted with the population of Minnesota, between the years of 1990 and 1999, it was observed that MP had an incidence of 32.6 cases per 100,000 patients/year [56]. On the other hand, data from the US military service indicate that the rate of MP has an incidence of 62 cases/100,000/year [57].

Numerous risk factors for this neuropathy have been described in the literature: pregnancy, DM, long-shafted footwear, obesity with a body mass index (BMI) ≥ 30, Hansen's disease, acquired immunodeficiency syndrome, iatrogenesis, long period in prone position, direct local trauma, toxins (alcohol, lead), intra-abdominal tumors, and tight clothing such as police uniforms and belt use [58–72].

Patients in the prone position for lumbar or thoracic laminectomy have a higher risk of developing this neuropathy postoperatively, especially if they have a high BMI and if the surgery lasts longer than 3.5 hours [61, 73, 74]. Gupta et al. (2004) revealed that the prevalence of MP in 110 patients who underwent posterior lumbar surgery was 12% [75]. In addition to spine surgery, MP is described as a complication resulting from gynecological-obstetric surgery, endoscopic laparoscopy, cesarean delivery, and bone grafting from the anterosuperior iliac crest [76–79].

Neuropathy of the lateral femoral cutaneous nerve is also described in hip arthroplasty surgeries. Goulding et al. (2010) described that among the 132 patients who underwent two different hip arthroplasty techniques ($N = 55$) total hip arthroplasty via anterior ($N = 77$) hip resurfacing (N=107) 81% developed MP. This author identified among the patients a neuropathic pain score of 2.42/10 [80].

1.4 Epidemiology of Piriformis Syndrome

This is a syndrome described in which the sciatic nerve (SN) in its course under the piriformis muscle/level of the ischial tuberosity undergoes compressive process usually triggering painful symptoms in the patient. There are several eponyms for this disease in the literature, such as deep gluteal syndrome, pelvic outlet syndrome, and infrapiriform foramen syndrome [81, 82].

The first case of sciatica associated with the piriformis muscle was described by Yeoman (1928) when analyzing 100 cases of arthritis of the sacroiliac joint [83]. Only 6 years later, Mixter and Barr (1934) described the association of sciatica with intervertebral disc herniation [84]. However, it was only later, in 1947 that Robson DR first coined the term "piriformis syndrome" (PS) for patients who had pain in the region of the sacroiliac joint and piriformis muscle [85].

PS is a controversial disease that still sparks heated discussions among scholars of peripheral nerve diseases. Strong skepticism exists about PS among health professionals. A survey conducted in the USA, involving 75 physiatrists, revealed that 72% were confident in the existence of the disease, 55% reported that the diagnosis was overestimated, and 38% believed that the disease was underdiagnosed [86–88]. Several authors believe that PS would result more from a disorder myofascial rather than a compressive neuropathy [86–88].

It is noted that its clinical manifestations are not very consistent, and can present as pain in the gluteal region, as well as symptoms similar to those identified in lumbosciatalgia, with pain radiating distally to the ipsilateral lower limb.

Chang et al. (2023) state that SP is responsible for 0.3–6% of all cases of low back pain and lumbosciatalgia [89]. Shane and Cass (2015) believe that this syndrome occurs in a ratio of 1:6 men/women and is more common in middle-aged adults [90]. Other authors show that its prevalence as a cause of sciatica would be around 5–6% [91, 92]. Hopayan et al. (2010) revealed in their systematic review that the average age of patients with SP is 43 years [93].

1.5 Epidemiology of Compressive Syndrome of the Peroneal Nerve

Compressive neuropathy of the peroneal nerve (CNPN) is the most common compressive neuropathy of the lower limb and the third most common neuropathy of the limbs, right after carpal tunnel syndrome and cubital tunnel syndrome. Its clinical importance also arises due to paresis of foot dorsiflexion, causing the patient to develop "foot drop." It is important to note that diseases located far from the peroneal nerve can lead the patient to develop a clinical picture similar to CNPN, such as a herniated disc compressing an L5 spinal nerve.

Among the oldest known descriptions of CNPN is the work of Sultan (1921) on a ganglion cyst as the cause of CNPN. Brooks (1952) described a series of cases of this neuropathy caused by the ganglion cyst. In 1966, Noble described two case reports where the peroneal nerve injury was caused by trauma, in which the patient presented inversion of the ankle resulting in intraneural hemorrhage from the injury of the vasa nervorum. In 1966, White also published a case report, in which the peroneal nerve injury occurred due to traumatic injury, whose mechanism involved traction of the affected limb. Cobb et al. (1974) described two case reports of ganglion cyst also as etiology of CNPN [94–97].

Few studies describe the incidence of CNPN in the general population. Studies conducted in Egypt revealed that the annual incidence of this neuropathy is around 19–40/100,000 inhabitants, totaling between 0.6% and 1.2% of all identified neuropathies [98, 99].

The medical literature has several articles where CNPN can arise as a result of complications from orthopedic procedures. Marciniak et al. (2013) suggest that this mononeuropathy is identified in 2–27% of patients who underwent high osteotomies of the tibia/fibula. Bouche et al. (2013), in their work, identified that 0.3–1.3% of patients who underwent knee arthroplasty developed this neuropathy [100, 101].

Patients also with clinical picture of knee trauma associated with dislocation can develop this neuropathy. Moatshe et al. (2017) in a prospective study, involving 303 patients, observed that peroneal neuropathy was diagnosed in 16–40% of cases [102].

1.6 Epidemiology of Compressive Syndrome of the Anterior Tarsal Tunnel

The anterior tarsal tunnel syndrome or compressive syndrome of the deep peroneal nerve (DPN) is defined as a chronic compressive neuropathy of this nerve, when it runs the path inside the inferior extensor retinaculum, at the ankle level [103, 104].

The first description of this compressive syndrome was made by authors Kopell and Thompson in 1963. In 1968, Marinacci named this syndrome and established its electrophysiological diagnosis [105, 106].

The anterior tarsal tunnel syndrome is a rare entity when compared to other neuropathies present in the lower limb, such as, the CNPN and posterior tarsal tunnel syndrome [103]. It is estimated that this mononeuropathy is present in 5% of patients with complaints of numbness in the feet [105, 107].

Patients with this mononeuropathy usually have symptoms of pain, paresthesias, hypoesthesia, foot weakness, and more rarely with paresis for extension of the toes [108]. Symptoms tend to occur in the space located between the first and second toes of the foot (first interdigital space), since the deep peroneal nerve is responsible for sensory innervation in this skin territory [109].

1.7 Epidemiology of Compressive Syndrome of the Posterior Tarsal Tunnel

The posterior tarsal tunnel syndrome (PTTS) is defined as a compressive neuropathy of the tibial nerve or its plantar branches within the tarsal tunnel that can be idiopathic or present diverse etiology, often associated with lesions that occupy the space of this osteofibrous tunnel [110–113]. The first historical description of this neuropathy was made by Pollock and Davis in 1933, in which a patient presented symptoms of the syndrome after a traumatic compression of the tibial nerve [114]. In 1960, Koppel and Thompson described the clinical characteristics resulting from the posterior tarsal tunnel syndrome, and in 1962, Keck coined the term "tarsal tunnel syndrome" when publishing a case report [115, 116].

As with other lower limb neuropathies, the etiologies associated with posterior tarsal tunnel syndrome are varied. Among the most cited causes in the literature are those of traumatic, infectious, inflammatory, tumoral, vascular, and idiopathic origin [117]. In a systematic review conducted in 1990, Cimino WR observed that in 20% of PTTS cases, the etiology is idiopathic, in the remaining cases, it was possible to identify an underlying etiology [118].

The sustentaculum tali is an accessory bone located in the foot that connects through a fibrotic or fibrocartilaginous band to the talus. This accessory bone is positioned between the talus and the calcaneus, which can cause compression of the posterior tibial nerve and/or its branches located inside the tarsal tunnel [119–121].

Tarsal coalition is a cause of PTTS described in the literature. It is a bridge of bone, fibrous, or cartilaginous origin that unites two or more tarsal bones. It is estimated that the incidence in the general population is around 1%. It is known that calcaneonavicular and talocalcaneal coalitions are the most frequently identified. The diagnosis can be made by radiography [122, 123].

A Baker's cyst develops from the growth of the gastrocnemio-semimembranosus bursa. It is a usually asymptomatic lesion that presents in the popliteal fossa region and can be the cause of thrombophlebitis, compartment syndrome, and compressive neuropathy. The literature describes the rupture of a Baker's cyst with extravasation of the cystic content to the calf region with compression of the tibial nerve [124]. The initial symptom is described as abrupt intense pain located in the popliteal fossa region [124].

The presence of accessory muscles in the ankle region as a risk factor for PTTS is described in the literature. It is believed that these muscles act as an expansive lesion that would trigger the neuropathy [125]. The accessory muscle most associated with this compressive neuropathy is the flexor digitorum accessorius longus; however, the tibiocalcaneus internus and accessory soleus are also described [125].

Between 17% and 43% of patients can identify in their histories some type of local trauma to the ankle/foot such as fractures, ankle sprains, and ligament injuries [126]. Chronic instability of the medial ankle is described as a risk factor for PTTS and may be associated with frequent sprains that can lead to ligament laxity [127].

In 10% of PTTS cases, it is possible to identify a history of inflammatory processes such as osteoarthritis, rheumatoid arthritis, and tenosynovitis [128–130].

The medical literature describes the onset of PTTS after surgical procedures to correct foot deformities such as cavovarus feet. It is believed that the reduction of the posterior tarsal tunnel after the procedure would lead to compression of the tibial nerve by the flexor retinaculum [130–132].

Tumors like schwannoma can be an etiology of PTTS. This tumor is most commonly identified in the skull, spinal nerve, brachial plexus, and rarely affects nerves in the lower limb. The lower limb nerve most affected by schwannoma is the tibial nerve. Generally, tumors of this nature grow slowly and produce non-painful asymptomatic masses. When symptomatic, they produce symptoms of numbness and pain [133–135].

The medical literature describes distinct tumors from the nerve lineage, as a cause of tibial neuropathy, such as B cell lymphoma [136].

Intraneural ganglion cyst can lead to PTTS, especially when it affects the tibial nerve at the level of the tarsal tunnel. Intraneural ganglion cysts originate within the nerve, from the epineurium. There is a fibrous capsule filled with a thick mucinous fluid. They occur most commonly between the third and fourth decade of life. It is believed to originate from the degeneration of perineural connective tissue, more rarely its expansion is caused by the joint synovial fluid that fills it via the articular branch [137–139].

Among the bone tumors that can cause PTTS, osteochondroma stands out. This lesion is the most common benign tumor, accounting for about 30% of all benign bone tumors. It usually presents as a bulge on the surface of the bone that has a medullary cavity inside with continuity with the medullary structure of the bone. Despite being the most common benign bone tumor, its location in the foot is rare. It does not show gender preference and occurs most commonly in children and adolescents [140, 141].

Other causes of PTTS are endocrine diseases such as hypothyroidism, mucopolysaccharidoses, gout, and dyslipidemias. It is also described, PTTS after intense physical activities, such as those present in the sports activities of marathon runners [142].

1.8 Conclusions

The most prevalent compressive neuropathy of the lower limb involves the peroneal nerve, at the level of the neck of the fibula. The medical literature has few studies that assess the incidence and prevalence of compressive neuropathies of these limbs. The most commonly identified risk factors associated with these compressive neuropathies are common diseases and relatively uncomplicated for diagnosis, such as DM, connective tissue diseases, vitamin B12 deficiency, and alcoholism.

References

1. Hughes RA. Peripheral neuropathy. BMJ. 2002;324(7335):466–9.
2. Trivedi S, Pandit A, Ganguly G, Das SK. Epidemiology of peripheral neuropathy: an Indian perspective. Ann Indian Acad Neurol. 2017;20(3):173–84. https://doi.org/10.4103/aian.AIAN_470_16. PMID: 28904445; PMCID: PMC5586108.
3. Ghosh B, Sengupta S, Bhattacharjee R, Pal S, Saha SP, Ganguly G, et al. Spectrum of peripheral neuropathy in eastern India. J Indian Med Assoc. 2006;104:168, 170–3.
4. Hicks CW, Wang D, Windham BG, et al. Prevalence of peripheral neuropathy defined by monofilament insensitivity in middle-aged and older adults in two US cohorts. Sci Rep. 2021;11:19159. https://doi.org/10.1038/s41598-021-98565-w.
5. Bowley MP, Doughty CT. Entrapment neuropathies of the lower extremity. Med Clin North Am. 2019;103(2):371–82.
6. Hammi C, Yeung B. Neuropathy. [Updated 2022 Oct 15]. In: StatPearls [Internet]. Treasure Island: StatPearls Publishing; 2024. Available from: https://www.ncbi.nlm.nih.gov/books/NBK542220/.
7. Donofrio PD. Peripheral neuropathy. 1st ed. New York: Demos Medical; 2012.
8. Kazamel M, Stino AM, Smith AG. Metabolic syndrome and peripheral neuropathy. Muscle Nerve. 2021;63(3):285–93.
9. Liampas A, Parperis K, Erotocritou MF, Nteveros A, Papadopoulou M, Moschovos C, Akil M, Coaccioli S, Hadjigeorgiou GM, Hadjivassiliou M, Zis P. Primary Sjögren syndrome-related peripheral neuropathy: a systematic review and meta-analysis. Eur J Neurol. 2023;30(1):255–65.
10. Chen GY, Tang ZQ, Bao ZX. Vitamin B12 deficiency may play an etiological role in atrophic glossitis and its grading: a clinical case-control study. BMC Oral Health. 2022;22(1):456. https://doi.org/10.1186/s12903-022-02464-z. PMID: 36307840; PMCID: PMC9617421.
11. Morgello S. HIV neuropathology. Handb Clin Neurol. 2018;152:3–19. https://doi.org/10.1016/B978-0-444-63849-6.00002-5. PMID: 29604982.
12. Kaku M, Berk JL. Neuropathy associated with systemic amyloidosis. Semin Neurol. 2019;39(5):578–88. https://doi.org/10.1055/s-0039-1688994. Epub 2019 Oct 22.
13. Crissinger T, Baldwin K. Early disseminated Lyme disease: cranial neuropathy, meningitis, and polyradiculopathy. Infect Dis Clin N Am. 2022;36(3):541–51.
14. Reñé R, Salazar A, Ferrer X. Complicaciones neurológicas por citomegalovirus en pacientes con SIDA [Neurological complications caused by cytomegalovirus in patients with AIDS]. Rev Neurol. 1996;24(136):1590–6.
15. Shang P, Zhu M, Wang Y, Zheng X, Wu X, Zhu J, Feng J, Zhang HL. Axonal variants of Guillain-Barré syndrome: an update. J Neurol. 2021;268(7):2402–19. https://doi.org/10.1007/s00415-020-09742-2.
16. Finsterer J. Small fiber neuropathy underlying dysautonomia in COVID-19 and in post-SARS-CoV-2 vaccination and long-COVID syndromes. Muscle Nerve. 2022;65(6):E31–2.
17. Shahrizaila N, Lehmann HC, Kuwabara S. Guillain-Barré syndrome. Lancet. 2021;397(10280):1214–28. https://doi.org/10.1016/S0140-6736(21)00517-1.
18. Roa BB, Garcia CA, Lupski JR. Charcot-Marie-Tooth disease type 1A: molecular mechanisms of gene dosage and point mutation underlying a common inherited peripheral neuropathy. Int J Neurol. 1991;25–26:97–107. PMID: 11980069.
19. Plante-Bordeneuve V, Said G. Dejerine-Sottas disease and hereditary demyelinating polyneuropathy of infancy. Muscle Nerve. 2002;26(5):608–21. https://doi.org/10.1002/mus.10197. PMID: 12402282.
20. Attarian S, Fatehi F, Rajabally YA, Pareyson D. Hereditary neuropathy with liability to pressure palsies. J Neurol. 2020;267(8):2198–206. https://doi.org/10.1007/s00415-019-09319-8.
21. Tavee J. Peripheral neuropathy in sarcoidosis. J Neuroimmunol. 2022;368:577864. https://doi.org/10.1016/j.jneuroim.2022.577864.

22. Kramarz C, Murphy E, Reilly MM, Rossor AM. Nutritional peripheral neuropathies. J Neurol Neurosurg Psychiatry. 2023;95(1):61–72. https://doi.org/10.1136/jnnp-2022-329849.
23. Misumi J, Nagano M, Kaisaku J, Hitoshi T. Effects of vitamin B12 and B6 on 2,5-hexanedione-induced neuropathy. Arch Toxicol. 1985;56(3):204–6. https://doi.org/10.1007/BF00333428.
24. Shachaf S, Yair M. The correlation between antiphospholipid syndrome and cryoglobulinemia: case series of 4 patients and review of the literature. Rev Bras Reumatol Engl Ed. 2016;56(1):2–7. English, Portuguese. https://doi.org/10.1016/j.rbre.2014.09.007. Epub 2015 Jan 7. PMID: 27267327.
25. Gondin FAA, Freitas MRG, Pereira RC. Neuropatias periféricas. 1ª ed. São Paulo: Ominifarma; 2020.
26. Levin SN, Lyons JL. Infections of the nervous system. Am J Med. 2018;131(1):25–32.
27. Querol L, Siles AM, Alba-Rovira R, et al. Antibodies against peripheral nerve antigens in chronic inflammatory demyelinating polyradiculoneuropathy. Sci Rep. 2017;7(1):14411.
28. Neundörfer B. Toxische polyneuropathien [Toxic polyneuropathies]. Versicherungsmedizin. 1992;44(4):119–25. German. PMID: 1509644.
29. Papantoniou M, Zampelis T, Rentzos M, et al. Anti-Hu antibody seropositive neuropathy with large and small fiber involvement mimicking alcoholic neuropathy: a case report. Egypt J Neurol Psychiatry Neurosurg. 2023;59:161. https://doi.org/10.1186/s41983-023-00763-y.
30. Bhandari J, Awais M, Aeddula NR. Cryoglobulinemia. [Updated 2022 Aug 10]. In: StatPearls [Internet]. Treasure Island: StatPearls Publishing; 2024. Available from: https://www.ncbi.nlm.nih.gov/books/NBK557606/.
31. Justiz Vaillant AA, Goyal A, Varacallo M. Systemic lupus erythematosus. [Updated 2023 Aug 4]. In: StatPearls [Internet]. Treasure Island: StatPearls Publishing; 2024. Available from: https://www.ncbi.nlm.nih.gov/books/NBK535405/.
32. Olney RK. Neuropathies associated with connective tissue disease. Semin Neurol. 1998;18(1):63–72. https://doi.org/10.1055/s-2008-1040862. PMID: 9562668.
33. Chauhan K, Jandu JS, Brent LH, et al. Rheumatoid arthritis. [Updated 2023 May 25]. In: StatPearls [Internet]. Treasure Island: StatPearls Publishing; 2024. Available from: https://www.ncbi.nlm.nih.gov/books/NBK441999/.
34. Pop-Busui R, Boulton AJ, Feldman EL, Bril V, Freeman R, Malik RA, et al. Diabetic neuropathy: a position statement by the American Diabetes Association. Diabetes Care. 2017;40(1):136–54. https://doi.org/10.2337/dc16-2042.
35. Young MJ, Boulton AJ, MacLeod AF, Williams DR, Sonksen PH. A multicentre study of the prevalence of diabetic peripheral neuropathy in the United Kingdom hospital clinic population. Diabetologia. 1993;36:150–4.
36. Cabezas-Cerrato J. The prevalence of clinical diabetic polyneuropathy in Spain: a study in primary care and hospital clinic groups. Neuropathy Spanish Study Group of the Spanish Diabetes Society (SDS). Diabetologia. 1998;41:1263–9.
37. Viswanathan V, Seena R, Nair MB, Snehalatha C, Bhoopathy RM, Ramachandran A. Nerve conduction abnormalities in different stages of glucose intolerance. Neurol India. 2004;52:466–9.
38. Babu MM, Kiran MR, Ravindra K, Srinivas V, Kandregula P, Vardhan RV, et al. Clinical manifestation and prevalence of peripheral neuropathy and nerve dysfunction in patients with chronic kidney disease. Int J Res Med Sci. 2015;3:451–5.
39. Nations SP, Katz JS, Lyde CB, Barohn RJ. Leprous neuropathy: an American perspective. Semin Neurol. 1998;18:113–24.
40. Global leprosy: update on the 2012 situation. Wkly Epidemiol Rec. 2013;88:365–79.
41. Global leprosy update, 2013; reducing disease burden. Wkly Epidemiol Rec. 2014;89:389–400.
42. Suneetha S, Arunthathi S, Chandi S, Kurian N, Chacko CJ. Histological studies in primary neuritic leprosy: changes in the apparently normal skin. Lepr Rev. 1998;69:351–7.
43. Mahajan PM, Jogaikar DG, Mehta JM. A study of pure neuritic leprosy: clinical experience. Indian J Lepr. 1996;68:137–41.

44. de Letter MA, Schmitz PI, Visser LH, Verheul FA, Schellens RL, Op de Coul DA, et al. Risk factors for the development of polyneuropathy and myopathy in critically ill patients. Crit Care Med. 2001;29:2281–6.
45. De Jonghe B, Sharshar T, Lefaucheur JP, Authier FJ, Durand-Zaleski I, Boussarsar M, et al. Paresis acquired in the intensive care unit: a prospective multicenter study. JAMA. 2002;288:2859–67.
46. Leijten FS, Harinck-de Weerd JE, Poortvliet DC, de Weerd AW. The role of polyneuropathy in motor convalescence after prolonged mechanical ventilation. JAMA. 1995;274:1221–5.
47. Snoussi M, Frikha F, Bahloul Z. Peripheral neuropathy in connective tissue diseases [Internet]. In: Demystifying polyneuropathy – recent advances and new directions. IntechOpen; 2019. https://doi.org/10.5772/intechopen.82271.
48. Matthew Grantz MD. Unusual peripheral neuropathies. Part II: Intrinsic reactive causes. Semin Neurol. 2010;30:396–404.
49. Ilniczky S, Kamondi A, Arányi Z, et al. Simultaneous central and peripheral nervous system involvement in systemic lupus erythematosus. Ideggyogy Sz. 2007;60:398–402.
50. Omdal R, Mellgren SI, Goransson L, et al. Small nerve fiber involvement in systemic lupus erythematosus: a controlled study. Arthritis Rheum. 2002;46:1228–32. https://doi.org/10.1002/art.10303.
51. Stein J, Geisel J, Obeid R. Association between neuropathy and B-vitamins: a systematic review and meta-analysis. Eur J Neurol. 2021;28(6):2054–64. https://doi.org/10.1111/ene.14786. Epub 2021 Mar 15. PMID: 33619867.
52. Gomez YC, Remotti E, Momah DU, Zhang E, Swanson DD, Kim R, Urits I, Kaye AD, Robinson CL. Meralgia paresthetica review: update on presentation, pathophysiology, and treatment. Health Psychol Res. 2023;11:71454. https://doi.org/10.52965/001c.71454. PMID: 36937080; PMCID: PMC10019995.
53. Madiraca Glasović D, Šlaus N, Šitum M, Pećina M. Meralgia paresthetica – lateral femoral cutaneous nerve entrapment. Rad Hrvatske akademije znanosti i umjetnosti Medicinske znanosti. 2021;54–55:56–63. https://doi.org/10.21857/mzvkptq6v9.
54. van Slobbe AM, Bohnen AM, Bernsen RM, et al. Incidence rates and determinants in meralgia paresthetica in general practice. J Neurol. 2004;251(3):294–7.
55. Harney D, Patijn J. Meralgia paresthetica: diagnosis and management strategies. Pain Med. 2007;8(8):669–77.
56. Parisi TJ, Mandrekar J, Dyck PJB, Klein CJ. Meralgia paresthetica: relation to obesity, advanced age, and diabetes mellitus. Neurology. 2011;77(16):1538–42. https://doi.org/10.1212/wnl.0b013e318233b356.
57. Knapik JJ, Reynolds KL, Orr R, Pope R. Load carriage-related paresthesias (part 2): meralgia paresthetica. J Spec Oper Med. 2017;17(1):94. https://doi.org/10.55460/6krp-71df.
58. Cheatham SW, Kolber MJ, Salamh PA. Meralgia paresthetica: a review of the literature. Int J Sports Phys Ther. 2013;8(6):883–93. PMID: 24377074; PMCID: PMC3867081.
59. Khalil N, Nicotra A, Rakowicz W. Treatment for meralgia paraesthetica. Cochrane Database Syst Rev. 2012;2012:CD004159.
60. Glasović DM, Šlaus N, Šitum M, Pećina M. Review article RAD 547. Med Sci. 2021;547:54–5.
61. Yoshida S, Oya S, Matsui T. Risk factors of meralgia paresthetica after prone position surgery: possible influence of operating position, laminectomy level, and preoperative thoracic kyphosis. J Clin Neurosci. 2021;89:292–6. https://doi.org/10.1016/j.jocn.2021.05.022.
62. Drăghici N, Vacaras V, Bolchis R, Bashimov A, Domnița D, Iluț S, Livinț Popa L, Lupescu T, Mureșanu D. Diagnostic approach to lower limb entrapment neuropathies: a narrative literature review. Diagnostics. 2023;13:3385. https://doi.org/10.3390/diagnostics13213385.
63. Beresford HR. Meralgia paresthetica after seat-belt trauma. J Trauma. 1971;11(7):629–30.
64. Blake SM, Treble NJ. Meralgia paraesthetica--an addition to "seatbelt syndrome". Ann R Coll Surg Engl. 2004;86(6):W6–7.
65. Fargo MV, Konitzer LN. Meralgia paresthetica due to body armor wear in U.S. soldiers serving in Iraq: a case report and review of the literature. Mil Med. 2007;172(6):663–5.

66. Goel A. Meralgia paresthetica secondary to limb length discrepancy: case report. Arch Phys Med Rehabil. 1999;80(3):348–9.
67. Haim A, Pritsch T, Ben-Galim P, et al. Meralgia paresthetica: a retrospective analysis of 79 patients evaluated and treated according to a standard algorithm. Acta Orthop. 2006;77(3):482–6.
68. Jiang GX, Xu WD, Wang AH. Spinal stenosis with meralgia paraesthetica. J Bone Joint Surg Br. 1988;70(2):272–3.
69. Korkmaz N, Ozcakar L. Meralgia paresthetica in a policeman: the belt or the gun. Plast Reconstr Surg. 2004;114(4):1012–3.
70. Mondelli M, Rossi S, Romano C. Body mass index in meralgia paresthetica: a case-control study. Acta Neurol Scand. 2007;116(2):118–23.
71. Moscona AR, Sekel R. Post-traumatic meralgia paresthetica--an unusual presentation. J Trauma. 1978;18(4):288.
72. Park JW, Kim DH, Hwang M, et al. Meralgia paresthetica caused by hip-huggers in a patient with aberrant course of the lateral femoral cutaneous nerve. Muscle Nerve. 2007;35(5):678–80.
73. Yang SH, Wu CC, Chen PQ. Postoperative meralgia paresthetica after posterior spine surgery: incidence, risk factors, and clinical outcomes. Spine (Phila Pa 1976). 2005;30:E547–50.
74. Ercan S, Ataizi ZS, Ertilav K. The correlation of meralgia paresthetica and spinal surgery in prone position. Turk Neurosurg. 2020;30:89–93.
75. Gupta A, Muzumdar D, Ramani PS. Meralgia paraesthetica following lumbar spine surgery: a study in 110 consecutive surgically treated cases. Neurol India. 2004;52:66.
76. Yamamoto T, Nagira K, Kurosaka M. Meralgia paresthetica occurring 40 years after iliac bone graft harvesting: case report. Neurosurgery. 2001;49(6):1455–7.
77. Kavanagh D, Connolly S, Fleming F, et al. Meralgia paraesthetica following open appendicectomy. Ir Med J. 2005;98(6):183–5.
78. Polidori L, Magarelli M, Tramutoli R. Meralgia paresthetica as a complication of laparoscopic appendectomy. Surg Endosc. 2003;17(5):832.
79. Paul F, Zipp F. Bilateral meralgia paresthetica after cesarian section with epidural analgesia. J Peripher Nerv Syst. 2006;11(1):98–9.
80. Goulding K, Beaule PE, Kim PR, et al. Incidence of lateral femoral cutaneous nerve neuropraxia after anterior approach hip arthroplasty. Clin Orthop Relat Res. 2010;468(9):2397–404.
81. Hopayian K. Sciatica in the community – not always disc herniation. Int J Clin Pract. 1999;53:197–8.
82. Reichel G, Gaerisch F Jr. Piriformis syndrome. A contribution to the differential diagnosis of lumbago and coccygodynia (German). Zentralbl Neurochir. 1988;49:178–84.
83. Yeoman W. The relation of arthritis of the sacroiliac joint to sciatica, with the analysis of 100 cases. Lancet. 1928;2:111922.
84. Mixter W, Barr J. Rupture of the intervertebral disc with involvement of the spinal canal. N Engl J Med. 1934;211:2105.
85. Robinson DR. Pyriformis syndrome in relation to sciatic pain. Am J Surg. 1947;73:3558.
86. McCrory P. The "piriformis syndrome"--myth or reality? Br J Sports Med. 2001;35(4):209–10.
87. Campbell WW, Landau ME. Controversial entrapment neuropathies. Neurosurg Clin N Am. 2008;19(4):597–608, vi–vii
88. Porta M. A comparative trial of botulinum toxin type A and methylprednisolone for the treatment of myofascial pain syndrome and pain from chronic muscle spasm. Pain. 2000;85(1–2):101–5.
89. Byrd JW. Piriformis syndrome. Oper Tech Sports Med. 2005;13:71–9.
90. Shane P, Cass DO. Piriformis syndrome: a cause of nondiscogenic sciatica. Curr Sports Med Rep. 2015;14(1):41–4.
91. Papadopoulos EC, Khan SN. Piriformis syndrome and low back pain: a new classification and review of the literature. Orthop Clin North Am. 2004;35(1):65–71.
92. Hallin RP. Sciatic pain and the piriformis muscle. Postgrad Med. 1983;74:69–72.

93. Hopayian K, Song F, Riera R, Sambandan S. The clinical features of the piriformis syndrome: a systematic review. Eur Spine J. 2010;19(12):2095–109.
94. Sultan C. Ganglion der nervenscheide des nervus peroneus. Zentralbl Chir. 1921;48:963–5.
95. Brooks DM. Nerve compression by simple ganglia: a review of thirteen collected cases. J Bone Joint Surg Br. 1952;34-B:391–400.
96. Cobb CA, Moiel RH. Ganglion of the peroneal nerve. Report of two cases. J Neurosurg. 1974;41:255–9.
97. Noble W. Peroneal palsy due to hematoma in the common peroneal nerve sheath after distal torsional fractures and inversion ankle sprains. J Bone Joint Surg Am. 1966;48-A:1484–95.
98. Khedr EM, Fawi G, Allah Abbas MA, El-Fetoh NA, Zaki AF, Gamea A. Prevalence of common types of compression neuropathies in Qena Governorate/Egypt: a population-based survey. Neuroepidemiology. 2016;46(4):253–60.
99. Kandil MR, Darwish ES, Khedr EM, Sabry MM, Abdulah MA. A community-based epidemiological study of peripheral neuropathies in Assiut, Egypt. Neurol Res. 2012;34(10):960–6.
100. Marciniak C. Fibular (peroneal) neuropathy: electrodiagnostic features and clinical correlates. Phys Med Rehabil Clin N Am. 2013;24(1):121–37. https://doi.org/10.1016/j.pmr.2012.08.016.
101. Bouche P. Compression and entrapment neuropathies. In: Handbook of clinical neurology, vol. 115. Amsterdam: Elsevier B.V.; 2013. p. 311–66. https://doi.org/10.1016/B978-0-444-52902-2.00019-9.
102. Moatshe G, Dornan GJ, Løken S, Ludvigsen TC, Laprade RF, Engebretsen L. Demographics and injuries associated with knee dislocation: a prospective review of 303 patients. Orthop J Sports Med. 2017;5(5):2325967117706521. https://doi.org/10.1177/2325967117706521.
103. DiDomenico LA, Masternick EB. Anterior tarsal tunnel syndrome. Clin Podiatr Med Surg. 2006;23(3):611–20. https://doi.org/10.1016/j.cpm.2006.04.007. PMID: 16958392.
104. Logullo F, Ganino C, Lupidi F, Perozzi C, Di Bella P, Provinciali L. Anterior tarsal tunnel syndrome: a misunderstood and a misleading entrapment neuropathy. Neurol Sci. 2014;35(5):773–5. https://doi.org/10.1007/s10072-013-1601-8. Epub 2013 Dec 12. PMID: 24337947.
105. Dreyer MA, Gibboney MD. Anterior tarsal tunnel syndrome. [Updated 2023 May 23]. In: StatPearls [Internet]. Treasure Island: StatPearls Publishing; 2023. Available from: https://www.ncbi.nlm.nih.gov/books/NBK538488/.
106. Adelman KA, Wilson G, Wolf JA. Anterior tarsal tunnel syndrome. J Foot Surg. 1988;27(4):299–302. PMID: 3225388.
107. Yassin M, Garti A, Weissbrot M, Heller E, Robinson D. Treatment of anterior tarsal tunnel syndrome through an endoscopic or open technique. Foot (Edinb). 2015;25(3):148–51.
108. Sarrafian S. The anatomy of the foot and ankle. Philadelphia: J.B. Lippincott; 1983.
109. Aktan Ikiz ZA, Ucerler H, Uygur M. Dimensions of the anterior tarsal tunnel and features of the deep peroneal nerve in relation to clinical application. Surg Radiol Anat. 2007;29(7):527–30. https://doi.org/10.1007/s00276-007-0229-x. Epub 2007 Jul 3. PMID: 17607504.
110. Bailie DS, Kelikian AS. Tarsal tunnel syndrome: diagnosis, surgical technique, and functional outcome. Foot Ankle Int. 1998;19:65–72.
111. Cimino WR. Tarsal tunnel syndrome: review of the literature. Foot Ankle. 1990;11:47–52.
112. Takakura Y, Kitada C, Sugimoto K, et al. Tarsal tunnel syndrome. Causes and results of operative treatment. J Bone Joint Surg. 1991;73:125–8.
113. Garchar DJ, Lewis JE, DiDomenico LA. Hypertrophic sustentaculum tali causing a tarsal tunnel syndrome: a case report. J Foot Ankle Surg. 2001;40:110–2.
114. Pollock L, Davis L. Peripheral nerve injuries. Am J Surg. 1932;18:361.
115. Koppel HP, Thompson WA. Peripheral entrapment neuropathies of the lower extremity. N Engl J Med. 1960;960(262):56–60.
116. Keck C. The tarsal-tunnel syndrome. J Bone Joint Surg. 1962;44A:180–2.

117. Dellon AL. The four medial ankle tunnels: a critical review of perceptions of tarsal tunnel syndrome and neuropathy. Neurosurg Clin N Am. 2008;19(4):629–48, vii. https://doi.org/10.1016/j.nec.2008.07.003. PMID: 19010287.
118. Cimino WR. Tarsal tunnel syndrome: a review of the literature. Foot Ankle Int. 1990;11:47–52.
119. Bencardino J, Rosenberg Z, Beltran J, et al. Os sustentaculi: depiction on MR images. Skeletal Radiol. 1997;26:505–6.
120. Kose O. The accessory ossicles of the foot and ankle; a diagnostic pitfall in emergency department in context of foot and ankle trauma/Ayak ve ayak bilegi cevresinde gorulen aksesuar kemikcikler; acil serviste ayak ve ayak bilegi travma hastalarinda tanisal tuzak. J Acad Emerg Med. 2012;11:106–15.
121. Kraft H. Assimilated accessory skeletal element of the foot (os sustentaculi) as cause for frequently recurring disorders. Arch Orthop Unfallchir. 1958;49:652.
122. Stormont DM, Peterson HA. The relative incidence of tarsal coalition. Clin Orthop Relat Res. 1983;(181):28–36.
123. Taniguchi A, Tanaka Y, Kadono K, et al. C sign for diagnosis of talocalcaneal coalition. Radiology. 2003;228:501–5.
124. Moon SH, Im S, Park GY, Moon SJ, Park HJ, Choi HS, Jo YR. Compressive neuropathy of the posterior tibial nerve at the lower calf caused by a ruptured intramuscular baker cyst. Ann Rehabil Med. 2013;37(4):577–81. https://doi.org/10.5535/arm.2013.37.4.577.
125. Cheung Y. Normal variants: accessory muscles about the ankle. Magn Reson Imaging Clin N Am. 2017;25(1):11–26. https://doi.org/10.1016/j.mric.2016.08.002.
126. Oh S, Meyer R. Entrapment neuropathies of the tibial nerve. Neurol Clin. 1999;17:593–615.
127. Alshalawi S, Galhoum AE, Alrashidi Y, et al. Medial ankle instability: the deltoid dilemma. Foot Ankle Clin. 2018;23(4):639–57. https://doi.org/10.1016/j.fcl.2018.07.008.
128. Mummenthaler M, Stöhr M, Müller-Vahl H, editors. Läsion peripherer Nerven und radikuläre Syndrome. Stuttgart: Thieme Verlag; 2003.
129. Tackmann W, Richter HP, Stöhr M, editors. Kompressionssyndrome peripherer Nerven. Heidelberg: Springer Verlag; 1989.
130. Stødle AH, Molund M, Nilsen F, Hellund JC, Hvaal K. Tibial nerve palsy after lateralizing calcaneal osteotomy. Foot Ankle Spec. 2019;12(5):426–31. https://doi.org/10.1177/1938640018816363.
131. Willis AR, Samad AA, Prado GT, Gabisan GG. Heterotopic ossification and entrapment of the tibial nerve within the tarsal tunnel: a case report. J Foot Ankle Surg. 2016;55(5):1106–9. https://doi.org/10.1053/j.jfas.2016.01.032.
132. Cody EA, Greditzer HG, Macmahon A, Burket JC, Sofka CM, Ellis SJ. Effects on the tarsal tunnel following Malerba Z-type osteotomy compared to standard lateralizing calcaneal osteotomy. Foot Ankle Int. 2016;37(9):1017–22. https://doi.org/10.1177/1071100716651966.
133. Albert P, Patel J, Badawy K, Weissinger W, Brenner M, Bourhill I, Parnell J. Peripheral nerve schwannoma: a review of varying clinical presentations and imaging findings. J Foot Ankle Surg. 2017;56:632–7. https://doi.org/10.1053/j.jfas.2016.12.003.
134. Nawabi DH, Sinisi M. Schwannoma of the posterior tibial nerve: the problem of delay in diagnosis. J Bone Joint Surg Br. 2007;89(6):814–6. https://doi.org/10.1302/0301-620X.89B6.19077.
135. Hallahan K, Vinokur J, Demski S, Faulkner-Jones B, Giurini J. Tarsal tunnel syndrome secondary to schwannoma of the posterior tibial nerve. J Foot Ankle Surg. 2014;53-1:79–82. https://doi.org/10.1053/j.jfas.2012.12.020.
136. Moussa A, Chakhachiro Z, Sawaya RA. Posterior tibial nerve lymphoma presenting as tarsal tunnel syndrome: a case report. J Foot Ankle Surg. 2018;57(1):167–9. https://doi.org/10.1053/j.jfas.2017.07.004.
137. Spinner RJ, Hébert-Blouin M-N, Maniker AH, Amrami KK. Clock face model applied to tibial intraneural ganglia in the popliteal fossa. Skeletal Radiol. 2009;38(7):691–6.
138. Spinner RJ, Atkinson JL, Tiel RL. Peroneal intraneural ganglia: the importance of the articular branch. A unifying theory. J Neurosurg. 2003;99(2):330–43.

139. Spinner RJ, Amrami KK, Wolanskyj AP, et al. Dynamic phases of peroneal and tibial intraneural ganglia formation: a new dimension added to the unifying articular theory. J Neurosurg. 2007;107:296–307.
140. Kitsoulis P, Galani V, Stefanaki K, Paraskevas G, Karatzias G, Agnantis NJ, Bai M. Osteochondromas: review of the clinical, radiological and pathological features. In Vivo. 2008;22(5):633–46.
141. Herrera-Perez M, Aciego De Mendoza M, De Bergua-Domingo JM, Pais-Brito JL. Osteochondromas around the ankle: report of a case and literature review. Int J Surg Case Rep. 2013;4(11):1025–7.
142. Hirose CB, McGarvey WC. Anterior tarsal tunnel syndrome. Foot Ankle Clin N Am. 2004;9:255–69.

Chapter 2
General Aspects of Neuropathies

2.1 Introduction

Neuropathies consist of a heterogeneous group of diseases whose etiologies are extremely numerous such as compressive syndromes, inflammatory diseases, genetic and paraneoplastic syndromes, infectious processes, and deficiency diseases. Neuropathies can be classified into mononeuropathy, radiculopathy, plexopathy, ganglionopathy, and multiple mononeuropathies.

In general, peripheral neuropathies are relatively common. The prevalence of these diseases in the population varies between 2.4% and 11%, and the prevalence, disregarding age, is 1–12% and among the elderly population around 30%. It is estimated that the incidence of this disease is 77 people/100,000 inhabitants per year [1–4].

Regarding the etiology, a patient may have more than one cause for their neuropathy. So, in this way, a patient could, for example, have diabetes mellitus (DM), vitamin B12 deficiency, and hypothyroidism concurrently [5]. Despite the existence of complementary tests available today, about a third of neuropathies do not have a defined diagnosis, a third present genetic etiology, and a third acquired character [6]. Table 2.1.

Mononeuropathies generally affect large nerves in the upper or lower limbs. The most common cause for this type of pathology is compressive syndromes, but vasculitis or local ischemia can also be the etiology in these cases. An example of mononeuropathy is compressive syndrome of the fibular nerve at the level of the fibula neck.

The term "multiple mononeuropathy" applies to mononeuropathies in which at least two nerves are compromised, in a short time interval. In this type of

---

Supplementary Information The online version contains supplementary material available at https://doi.org/10.1007/978-3-031-90058-7_2.

M. J. S. Magalhães, *Lower Extremity Nerve Entrapments*,
https://doi.org/10.1007/978-3-031-90058-7_2

Table 2.1 Etiology/risk factors of peripheral neuropathies and some complementary exams that assist in diagnosis

Name of neuropathy/ disease	Symptoms, signs, and laboratory findings	Complementary exams
Carpal tunnel syndrome [7]	Pain/paresthesia in the palmar region of the I, II, III digits of the hand and lateral face of the IV digit and thenar atrophy	Electroneuromyography of the upper limbs, wrist ultrasound
Cubital tunnel syndrome [7]	Pain/paresthesia in the palmar region on the medial side of the IV digit and V digit. Atrophy of the interosseous muscles	Electroneuromyography of the upper limbs, elbow ultrasound
Common peroneal nerve [7]	Pain/paresthesia in the region of the dorsum of the foot and lateral face of the leg. Paresis for dorsiflexion of the foot, eversion of the foot and extension of the toes and hallux	Electroneuromyography of the lower limbs. Ultrasound of the fibular tunnel
Piriformis syndrome [7]	Pain in the gluteal region, ipsilateral sciatica	Electroneuromyography of the lower limbs, pelvic MRI, lumbar spine MRI
Posterior tarsal tunnel syndrome [7]	Pain in the medial region of the foot, plantar region pain	Electroneuromyography of the lower limbs, foot X-ray, foot MRI, foot ultrasound
Anterior tarsal tunnel syndrome [7]	Pain in the region of the first interdigital space	Electroneuromyography of the lower limbs. MRI of the foot. X-ray of the foot
Hypothyroidism [8]	Neuropathy, fatigue, hair loss, edema in lower limbs, mood changes, weight gain, trophic skin changes, hoarseness, speech slowing, facial changes, and cold intolerance	TSH, Free T4. Electroneuromyography of the limbs
Diabetes mellitus [8]	Increased thirst, hyperphagia, weight loss, polyuria, neuropathy in lower limbs	Fasting blood glucose, HBA1C, glucose tolerance test, electroneuromyography
Sjögren's syndrome [9]	Xerostomia, dry eye, parotid enlargement, neuropathy	Anti-Ro, anti-La, electroneuromyography
Vitamin B12 deficiency [10]	Polyneuropathy, degeneration of the posterior funiculus, cognitive changes, megaloblastic anemia	Serum vitamin B12 dosage, methylmalonic acid, homocysteine, upper digestive endoscopy, Schilling test, electroneuromyography of the limbs
HIV [11]	Weight loss, recurrent infections, chronic diarrhea, polyneuropathy, fatigue, night sweats, persistent fever, oral candidiasis, lymphadenopathies, herpes zoster, anemia, thrombocytopenia, leukopenia, anorexia, Kaposi's sarcoma, oral hairy leukoplakia	HIV serology, complete blood count (lymphocyte count)

(continued)

Table 2.1 (continued)

Name of neuropathy/ disease	Symptoms, signs, and laboratory findings	Complementary exams
Amyloidosis [12]	Neuropathy, heart failure, nephrotic syndrome, painless hepatomegaly, dyspnea, hoarseness, cerebral hemorrhage, gastric atony, malabsorption, goiter	Genetic test for transthyretin, biopsy, electroneuromyography of the limbs
Lyme disease [13]	Erythema migrans, fatigue, chills, fever, headache, neck stiffness, myalgias, arthralgias, arthritis, polymorphic erythema, atrioventricular blocks, and rarely myopericarditis and cardiomegaly	Serology for *Borrelia* spp., electroneuromyography of the limbs
Cytomegalovirus [14]	Neuropathy, fever, flu-like symptoms	Serology for cytomegalovirus, electroneuromyography of the limbs
Zika virus [15]	Arthralgias, retroocular pain, polyneuropathy, fever, fatigue, maculopapular rash, conjunctivitis, headache	Serological test for Zika virus, electroneuromyography of the limbs
COVID-19 [16]	Fever, cough, diffuse myalgia, peripheral neuropathies, anosmia, and arthralgias	PCR for COVID-19, electroneuromyography of the limbs
Guillain-Barré syndrome [17]	Polyneuropathy, symmetric paresis, areflexia, and progressive usually started in the lower limbs, paresthesias, in severe cases respiratory failure and ocular involvement	Cerebrospinal fluid-cytoproteic dissociation, normal cellularity with elevated proteins, electroneuromyography of the limbs
Miller-Fisher syndrome [17]	Ataxia, ophthalmoplegia, areflexia, and diplopia	Cerebrospinal fluid—cytoproteic dissociation, normal cellularity with elevated proteins, electroneuromyography of the limbs
Charcot-Marie-Tooth disease [18]	Slow progressive paresis that starts in the lower limbs, "stork leg" deformity, thermal-painful and vibratory hypoesthesia in a glove-and-sock pattern, deep tendon reflexes are absent, foot deformity with hammertoes and high arches. Hand paresis starts later	Genetic test for the *PMP22* gene, electroneuromyography of the limbs
Dejerine-Sottas disease [19]	Symptoms start in childhood, progressive paresis, hypoesthesia, abolition of deep tendon reflexes, and thickening of nerves	Search for mutation in the genes *PMP22*, *MPZ*, *EGR2*, electroneuromyography of the limbs

(continued)

Table 2.1 (continued)

Name of neuropathy/disease	Symptoms, signs, and laboratory findings	Complementary exams
Hereditary motor neuropathy with susceptibility to pressure paralysis [20]	Development of multiple mononeuropathies after minor traumas, paresis, muscle hypotrophy, pain, and hypoesthesias	Search for mutation in the *PMP22* gene, electroneuromyography of the limbs
Sarcoidosis [21]	Dyspnea, cough, fatigue, weakness, weight loss, low fever, polyneuropathy, dacryocystitis, erythema nodosum, hypercalcemia, and skin changes	Biopsy of the affected site: lymph nodes, dermatological lesions, conjunctiva, etc. Serum ACE (angiotensin-converting enzyme) dosage, electroneuromyography of the limbs
Vitamin B1 deficiency [22]	Polyneuropathy predominantly in lower limbs, with burning pain, paresthesias, dysesthesias, cognitive changes, psychosis, cardiomyopathy, nystagmus, ataxia, and ophthalmoplegia	Serum vitamin B1 dosage, electroneuromyography of the limbs
Vitamin B6 intoxication [23]	Polyneuropathy affecting proprioceptive and vibratory sensitivity	Serum vitamin B6 dosage, electroneuromyography of the limbs
Hansen's disease [24–26]	Paucibacillary form—skin lesions, hypoesthetic macules, centrally hypopigmented, the lesions are not itchy, thickening of peripheral nerves Lepromatous form—papules, nodules, skin plaques, polyneuropathy, loss of eyebrows and eyelashes Complications: collapse of nasal cartilage, plantar ulcers, erectile dysfunction, glaucoma, iritis, and corneal insensitivity	Skin biopsy, IgM serology for *M. leprae*, electroneuromyography of the limbs
Chronic acquired demyelinating polyneuropathy; chronic relapsing polyneuropathy; CIDP [27]	Symptoms similar to Guillain-Barré syndrome, but with symptoms lasting more than 2 months	Cerebrospinal fluid—cytoproteic dissociation, normal cellularity with elevated proteins, electroneuromyography of the limbs
Lead poisoning [28]	Cognitive impairment, neuropathies, chronic renal dysfunction, abdominal cramps, constipation, mood changes, encephalopathy, and male infertility	Serum lead dosage, X-ray of long bones, electroneuromyography of the limbs

(continued)

Table 2.1 (continued)

Name of neuropathy/ disease	Symptoms, signs, and laboratory findings	Complementary exams
Paraneoplastic syndrome [29]	Polyneuropathy	Anti-Hu antibody, chest computed tomography to rule out lung cancer, electroneuromyography of the limbs
POEMS [30]	Polyneuropathy, organomegaly, endocrinopathy, monoclonal gammopathy, and skin changes	Protein electrophoresis, serum levels of VEGF (vascular endothelial growth factor), complete blood count, immunoglobulin electrophoresis (immunofixation), electroneuromyography of the limbs
Cryoglobulinemia [31, 32]	Polyneuropathy, purpura, arthralgias, and paresis	Serum cryoglobulin measurement, HIV, hepatitis C serology, rheumatoid factor, ANA, hepatitis B serology, and electroneuromyography of the limbs
Systemic lupus erythematosus [33, 34]	Fever, weight loss, arthralgias, arthritis, skin lesions, photosensitivity, oral ulcers, anemia, optic neuritis, myelitis, psychiatric changes, headache, neuropathy, pleural effusion, nephritis, alopecia, and pericarditis	ANA, anti-β2GP1 antibody, anti-dsDNA antibody, anti-Smith antibody, anticardiolipin antibody, complement C3, complement C4, electroneuromyography of the limbs
Rheumatoid arthritis [34]	Joint pain, morning joint stiffness, neuropathy, skin nodules, interstitial lung disease, and associated Sjögren's syndrome	Rheumatoid factor, anti-Ro, anti-La, electroneuromyography of the limbs

neuropathy, the etiology can be associated with infectious processes such as Hansen's disease, HIV, vasculitis, collagen diseases, sarcoidosis, paraneoplastic syndromes, and DM [7, 11, 29].

Ganglionopathies are severe neuropathies, in which the sensory loss identified in the neurological examination is profound and often does not produce a stocking-and-glove-type pattern. In this neuropathy, there is a compromise of proprioception and vibratory sensitivity. Among the most common etiologies of ganglionopathies are paraneoplastic syndrome due to lung carcinoma, Sjögren's syndrome, and pyridoxine poisoning.

Pure motor neuropathies are rare. Initially, they can be confused with syndromes that compromise the lower motor neuron, such as amyotrophic lateral sclerosis (ALS) and progressive muscular atrophy. Among the causes of purely motor neuropathies are lead poisoning, lymphoma, porphyria, and prolonged use of dapsone [35].

Lehmann et al. (2020) classify neuropathies into five patterns, which facilitate clinical reasoning for their management [1].

1. Predominantly sensory distal neuropathy, slowly progressive.
2. Slowly progressive neuropathy that compromises muscles with abnormalities in the feet.
3. Neuropathy with subacute onset and/or proximal motor involvement.
4. Subacute neuropathy, rapidly progressive, painful with autonomic dysfunction.
5. Neuropathy with sensory ataxia, loss of proprioception, and pseudoathetosis.

In the first group, diabetes mellitus (DM), alcoholism, and chemotherapy treatment are identified as etiology. In the exclusion of these etiologies, the patient probably has idiopathic axonal polyneuropathy.

In the second group of neuropathies, it is usually constituted by rarer diseases, in which symptoms can arise in adulthood or childhood. The genetic etiology in this group should be excluded.

In the third group, diabetic plexopathy, vasculitis, paraneoplastic syndromes, and chronic inflammatory demyelinating polyneuropathy (CIDP) can be identified as etiology.

In the fourth group, Guillain-Barré syndrome, vasculitis, hereditary amyloidosis by transthyretin, and paraneoplastic syndromes are identified.

In the fifth group, paraproteinemias, Sjögren's syndrome, paraneoplastic syndromes, and mitochondrial diseases exist as etiology.

The objective of this chapter is to review the main clinical aspects of neuropathies, emphasizing the anamnesis, clinical findings, physical examination of the patient, and complementary exams.

2.2 Anamnesis

2.2.1 History of Present Illness

The first step is to recognize what complaints the patient presents to you. The symptoms in neuropathies can be of a positive or negative type.

Among the positive sensory symptoms are paresthesia, allodynia, pain, and dysesthesia. Among the negative sensory symptoms are hypoesthesia and anesthesia. Regarding motor complaints, among the negative symptoms are paresis, hypotonia, and muscle hypotrophy and among the positives, myokymia, fibrillation, and cramps [7].

The most identified sensory pattern in polyneuropathy is the one in which the patient develops the clinical picture of sensory alterations in a stocking-and-glove pattern, which evolved from the toes to the thighs and fingers to the wrist and forearm. Usually, sensory symptoms are symmetrical. When a greater asymmetry is evidenced, radiculopathy, plexopathy, spinal cord injury, brainstem injury, or cerebral cortex should be suspected to be associated with polyneuropathy. When neuropathy evolves and compromises the knees, the patient usually reports the onset of symptoms in the hands. Among the symptoms described are neuropathic pain, paresthesia, thermal-algic hypoesthesia, and epicritic tactile, proprioceptive, and vibratory sensations. Only a small percentage of patients evolve with allodynia. A striking characteristic is that painful symptoms tend to accentuate during the night period. In the degeneration of the posterior funiculus due to vitamin B12 deficiency, there is a loss of vibratory sensitivity, epicritic tactile, and proprioceptive, with maintenance of thermal-algic sensitivity [22].

As nerves carry autonomic fibers in their structure, some patients may manifest autonomic symptoms in their neurological examination. Symptoms and signs of autonomic neuropathy may arise: dysfunction of pupil accommodation to light, reduction or abolition of sweating in the affected areas, intolerance to heat and cold, hypotension during orthostatic position, changes in bladder and intestinal control, erectile dysfunction, dizziness during position change, Charcot's joints, changes in skin and nail trophism, and hard-to-heal ulcers in the lower limbs.

Regarding motor symptoms, the first signs identified are gait instability, especially for walking in the dark or even maintaining static balance with eyes closed. It is not uncommon for the patient to report that initially they had stumbles when walking on irregular surfaces and stairs. With the progression of the disease, there may arise paresis for foot dorsiflexion, producing a steppage gait. Rarely do neuropathies present patterns of muscle weakness in which the manifestations begin proximally. Among these neuropathies, we can identify in a small percentage of patients with clinical picture of Guillain-Barré syndrome and patients with CIDP [1].

It is important to identify the presence of fever and night sweats, as these findings may suggest the presence of hematological diseases, oncological diseases, or chronic infections. It is important to assess whether there is involvement of sensitivity. Patients with only motor involvement may have diseases whose manifestations are similar to neuropathy, such as amyotrophic lateral sclerosis (ALS), spinal muscular atrophy, or myopathy [1].

2.2.2 *Past History*

During the collection of past history, clues about the etiology of the patient's neuropathy can be identified.

It is important to check if your patient has had previous contact with insecticides and herbicides, history of cancer, and chemotherapy treatment. It is known that some chemotherapeutic agents can cause peripheral neuropathy.

Past and present use of medications should be investigated. Antibiotics and various other medications can induce neuropathies, such as dapsone, amiodarone, cimetidine, chloroquine, gentamicin, and imipramine [28]. Among the most relevant metabolic diseases, we identify DM and hypothyroidism. Veganism is described as causing vitamin B12 deficiency [36]. Treatment with radiotherapy, especially in the cervical region, in some cases triggers actinic plexitis, which can occur years after the oncological treatment [37].

Some surgeries can lead to vitamin B12 deficiency, such as bariatric surgery. Prolonged period of immobility in ICU beds can promote the emergence of neuropathies [38]. The COVID-19 pandemic has also been associated with peripheral neuropathies [39]. HIV infection is also described in the literature as causing neuropathy [11].

2.2.3 *Social History*

Some types of employment can promote contact with chemical agents and heavy metals [28]. Excessive consumption of alcoholic beverages can also cause neuropathies due to deficiency of group B vitamins [22].

2.3 Physical Examination

2.3.1 *Inspection*

Evaluation of the oral mucosa can reveal the presence of ulcers that may suggest Behçet's disease. Patients with enlarged parotid gland, associated with dry eye, may suggest Sjögren's disease. Genital ulcers can be identified in patients with HIV and Behçet's disease [40]. In the oral mucosa, capillary leukoplakia and Kaposi can still be identified, which suggest HIV infection. The tongue without papillae suggests hypovitaminosis of the B complex [10]. In the hypopharynx, the presence of orange tonsils is identified in Tangier's disease [6]. The presence of bulging in the region of the nerve tunnels may indicate the presence of tumors such as schwannomas, lipomas, cysts, and other expansive lesions [41–44]. Dermatological changes in the face assist in the identification process of collagenoses [33]. In lupus erythematosus, some patients may have lesions caused by sun exposure [33]. In dermatomyositis, the heliotrope sign is identified on the face [45]. In Hansen's disease, the patient presents hypochromic lesions in which the thermal-algic sensitivity is compromised, in addition to anhidrosis [46]. The distal hypotrophic musculature in the lower limbs may suggest the Charcot-Marie-Tooth disease, especially when the signs are chronic [18, 47]. The hypotrophy of a muscle group may suggest a compressive neuropathy. In advanced carpal tunnel syndrome (CTS), thenar atrophy can be identified, in Guyon's syndrome and cubital syndrome, the patient may present with first interosseous atrophy. In lesions of the sciatic nerve due to a severe piriformis syndrome, the patient may evolve with calf atrophy. The identification of fasciculations during the physical examination suggests the presence of ALS (Figs. 2.1, 2.2, 2.3, 2.4, 2.5, 2.6a, b. Video 2.1—Patient diagnosed with ALS).

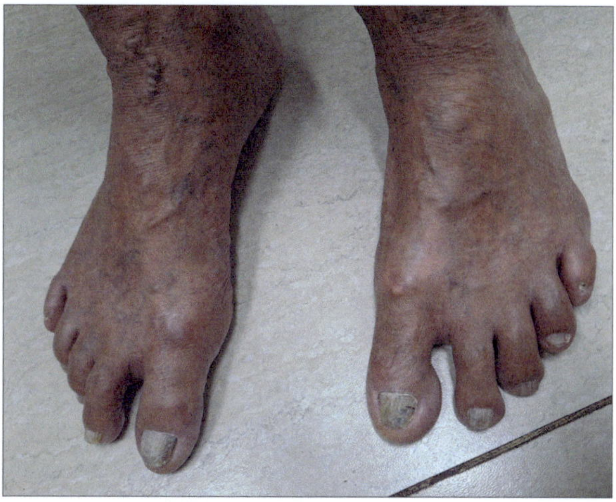

Fig. 2.1 Foot inspection showing nail hypotrophy and alopecia resulting from symmetric sensory motor polyneuropathy

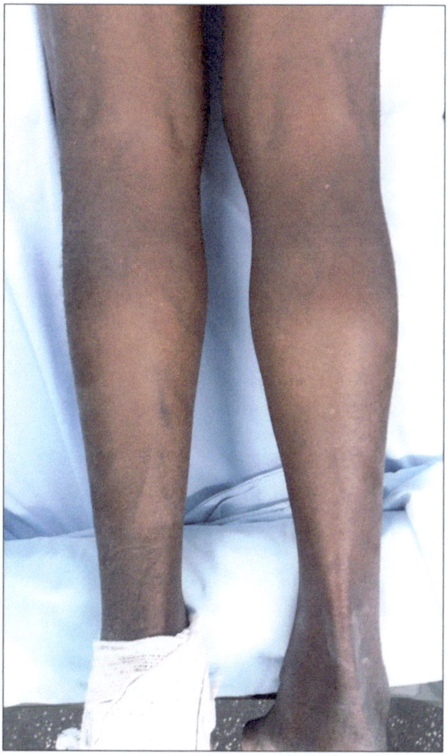

Fig. 2.2 Inspection of the lower limbs. Male patient, 63 years old, with clinical picture of piriformis syndrome in the left lower limb. The patient's main symptom is ipsilateral sciatica. In this clinical case, the etiology of the syndrome is associated with trauma in the gluteal region. Note the hypotrophy of the left calf

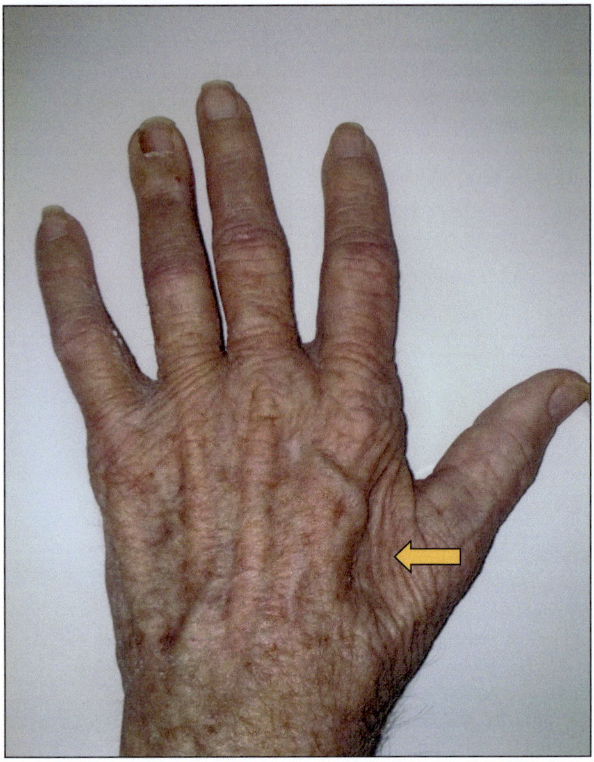

Fig. 2.3 Hand inspection showing hypotrophy of the first interosseous which is pointed out by the yellow arrow. This finding is typical of compressive lesions of the ulnar nerve in advanced stage

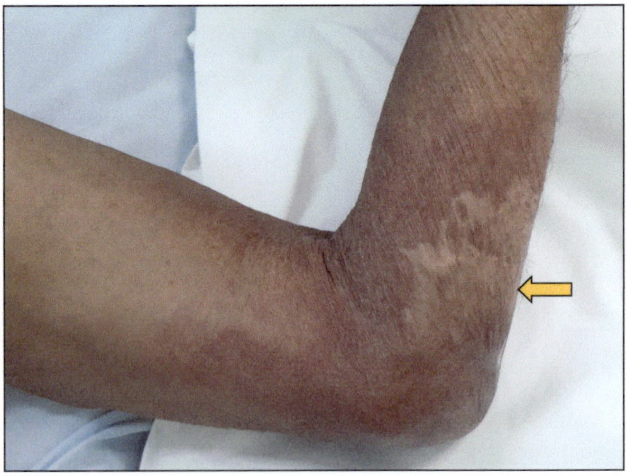

Fig. 2.4 Inspection of the medial face of the left elbow. The yellow arrow points to a hypochromic macule in a patient with Hansen's disease, with multiple compressive syndromes

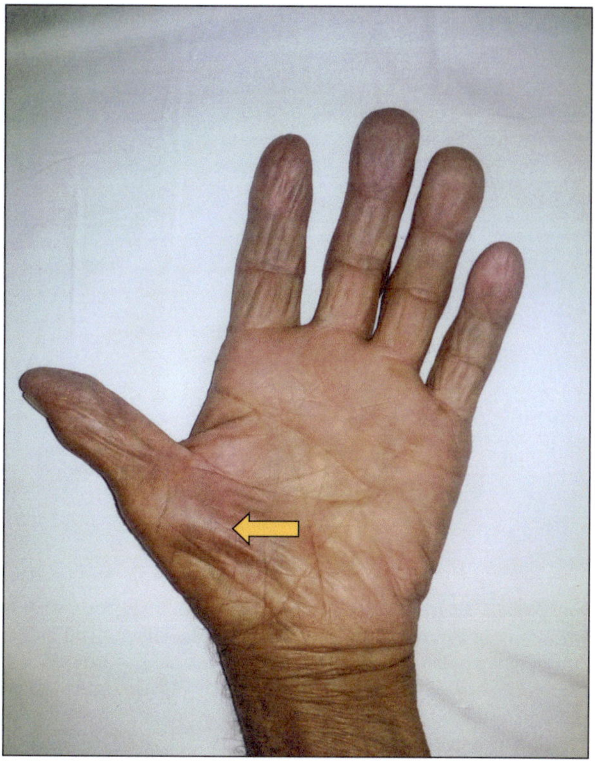

Fig. 2.5 Hand inspection showing hypotrophy of the thenar region (yellow arrow). Elderly patient with severe carpal tunnel syndrome

2.3.2 Gait Assessment

A patient who develops a steppage gait suggests paresis for dorsiflexion of the foot that is identified in compressive neuropathy of the common peroneal nerve and radiculopathy of the L5 spinal nerve. When the patient presents a heel gait, in which they spread their legs to walk and hit the feet on the ground during the march, indicates the involvement of thick axonal fibers, responsible for proprioceptive sensitivity. The inability to walk on the tips of the toes is identified in S1 radiculopathy, in which there may be paresis of the calf muscles. The inability to walk on the heel is identified in L5 radiculopathy and in peroneal nerve neuropathy [48]. It is important to mention that the Romberg sign may be positive when the patient has neuropathy in the lower limbs. However, it is worth remembering that other situations such as cerebellar and labyrinthine lesions can also alter this semiological maneuver [49] (Fig. 2.7a, b, Video 2.2).

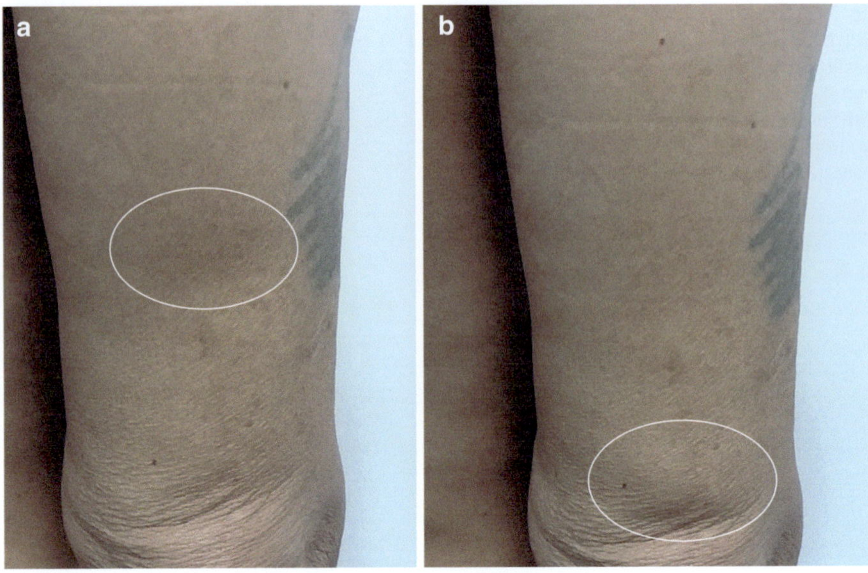

Fig. 2.6 (**a**, **b**) Inspection of the right arm in a patient with amyotrophic lateral sclerosis (ALS) whose initial symptoms of the disease were characterized by a progressive picture of tetraparesis and dysphagia. During the clinical examination, the presence of fasciculations in the triceps muscle was identified. The circles point to the muscle group contracted during the photo. ALS is a relevant differential diagnosis for patients with tetraparesis associated with fasciculations and preservation of sensitivity

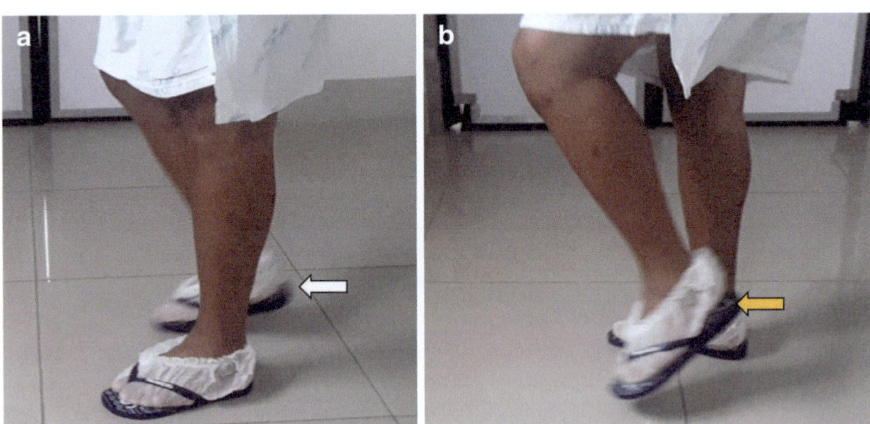

Fig. 2.7 (**a**, **b**) Evaluation of the gait of a patient with foot drop due to injury to the left peroneal nerve. The white arrow reveals that the right foot to move raises a few centimeters from the ground, but the left one during the walk raises several centimeters from the ground to compensate for the loss of dorsiflexion of the foot (yellow arrow)

2.3.3 Evaluation of Reflexes

It is important to remember that neuropathy involving motor nerve fibers is also classified as lower motor neuron syndrome; consequently, the patient may present hyporeflexia or areflexia in their neurological physical examination. Generally, distal reflexes will be compromised first, and later, proximal ones will be affected. It is worth remembering that the Achilles reflex will be abolished in lesions of the S1 spinal nerve; however, the L5 spinal nerve when injured, does not compromise this reflex. Lesions that compromise the L4 spinal nerve can reduce the patellar reflex [48].

The Babinski sign is identified in patients with upper neuron injury and therefore is not identified in patients with polyneuropathy, unless there is an overlap of disease involving the lower and upper motor neuron. Clonus is also identified in upper neuron lesions (Videos 2.3 and 2.4).

2.3.4 Palpation of Nerves and Osteofibrous Tunnels

Palpation of the nerves can assist in the process of identifying the etiology of neuropathy. Thickening of the peroneal and ulnar nerves can be identified in Charcot-Marie-Tooth type I neuropathy and Degerine-Sotas disease type III. Another disease that causes thickening of peripheral nerves is amyloidosis [1].

Other diseases can cause thickening of nerve trunks, such as familial amyloidotic polyneuropathy, neurofibromatosis, Refsum's disease, and chronic inflammatory demyelinating polyneuropathy.

In Hansen's disease, the patient in some cases develops thickening of nerves such as the ulnar and auricular magnus, among other nerves [46]. The presence of a positive Tinel's sign over the nerve tunnels helps to identify which nerve is compromised. Palpation of expansive lesions in the osteofibrous tunnels assists in the process of identifying the etiology of neuropathy. In these cases, the imaging exam will be of great value for better clarification and surgical planning [41–44, 50]. Patients with piriformis syndrome may present a point of pain in the buttock region that triggers local pain associated or not with sciatica [5] (Fig. 2.8).

2.3.5 Evaluation of Muscle Trophism

Inspection of the muscles gives clues about the patient's diagnosis. In deep peroneal neuropathy, some patients develop hypotrophy of the short extensor muscle of the hallux and toes. In Charcot-Marie-Tooth disease, symmetrical distal hypotrophy in the limbs is identified. The pes cavus may be present in patients with hereditary

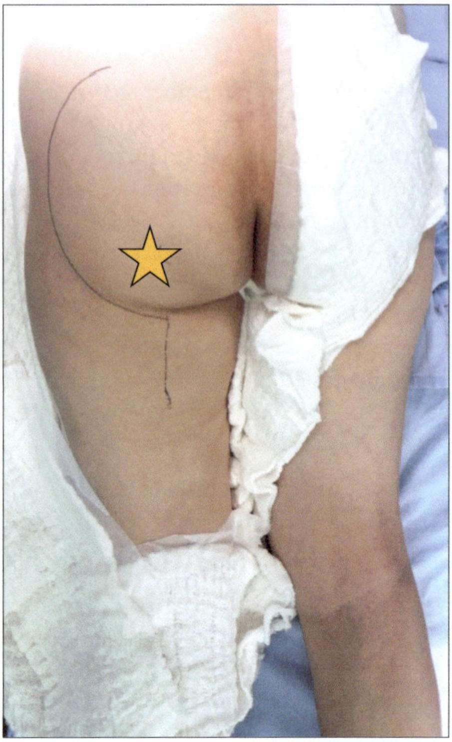

Fig. 2.8 Palpation in the region indicated by the yellow star on the left buttock caused intense pain. Middle-aged female patient, with a history of idiopathic piriformis syndrome. She underwent surgical treatment with resolution of symptoms

neuropathy with susceptibility to pressure paralysis. Thenar hypotrophy is identified in patients with advanced carpal tunnel syndrome. Hypotrophy of the first interosseous is typical of ulnar nerve injury, most commonly at the elbow level and more rarely by Guyon's syndrome (Figs. 2.2, 2.3, and 2.5). Inspection of the muscles of a pediatric or adolescent patient who shows an increase in calf volume, but with motor weakness in the lower limbs, may suggest the presence of dystrophies such as Duchene or Becker. Hypotrophy of the shoulder girdle associated with paresis of the upper limbs may suggest the presence of scapulo-humeral dystrophy.

2.3.6 Evaluation of Muscle Strength

The strength of each muscle group should be evaluated and in case of deficit, it should be classified on the Medical Research Council (MRC) scale with scores ranging from 0 to 5. Each compressive neuropathy can cause specific paresis when the compromised nerve has motor fibers in its composition. In median nerve neuropathy at the level of the carpal tunnel, it can result in weakness for digital grip [42]. In ulnar neuropathy, the patient may have paresis for thumb adduction resulting in Froment's sign. Still in the ulnar syndrome, the patient may develop an ulnar deviation of the fifth digit that receives the denomination of Wartenberg's sign. In the compressive syndrome of the common peroneal nerve, the patient may have paresis for dorsiflexion and eversion of the foot [51]. In meralgia paresthetica, the patient does not have paresis since the nerve is purely sensitive [52].

2.3.7 Evaluation of Sensitivity

During the sensitivity exam, the patient should close their eyes to increase the sensitivity of the semiological test. To perform the tactile sensitivity test, an esthesiometer can be used. However, cotton can be used for the test of epicritic tactile sensitivity. For the pain test, disposable pins or even a broken wooden spatula can be used, which can be found in virtually all medical offices. The 128 Hz or 64 Hz tuning fork is used for the evaluation of vibratory sensitivity, and passive finger movement will be used for proprioception assessment.

Hypoesthesia/pain on the lateral side of the thigh is a typical finding in lateral femoral cutaneous nerve compressive neuropathy [52]. In common peroneal nerve compressive neuropathy, patients tend to develop hypoesthesia, paresthesias, and pain in the lateral region of the leg and dorsum of the foot [51]. When only the deep peroneal nerve is compromised, sensory symptoms are located only in the first digital space of the toes [53]. In tibial nerve neuropathy, at the level of the posterior tarsal tunnel, the patient presents with sensory symptoms in the medial region of the foot and plantar region [50]. Sensitivity changes in the median nerve region that spare the skin of the thenar region may suggest carpal tunnel syndrome [42]. On the other hand, sensitivity changes in the ulnar nerve region in the hand may suggest the presence of a compressive neuropathy of the ulnar at the level of the elbow or wrist [44] (Fig. 2.9a, b).

The presence of vibratory and proprioceptive hypoesthesia suggests the involvement of large caliber myelinated fibers, and hypoesthesia for thermo-algic sensitivity suggests the involvement of small caliber unmyelinated and myelinated fibers. Conversely, the presence of epicritic tactile hypoesthesia suggests the involvement of large and small caliber myelinated fibers. Usually, in polyneuropathies, there is the involvement of fibers of both calibers [7].

The symptom of hyperesthesia, in general, is rare to be identified in neuropathies. In patients with severe sensory polyneuropathy or severe sensory mononeuropathy, involuntary movements in the fingers or hands called pseudoathetosis may be present [7].

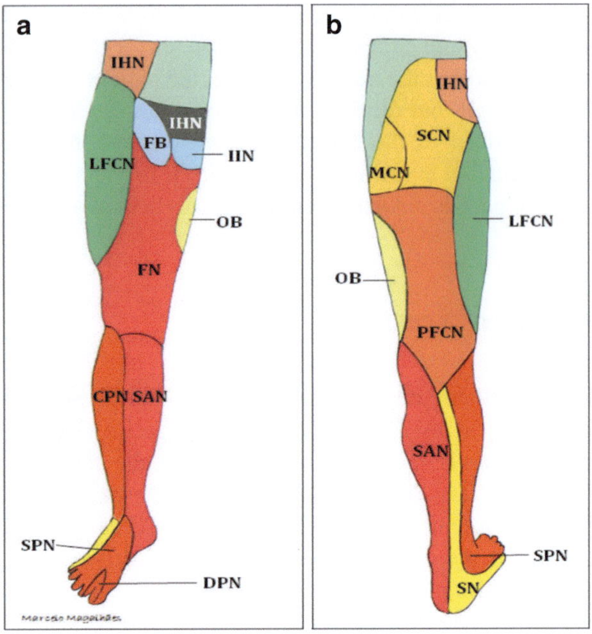

Fig. 2.9 (**a**, **b**) Anterior and posterior view of the sensory territories of the main nerves of the lower limb. *CPN* = common peroneal nerve, *DPN* = deep peroneal nerve, *FB* = femoral branch—genitofemoral nerve, *FN* = femoral nerve, *IHN* = ilihypogastric nerve, *IIN* = ilioinguinal nerve, *LFCN* = lateral femoral cutaneus nerve, *MCN* = medial cluneal nerve, *OB* = obturator nerve, *SAN* = saphenous nerve, *SCN* = superior cluneal nerve, *SPN* = superficial peroneal nerve, *SN* = sural nerve. *The sensory area of the ilioinguinal nerve also presents sensory fibers from the genital branch of the genitofemoral nerve

2.4 Complementary Exams

2.4.1 Electroneuromyographic Studies

The electroneuromyography (ENM) exam allows to define through nerve conduction studies and needle electromyography whether the symptoms/signs result from a neuropathy, radiculopathy, myopathy, and ganglionopathy or even overlap of more than one of these diseases. The ENM also allows to determine the severity of the disease, as well as, classify the neuropathy as axonal versus demyelinating [1]. This complementary exam also contributes to determine the temporality of neural damage, classifying it as acute, subacute, or chronic (Figs. 2.10, 2.11, 2.12, 2.13, 2.14, 2.15, 2.16, and 2.17).

In axonal involvement of a nerve, a reduction in the amplitude of the waves of the compound muscle action potential (CMAP), as well as sensory potentials, is expected, but with preservation of nerve conduction velocity or minimal compromise of these [25].

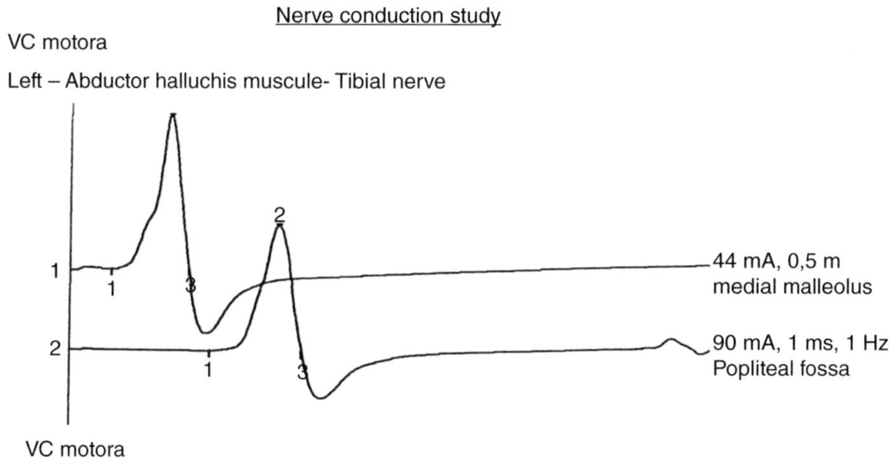

Fig. 2.10 Electroneuromyography of the lower limbs. Examination of a patient with preserved motor conduction of the tibial nerve from the evaluation of the abductor hallucis muscle

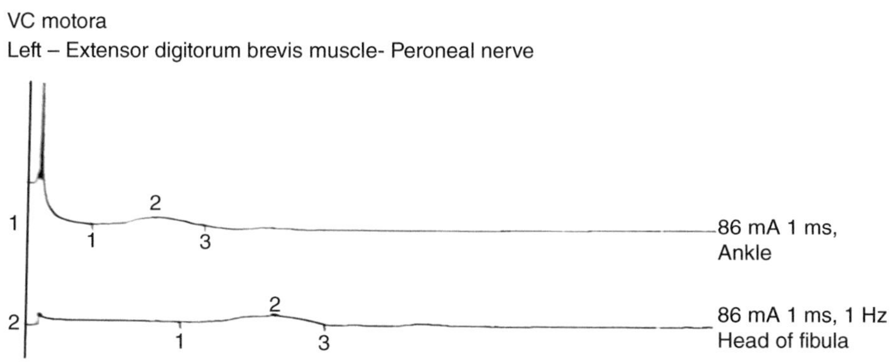

Fig. 2.11 Electroneuromyography of the lower limbs. Examination of a patient with motor conduction of the peroneal nerve revealing axonal type lesion from the evaluation of the extensor digitorum brevis muscle. Note the flattening of the wave when compared to a normal examination present in Fig. 2.10

Observe in Fig. 2.10 that the CMAP waves have a normal amplitude; however, in Fig. 2.11, it is possible to identify a typical flattening that is seen in patients with axonal type nerve lesions.

It is emphasized that in axonal lesions there is a technical difficulty to perform the topography of the point of involvement, since there is a decrease in motor responses in the studied nerve as a whole [25].

The block type lesion is observed when there is a significant reduction in the amplitude of the CMAP in proximal stimuli, however, without an increase in its duration [25]. This type of alteration can be identified in exams of patients with

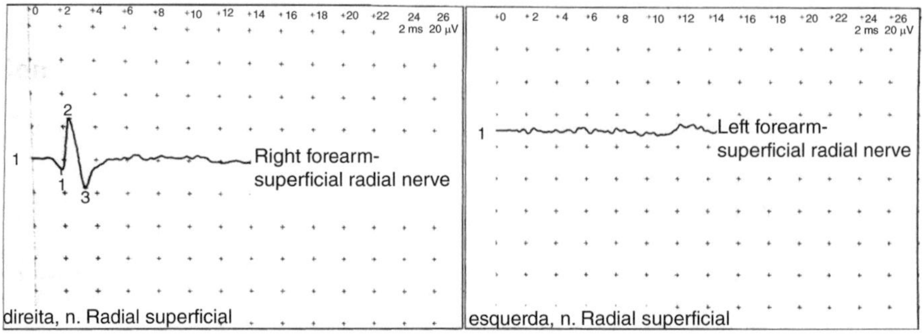

Fig. 2.12 Electroneuromyography of the upper limbs. Examination of a patient with severe neuropathy of the radial nerve in the left upper limb. Note the findings on the right, where the sensory conduction of the left radial nerve presents an indeterminable potential. The graph on the left represents the right radial nerve where the sensory conduction is preserved

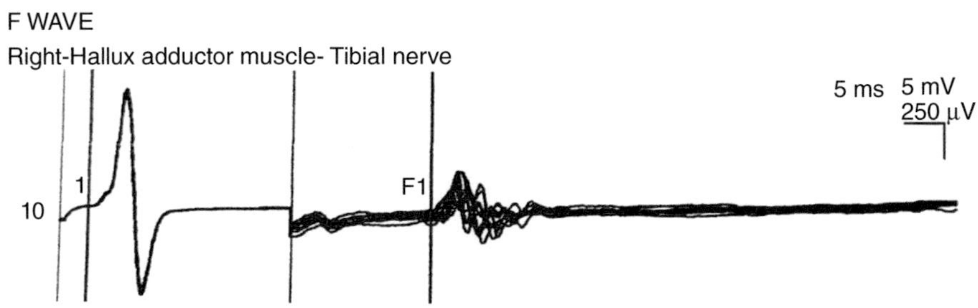

F WAVE ANALYSIS

M lat, ms	Lat F, ms	Lat. perif., ms	Fmin-M lat., ms	V pr., m/s	Dist. Vértebra-pto. estím., mm
3,1	40,2	21,2	37,1		0

Fig. 2.13 Electroneuromyography of the lower limbs. Examination revealing F wave with preserved latency

compressive neuropathies. Conduction block usually refers to a focal demyelination, therefore, a typically myelinic lesion.

See the exam present in Fig. 2.16, where there is a reduction in the amplitude of the CMAP wave of the peroneal nerve in the popliteal fossa. In this specific case, the patient had a diagnosis of compressive syndrome of the peroneal nerve.

Other electrophysiological findings that may be present in demyelinating type lesions are greater temporal dispersion of the CMAP and conduction velocity lower than the limit of normality [25].

It is important to remember that muscles at rest do not have electrical activity, except for the segment near the motor plate. The presence of electrical activity of the musculature at rest may suggest denervation due to nerve injury or myopathies [25].

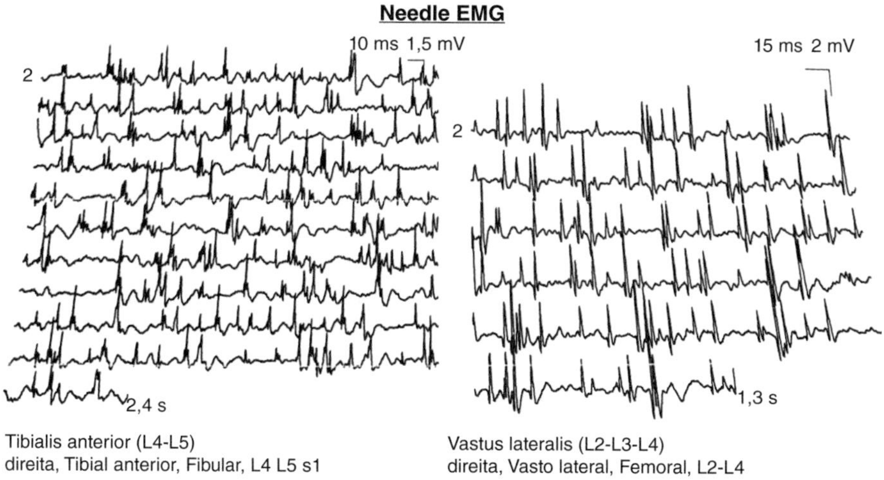

Fig. 2.14 Electroneuromyography of the lower limbs. During the study of voluntary isometric contraction, traces composed of action potentials from motor units with abnormal morphology/recruitment were obtained in the right vastus lateralis and right tibialis anterior muscles

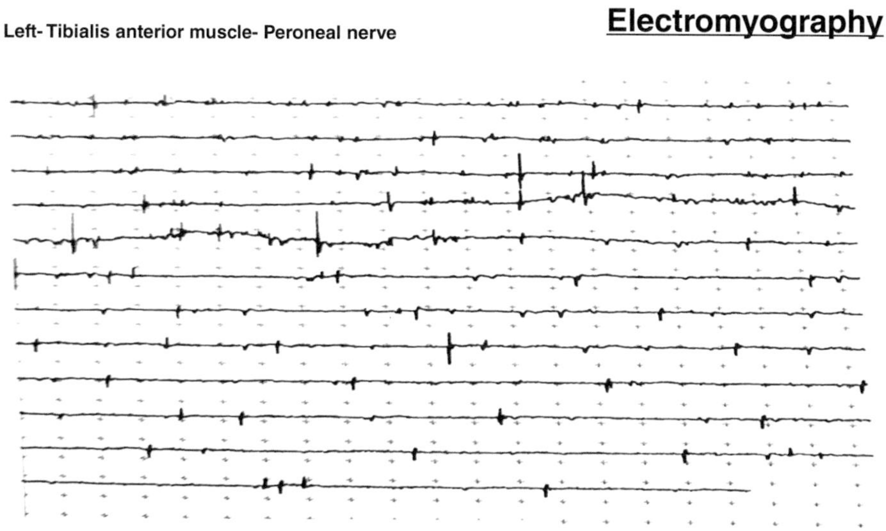

Fig. 2.15 Electromyography of the lower limbs of a patient with a clinical picture of common peroneal nerve neuropathy in the left lower limb. EMG (rest): presence of sharp waves and fibrillations in the left anterior tibial muscle at rest

Observe in Fig. 2.15, in which the patient presents a picture of electrical activity at rest of the tibialis anterior muscle, due to the clinical picture of compressive neuropathy of the peroneal nerve.

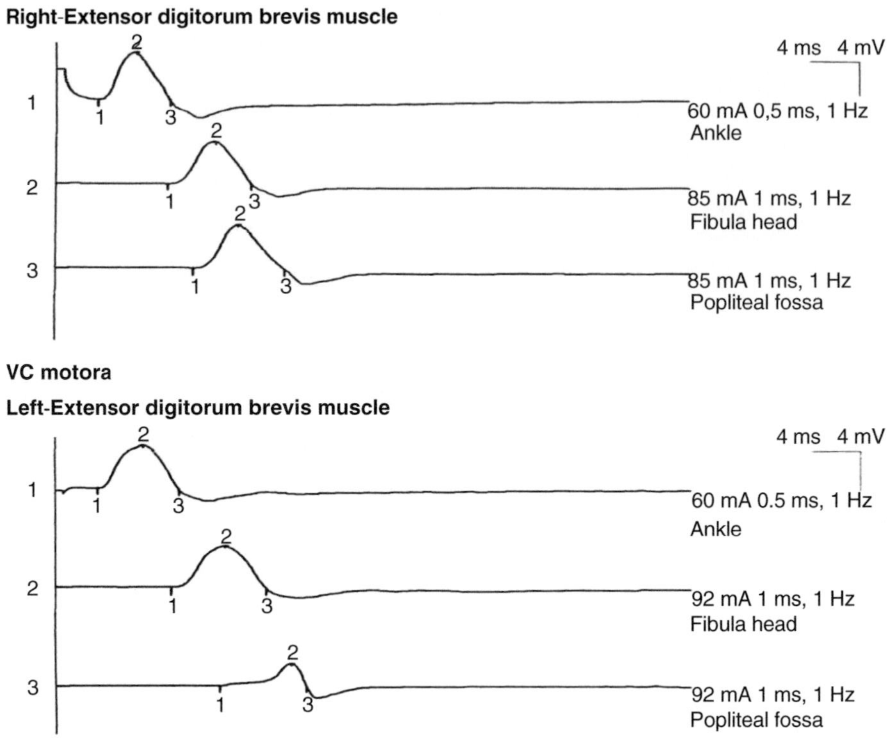

Fig. 2.16 Electroneuromyography of the lower limbs of a patient with a clinical picture of foot drop resulting from common peroneal nerve neuropathy in the left lower limb. The upper graph reveals motor neuroconduction with compound muscle action potentials (CMAPs) of the left deep peroneal nerve with reduced amplitude and speeds in the popliteal fossa proximal to the compression point, which is at the head of the fibula (conduction block). The upper graph reveals compound muscle action potentials (CMAPs) of the right deep peroneal nerve with preserved amplitudes and speeds

The electromyography study with muscle contraction allows to evaluate the form and the pattern in which the recruitment of motor unit potentials occurs. In lesions resulting from a myopathy, generally, the most observed pattern is reduction of amplitude and duration of potentials. From another perspective, in axonal lesions, usually, the potentials of motor units exhibit high amplitude and prolonged duration [25].

Refer to Fig. 2.14, which reveals the electromyography examination during voluntary isometric muscle contraction where traces composed of action potentials from motor units with abnormal morphology/recruitment in the right vastus lateralis and right tibialis anterior muscles were obtained. Note in this examination the increase in wave amplitudes, a finding that is compatible with axonal type neuropathy.

In Fig. 2.17, an electromyography examination of the lower limbs of a patient with a clinical picture of tibial nerve neuropathy at the level of the posterior tarsal tunnel is identified. It is possible to identify that voluntary activation presented motor unit potentials (MUPs) with normal recruitment and morphological

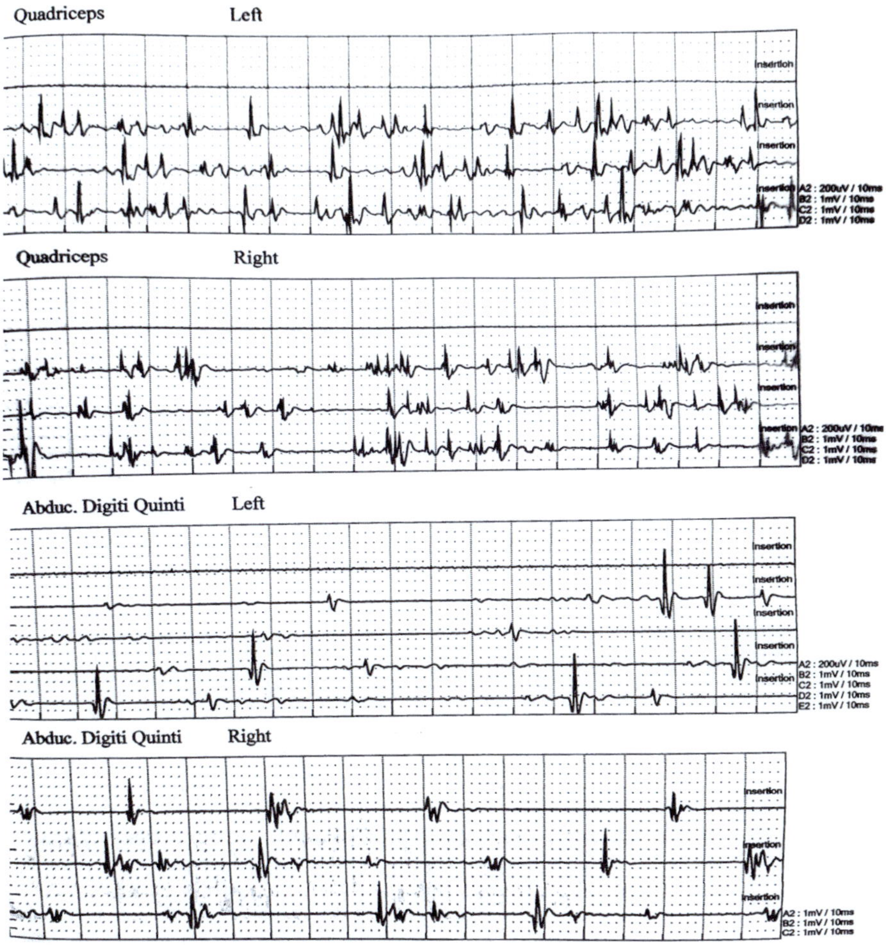

Fig. 2.17 Electromyography of the lower limbs of a patient with a clinical picture of tibial nerve neuropathy at the level of the posterior tarsal tunnel. EMG (with muscle contraction): Voluntary activation showed motor unit potentials (MUP) with normal recruitment and morphological characteristics in the quadriceps femoris muscle, except in the abductor digiti minimi muscle, whose MUPs are with neuropathic characteristics and reduced recruitment

characteristics in the quadriceps femoris muscle; however, in the abductor digiti minimi muscle, the MUPs are found with neuropathic characteristics and reduced recruitment.

Axonal injury findings are commonly identified in neuropathies with clinical pattern 1 [1]. On the other hand, in demyelinating neuropathy, there is a reduction in nerve conduction velocity or even conduction block, temporally dispersed potentials and absent or delayed late responses (e.g., absence of F wave) [1] (Fig. 2.13).

In clinical pattern 2, both demyelinating and axonal neuropathies are present. Neuropathy with uniform demyelination is suggestive of Charcot-Marie-Tooth disease (CMT) type 1A [47].

In clinical patterns 3 and 4, where irregular demyelinating neuropathy occurs, with different nerve conduction velocities, suggesting an immune-mediated etiology.

Clinical pattern 4, may present a pattern of axonal damage or demyelination.

Clinical pattern 5, mostly, presents reduced or absent SNAPs, with normal motor CMAPs [1].

2.4.2 Imaging Exam

Ultrasonography (US) can assist in the process of identifying a compressive neuropathy in which the nerve may present an increased transection area at a point proximal to the compression point. Patients with Charcot-Marie-Tooth disease 1A may present uniformly enlarged nerves. In immune-mediated neuropathies, the US can reveal an asymmetrically increased cross-sectional area among the compromised nerves. Another point of relevance is the identification of tumoral etiologies within the osteofibrous tunnels, as well as, cysts and anatomical variations.

Magnetic resonance imaging can reveal the presence of hyperintensity in the nerve compromised by neuropathy and can also reveal changes in the musculature compromised by the denervation process (Figs. 2.18, 2.19, and 2.20).

2.4.3 Cerebrospinal Fluid Exam

Patients with an acute picture of paresis, areflexia/hyperreflexia associated with sensory changes, should undergo lumbar puncture. The cytoproteic dissociation in which there is an elevation of protein values with normal cellularity values are

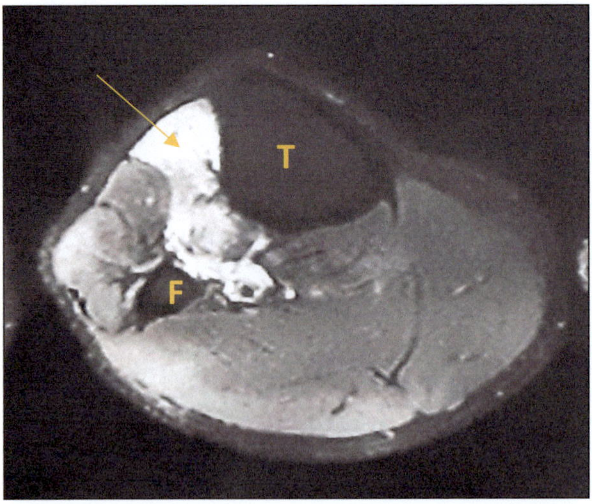

Fig. 2.18 Magnetic resonance imaging of the right leg of a patient with a picture of compressive neuropathy of the right peroneal nerve. The yellow arrow points to the anterior compartment muscle of the leg with a hyperintense appearance due to denervation. Legend: T = tibia, F = fibula

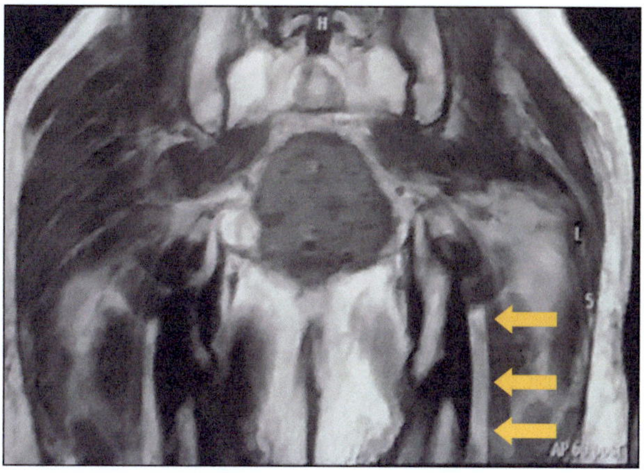

Fig. 2.19 Magnetic resonance imaging of the pelvis in coronal incidence. On the left, the thickened sciatic nerve (yellow arrows) is noted. Patient victim of trauma in the gluteal region, evolving with left piriformis syndrome

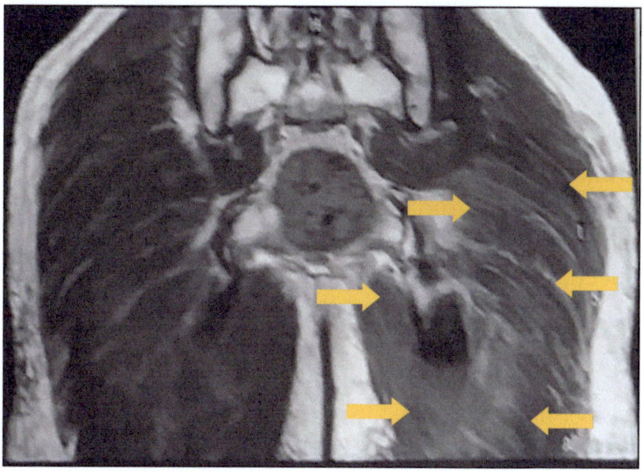

Fig. 2.20 Magnetic resonance imaging of the pelvis in coronal incidence. On the left, the presence of hypersignal in the gluteus maximus muscle resulting from its denervation (yellow arrows) after local trauma that occurred many months ago is noted

suggestive of Guillain-Barré syndrome [54]. The alteration of protein levels in the first week can be observed in 50% of patients with Guillain-Barré syndrome and in the second week in 80%. When the Miller-Fisher variant is present, the anti-GQ1b antibody can be identified in 80–90% of patients [55]. The entity motor axonal neuropathy (AMAN) has been associated with antibodies against GM1, GD1a, GalNac-GD1a, and GD1b [56].

Generally, only patients with clinical patterns of neuropathy type 3 and 5 may benefit from the lumbar puncture examination, allowing the identification of infectious, paraneoplastic [57], and vasculitic processes [58].

In infectious neuropathies, pleocytosis can be identified and the presence of oligoclonal bands is usually found in sarcoidosis, Behçet's disease, paraneoplastic syndromes and borreliosis, as well as inflammatory processes [1, 57, 59, 60].

2.4.4 Laboratory Tests

Patients with clinical patterns of neuropathy type 1 and 2 should undergo the following tests: complete blood count, HBA1c, kidney function, vitamin B12, liver function, methylmalonic acid, and homocysteine.

Among patients who develop clinical pattern type 3, they should undergo the following tests: anti-ganglioside GM1, GD1a, neurofascin (NF155, NF186), Caspr1, anti-myelin associated glycoprotein (MAG) antibody, and contactin-1.

Patients with neuropathy pattern type 4 may benefit from the research of the following tests for vasculitis: ACE, ANA, rheumatoid factor, anti-Ro/SSA, anti-La/SSB, ANCA, and cryoglobulins [1].

The serum vitamin B12 dosage test should always be requested, especially in patients with predominantly sensory distal symmetric chronic polyneuropathy. It is important to remember that serum homocysteine and methylmalonic acid (MMA) levels are elevated in patients with vitamin B12 deficiency. The request for the serum homocysteine and MMA dosage test increases the sensitivity of the evaluation of vitamin B12 [61]. Elevated serum homocysteine levels in patients with low normal serum values of vitamin B12 may be associated with polyneuropathy [61]. It is essential not to prescribe B complex vitamin-based medications for the treatment of polyneuropathy before investigating vitamin B12 deficiency, to avoid compromising the patient's actual serum result.

Protein electrophoresis is important for identifying numerous diseases potentially associated with neuropathy. This test quantifies the immunoglobulins produced, which when present in excess, may be associated with monoclonal gammopathy. Gammopathy can be present in patients suffering from a wide variety of diseases such as cryoglobulinemia, lymphomas, amyloidosis, multiple myeloma, Waldenström's macroglobulinemia, and POEMS (polyneuropathy, organomegaly, endocrinopathy, and skin manifestations) [61].

Patients with neuropathy associated with joint pain should undergo tests for antinuclear antibody (ANA), rheumatoid factor, aldolase, and creatine phosphokinase. For those who present with reduced tearing and xerostomia, a diagnosis of Sjögren's syndrome should be evaluated, for this, anti-SSA-Ro and anti-SSB-La antibodies can be requested.

Patients with progressive weight loss associated with night sweat, with tests showing lymphocyte counts below reference values, should be tested for HIV.

When the patient's history includes travel to rural areas endemic for ticks, Lyme disease serology should be requested.

In cases of chronic neuropathy, with recurrent episodes, where the symptoms are compatible with CIDP, a lumbar puncture should be performed to confirm the presence of elevated protein levels (>45 mg/dL) however, without abnormal cellularity values. Other antibodies that may be positive in CIDP are anti-ganglioside 18.6%, anti-contactin-1 6.2%, neurofascin 4.6%, and anti-peripheral myelin protein antibody 1.6% [27].

Patients suspected of multifocal motor neuropathy typically present with asymmetric, distal symptoms affecting the upper limbs. In these cases, anti-GM1 antibody should be requested. Other antibodies can be requested, such as anti-GM1:GalC complex [62] and anti-NS6S [63].

Charcot-Marie-Tooth disease is a chronic neuropathy in which the patient presents with pes cavus and "stork legs," especially when there is a positive family history. For these patients, a genetic test for PMP22 duplication should be requested [64]. The duplication of PMP22 can be identified in 70%, followed by the MPZ mutation with 5% [65].

In the suspicion of multiple mononeuropathies, HIV, cytomegalovirus, Lyme disease, hepatitis, ANA, C-reactive protein, angiotensin-converting enzyme (investigation of sarcoidosis), transthyretin (investigation of amyloidosis), erythrocyte sedimentation rate [66] should be investigated. In neuropathy that compromises the radial nerve alone, the serum level of lead should be investigated. In the suspicion of hereditary neuropathy, with predisposition to pressure paralysis, the genetic test for the deletion of the PMP22 gene should be requested.

Patients with acute or subacute axonal polyneuropathy may present porphyria as etiology. In this disease, the quantification of porphobilinogen and porphyrin excretion should be requested. In the suspicion of heavy metal poisoning, these can be detected in the urine test.

If the patient with neuropathy has small cell lung cancer, the anti-Hu antibody test should be requested as the chances of being a case of paraneoplastic syndrome are high [29].

2.4.5 *Nerve Biopsy*

A nerve biopsy brings some benefit only in cases where the patient presents a neuropathy of inflammatory etiology, such as a neuropathy due to non-systemic vasculitis. Another indication for biopsy would be CIDP. These are patients with a clinical picture compatible with type 4 pattern [67].

2.5 Conclusions

As neuropathies are made up of a heterogeneous group of diseases with dozens of etiologies, conducting anamnesis and physical examination of the patient with clinical neuropathy is fundamental for the correct identification of the etiology. Despite the available complementary tests and the expertise of the health professional, a considerable fraction of patients cannot adequately define the etiology of their neuropathy.

References

1. Lehmann HC, Wunderlich G, Fink GR, Sommer C. Diagnosis of peripheral neuropathy. Neurol Res Pract. 2020;2:20.
2. Visser NA, et al. Incidence of polyneuropathy in Utrecht, the Netherlands. Neurology. 2015;84(3):259–64.
3. Hanewinckel R, et al. Prevalence of polyneuropathy in the general middle-aged and elderly population. Neurology. 2016;87(18):1892–8.
4. Hanewinckel R, et al. The epidemiology and risk factors of chronic polyneuropathy. Eur J Epidemiol. 2016;31(1):5–20.
5. Probst D, Stout A, Hunt D. Piriformis syndrome: a narrative review of the anatomy, diagnosis, and treatment. PM R. 2019;11(Suppl 1):S54–63.
6. Burnett JR, Hooper AJ, McCormick SPA, et al. Tangier disease. In: Adam MP, Feldman J, Mirzaa GM, et al., editors. GeneReviews® [Internet]. Seattle: University of Washington, Seattle; 1993–2024; 2019.
7. Donofrio PD. Peripheral neuropathy. 1st ed. Demos Medical; 2012.
8. Kazamel M, Stino AM, Smith AG. Metabolic syndrome and peripheral neuropathy. Muscle Nerve. 2021;63(3):285–93.
9. Liampas A, Parperis K, Erotocritou MF, Nteveros A, Papadopoulou M, Moschovos C, Akil M, Coaccioli S, Hadjigeorgiou GM, Hadjivassiliou M, Zis P. Primary Sjögren syndrome-related peripheral neuropathy: a systematic review and meta-analysis. Eur J Neurol. 2023;30(1):255–65.
10. Chen GY, Tang ZQ, Bao ZX. Vitamin B12 deficiency may play an etiological role in atrophic glossitis and its grading: a clinical case-control study. BMC Oral Health. 2022;22(1):456.
11. Morgello S. HIV neuropathology. Handb Clin Neurol. 2018;152:3–19.
12. Kaku M, Berk JL. Neuropathy associated with systemic amyloidosis. Semin Neurol. 2019;39(5):578–88.
13. Crissinger T, Baldwin K. Early disseminated Lyme disease: cranial neuropathy, meningitis, and polyradiculopathy. Infect Dis Clin N Am. 2022;36(3):541–51.
14. Reñé R, Salazar A, Ferrer X. Complicaciones neurológicas por citomegalovirus en pacientes con SIDA [Neurological complications caused by cytomegalovirus in patients with AIDS]. Rev Neurol. 1996;24(136):1590–6.
15. Shang P, Zhu M, Wang Y, Zheng X, Wu X, Zhu J, Feng J, Zhang HL. Axonal variants of Guillain-Barré syndrome: an update. J Neurol. 2021;268(7):2402–19.
16. Finsterer J. Small fiber neuropathy underlying dysautonomia in COVID-19 and in post-SARS-CoV-2 vaccination and long-COVID syndromes. Muscle Nerve. 2022;65(6):E31–2.
17. Shahrizaila N, Lehmann HC, Kuwabara S. Guillain-Barré syndrome. Lancet. 2021;397(10280):1214–28.
18. Roa BB, Garcia CA, Lupski JR. Charcot-Marie-Tooth disease type 1A: molecular mechanisms of gene dosage and point mutation underlying a common inherited peripheral neuropathy. Int J Neurol. 1991;25–26:97–107.
19. Plante-Bordeneuve V, Said G. Dejerine-Sottas disease and hereditary demyelinating polyneuropathy of infancy. Muscle Nerve. 2002;26(5):608–21.
20. Attarian S, Fatehi F, Rajabally YA, Pareyson D. Hereditary neuropathy with liability to pressure palsies. J Neurol. 2020;267(8):2198–206.
21. Tavee J. Peripheral neuropathy in sarcoidosis. J Neuroimmunol. 2022;368:577864.
22. Kramarz C, Murphy E, Reilly MM, Rossor AM. Nutritional peripheral neuropathies. J Neurol Neurosurg Psychiatry. 2023;95(1):61–72.
23. Misumi J, Nagano M, Kaisaku J, Hitoshi T. Effects of vitamin B12 and B6 on 2,5-hexanedione-induced neuropathy. Arch Toxicol. 1985;56(3):204–6.
24. Bhandari J, Awais M, Robbins BA, et al. Leprosy. [Updated 2023 Sep 15]. In: StatPearls [Internet]. Treasure Island: StatPearls Publishing; 2024. Available from: https://www.ncbi.nlm.nih.gov/books/NBK559307/.

25. Gondin FAA, Freitas MRG, Pereira RC. Neuropatias periféricas. 1ª ed. São Paulo: Ominifarma; 2020.
26. Levin SN, Lyons JL. Infections of the nervous system. Am J Med. 2018;131(01):25–32.
27. Querol L, Siles AM, Alba-Rovira R, et al. Antibodies against peripheral nerve antigens in chronic inflammatory demyelinating polyradiculoneuropathy. Sci Rep. 2017;7(01):14411.
28. Neundörfer B. Toxische polyneuropathien [Toxic polyneuropathies]. Versicherungsmedizin. 1992;44(4):119–25. German.
29. Papantoniou M, Zampelis T, Rentzos M, et al. Anti-Hu antibody seropositive neuropathy with large and small fiber involvement mimicking alcoholic neuropathy: a case report. Egypt J Neurol Psychiatr Neurosurg. 2023;59:161.
30. Dispenzieri A. POEMS syndrome: 2019 update on diagnosis, risk-stratification, and management. Am J Hematol. 2019;94(7):812–27.
31. Bhandari J, Awais M, Aeddula NR. Cryoglobulinemia. [Updated 2022 Aug 10]. In: StatPearls [Internet]. Treasure Island: StatPearls Publishing; 2024. Available from: https://www.ncbi.nlm.nih.gov/books/NBK557606/.
32. Justiz Vaillant AA, Goyal A, Varacallo M. Systemic lupus erythematosus. [Updated 2023 Aug 4]. In: StatPearls [Internet]. Treasure Island: StatPearls Publishing; 2024. Available from: https://www.ncbi.nlm.nih.gov/books/NBK535405/.
33. Olney RK. Neuropathies associated with connective tissue disease. Semin Neurol. 1998;18(1):63–72.
34. Chauhan K, Jandu JS, Brent LH, et al. Rheumatoid arthritis. [Updated 2023 May 25]. In: StatPearls [Internet]. Treasure Island: StatPearls Publishing; 2024. Available from: https://www.ncbi.nlm.nih.gov/books/NBK441999/.
35. Nagy H, Veerapaneni KD. Myopathy. [Updated 2023 Aug 14]. In: StatPearls [Internet]. Treasure Island: StatPearls Publishing; 2024. Available from: https://www.ncbi.nlm.nih.gov/books/NBK562290/.
36. Huang-Link Y, Mirabelli P, Lindehammar H, Link H. Retinal changes associated with multivitamin deficiency before and after supplementation. Acta Neurol Scand. 2021;144(2):209–15.
37. Tairych G, Todoroff B, Sedivy R, Eberhard D, Deutinger M, Meissl G, Millesi H. Aktinische plexus brachialis-Läsion [Actinic brachial plexus lesion]. Handchir Mikrochir Plast Chir. 1998;30(4):254–7. German.
38. Hermans G, Van den Berghe G. Clinical review: intensive care unit acquired weakness. Crit Care. 2015;19(1):274.
39. Taga A, Lauria G. COVID-19 and the peripheral nervous system. A 2-year review from the pandemic to the vaccine era. J Peripher Nerv Syst. 2022;27(1):4–30.
40. Akbulut L, Gur G, Bodur H, Alli N, Borman P. Peripheral neuropathy in Behçet disease: an electroneurophysiological study. Clin Rheumatol. 2007;26(8):1240–4.
41. Magalhães MJS, Freire ALS, Souza CF, Fernandes CF, Alves CM, et al. Thoracic outlet syndrome caused by Hodgkin's lymphoma – case report. Open Access J Neurol Neurosurg. 2018;7(1):555701.
42. Magalhães MJS, Fujioka AJ, Chaves RB. Schwannoma como etiologia de síndrome do túnel do carpo – relato de caso. Arq Bras Neurocir Braz Neurosurg. 2015;34(04):309–12.
43. Magalhães MJS, Pereira DVM, Oliva HNP, Durães DTS, Caiado FL, Araújo GM, Freitas Junior ET. Peripheral nerve schwannomas: a literature review. Arq Bras Neurocir Braz Neurosurg. 2019;38(04):308–14.
44. Magalhães MJS, Hen Oliva HNP, Nunes BL. Compressive neuropathy of the ulnar nerve in the hypothenar region by lipoma: case report. Arq Bras Neurocir Braz Neurosurg. 2020;39(01):049–53.
45. Magalhaes MJS, Ferreira VM. Multiple nerve compression syndrome in dermatopolymyositis: case report. Arq Bras Neurocir Braz Neurosurg. 2016;35(01):85–8.
46. Gilmore A, Roller J, Dyer JA. Leprosy (Hansen's disease): an update and review. Mo Med. 2023;120(1):39–44.
47. Freitas MR, Nascimento OJ, Nevares MT, Escada TM. Doença de Charcot-Marie-Tooth. Estudos eletromiográficos em 45 pacientes [Charcot-Marie-Tooth disease. Electromyographic studies in 45 patients]. Arq Neuropsiquiatr. 1995;53(3-B):552–9. Portuguese.

48. Al Qaraghli MI, De Jesus O. Lumbar disc herniation. [Updated 2023 Aug 23]. In: StatPearls [Internet]. Treasure Island: StatPearls Publishing; 2024. Available from: https://www.ncbi.nlm.nih.gov/books/NBK560878/.
49. Forbes J, Munakomi S, Cronovich H. Romberg test. [Updated 2023 Aug 13]. In: StatPearls [Internet]. Treasure Island: StatPearls Publishing; 2024. Available from: https://www.ncbi.nlm.nih.gov/books/NBK563187/.
50. Magalhães MJS, Ribeiro ICV, Cardoso MM, Gepp RA. Surgical treatment compared to conservative treatment in remission of pain and hyposthesia in tarsal tunnel syndrome – systematic review. Arq Bras Neurocir Braz Neurosurg. 2022;41(02):e145–52.
51. Capodici A, Hagert E, Darrach H, Curtin C. An overview of common peroneal nerve dysfunction and systematic assessment of its relation to falls. Int Orthop. 2022;46(12):2757–63.
52. Gomez YC, Remotti E, Momah DU, Zhang E, Swanson DD, Kim R, Urits I, Kaye AD, Robinson CL. Meralgia paresthetica review: update on presentation, pathophysiology, and treatment. Health Psychol Res. 2023;11:71454.
53. Dreyer MA, Gibboney MD. Anterior tarsal tunnel syndrome. [Updated 2023 May 23]. In: StatPearls [Internet]. Treasure Island: StatPearls Publishing; 2024. Available from: https://www.ncbi.nlm.nih.gov/books/NBK538488/.
54. Illes Z, Blaabjerg M. Cerebrospinal fluid findings in Guillain-Barré syndrome and chronic inflammatory demyelinating polyneuropathies. Handb Clin Neurol. 2017;146:125–38.
55. Teener JW. Miller Fisher's syndrome. Semin Neurol. 2012;32(05):512–6.
56. Ogawara K, Kuwabara S, Mori M, Hattori T, Koga M, Yuki N. Axonal Guillain-Barré syndrome: relation to anti-ganglioside antibodies and Campylobacter jejuni infection in Japan. Ann Neurol. 2000;48(04):624–31.
57. Vicent-Lau KHV. Laboratory evaluation of peripheral neuropathy. Semin Neurol. 2019;39(5):531–41. https://doi.org/10.1055/s-0039-1691749. Epub 2019 Oct 22.
58. Godasi R, Pang G, Chauhan S, et al. Primary central nervous system vasculitis. [Updated 2023 Jun 19]. In: StatPearls [Internet]. Treasure Island: StatPearls Publishing; 2024. Available from: https://www.ncbi.nlm.nih.gov/books/NBK482476/.
59. Vegezzi E, Gastaldi M, Cortese A. Towards a standardised analysis of CSF in inflammatory neuropathies. J Neurol Neurosurg Psychiatry. 2021;92:916.
60. Kaminsky AL, Maisonobe T, Lenglet T, Psimaras D, Debs R, Viala K. Confirmed cases of neuroborreliosis with involvement of peripheral nervous system: description of a cohort. Medicine (Baltimore). 2020;99(40):e21986. https://doi.org/10.1097/MD.0000000000021986. PMID: 33019390; PMCID: PMC7535703.
61. Callaghan BC, Price RS, Feldman EL. Distal symmetric polyneuropathy: a review. JAMA. 2015;314(20):2172–81. https://doi.org/10.1001/jama.2015.13611. PMID: 26599185; PMCID: PMC5125083.
62. Galban-Horcajo F, Vlam L, Delmont E, Halstead SK, van den Berg L, van der Pol WL, Willison HJ. The diagnostic utility of determining anti-GM1: GalC complex antibodies in multifocal motor neuropathy: a validation study. J Neuromuscul Dis. 2015;2(2):157–65.
63. Pestronk A, Chuquilin M, Choksi R. Motor neuropathies and serum IgM binding to NS6S heparin disaccharide or GM1 ganglioside. J Neurol Neurosurg Psychiatry. 2010;81(7):726–30.
64. van Paassen BW, van der Kooi AJ, van Spaendonck-Zwarts KY, Verhamme C, Baas F, de Visser M. PMP22 related neuropathies: Charcot-Marie-Tooth disease type 1A and hereditary neuropathy with liability to pressure palsies. Orphanet J Rare Dis. 2014;9:38. https://doi.org/10.1186/1750-1172-9-38. PMID: 24646194; PMCID: PMC3994927.
65. Nakamura N, Kawamura N, Tateishi T, Doi H, Ohyagi Y, Kira J. [Predominant parasympathetic involvement in a patient with Charcot-Marie-Tooth disease caused by the MPZ Thr124Met mutation]. Rinsho Shinkeigaku. 2009;49(9):582–5. Japanese.
66. Hehir MK II, Logigian EL. Infectious neuropathies. Continuum (Minneap Minn). 2014;20(5):1274–92.
67. Moise ES, Bratu RM, Hanganu A, Sajin M. Relevance of nerve biopsy in the diagnosis of chronic inflammatory demyelinating polyneuropathy-a systematic review. Diagnostics (Basel). 2022;12(7):1691.

Chapter 3
Anatomy of the Lower Limb Nerves

3.1 Anatomy of the Sciatic Nerve

The sciatic or ischiadic nerve (SN) is the peripheral nerve with the largest diameter in the human body, about 2 cm [1]. It is made up of the posterior and anterior divisions of the spinal nerves L4, L5, S1, and S2, in addition to the anterior division of the spinal nerve S3. Anatomically, the posterior divisions are responsible for the formation of the peroneal nerve and the anterior ones for the tibial nerve [2]. Proximal injuries to this nerve are usually very severe and cause plegia of all muscles distal to the knee and significant sensory deficits involving the plantar region, lateral face of the leg, and dorsum of the foot (Fig. 3.1).

The sciatic nerve leaves the pelvis through the greater sciatic foramen to present a trajectory under the piriformis muscle. Beaton and Anson (1937) described six possible anatomical variations between the sciatic nerve and the piriformis muscle [3] (Fig. 3.2). It is important to mention that in the medical literature, there is the description of anatomical variation of the piriformis muscle in which the classification of Beaton and Anson is not possible to be applied [4]. Below is the classification of Beaton and Anson.

Type I—This is the most commonly identified anatomical variation, in which the nerve with a single bundle structure presents a trajectory below the piriformis muscle.

Type II—In this pattern, the nerve has two bundles, one of them presents a trajectory through the fibers of the muscle and another over the muscle.

Type III—Anatomical pattern in which the nerve in a single bundle emerges above the piriformis muscle.

Type IV—The nerve is divided into two bundles, one transits through the fibers of the piriformis muscle and the other division, passes below the muscle.

M. J. S. Magalhães, *Lower Extremity Nerve Entrapments*,
https://doi.org/10.1007/978-3-031-90058-7_3

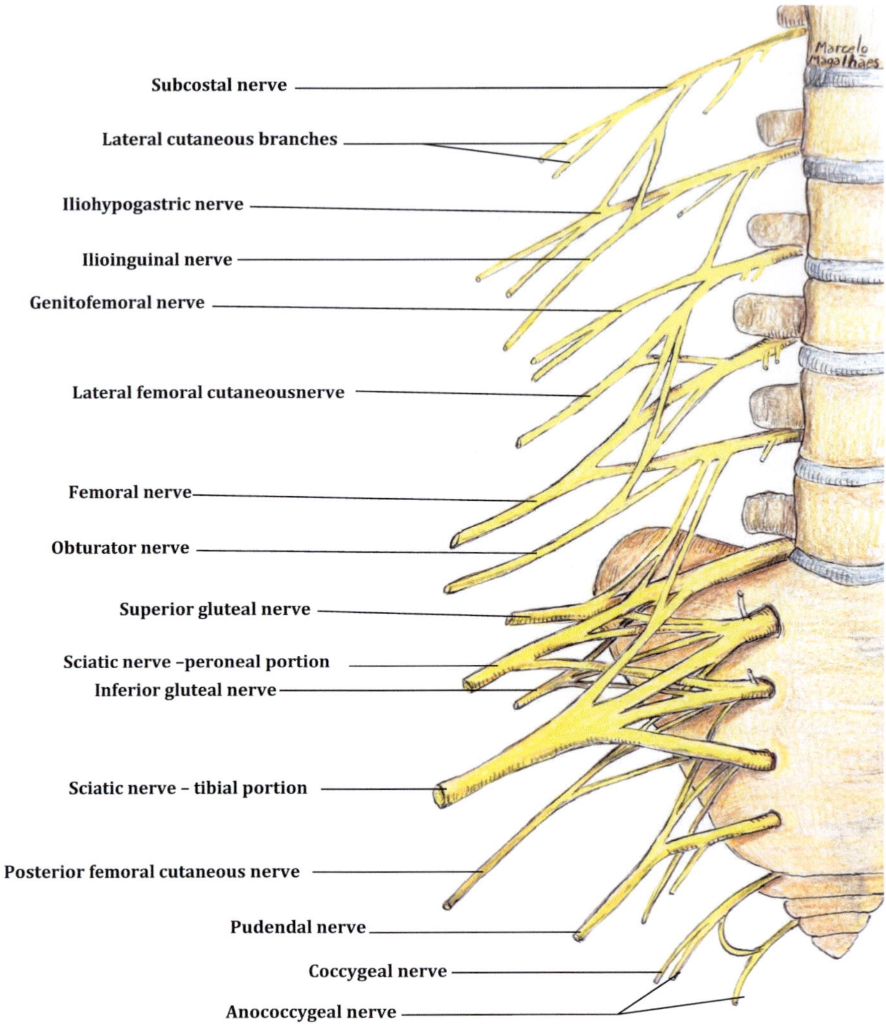

Fig. 3.1 Nerves and branches of the lumbosacral plexus

Type V—Anatomical variation in which the nerve in a single bundle emerges through the fibers of the muscle.

Type VI—In this anatomical pattern, the nerve presents two bundles that pass respectively below and above the muscle [5].

It is emphasized that the most commonly identified variations in the American population [6] and Eastern Europe are those of type I–IV [7], types I and II predominate among Indians [8] and Japanese [9, 10], and types IV, V, and VI predominate in the Ethiopian population [11] (Fig. 3.3). The piriformis muscle has great

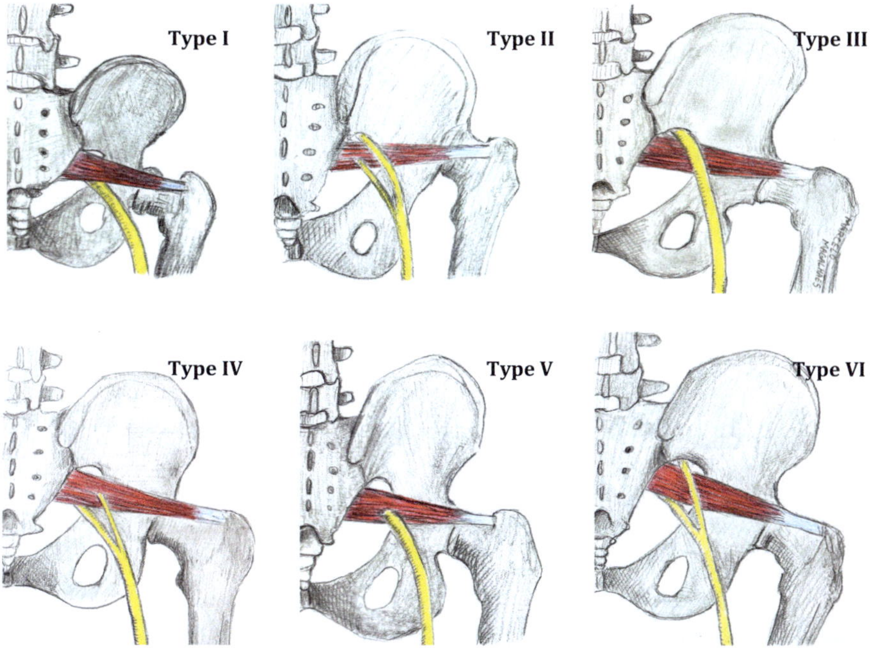

Fig. 3.2 Anatomical variation of the sciatic nerve and its relationship with the piriformis muscle

Fig. 3.3 View of the right gluteal region, with exposure of the posterior femoral cutaneous nerve. *BFM* = biceps femoris muscle, *GMM* = gluteus maximus muscle, *PFCN* = posterior femoral cutaneous nerve, *STM* = semitendinosus muscle

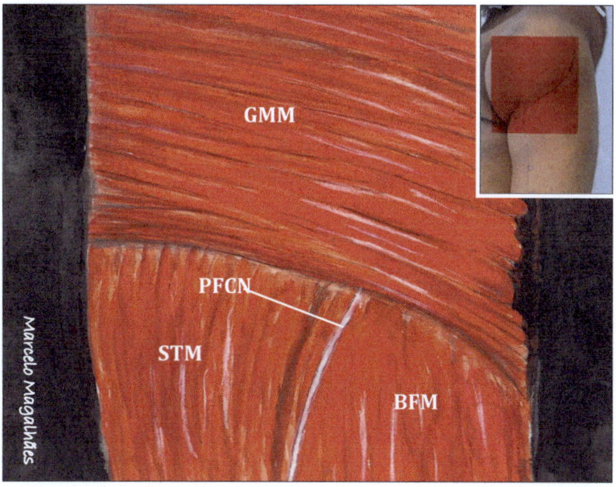

clinical relevance, as it is a compression point of the SN causing the piriformis syndrome.

After leaving the piriformis muscle and still under the gluteus maximus muscle, the nerve presents a trajectory over the superior gemellus, obturator internus, inferior gemellus, quadratus femoris, and adductor minimus muscles. Distal to the gluteal region, the nerve is positioned posterior to the femur, lateral to the biceps femoris muscle, and medial to the iliotibial tract. More distally, the biceps femoris muscle crosses over the sciatic nerve to position itself laterally to the nerve and the semitendinosus muscle positions itself medially to the SN [2] (Figs. 3.3, 3.4, and 3.5).

At the level of the thigh, the tibial division of the sciatic nerve produces branches for motor innervation of the semitendinosus, semimembranosus, and long head of the biceps femoris muscles and sciatic part of the adductor magnus muscle. The peroneal division, in turn, innervates the short head of the biceps femoris muscle.

It is important to remember that all motor and sensory innervation below the knee is performed by the branches of the sciatic nerve, with the exception of a medial skin extension that is performed by the saphenous nerve which is a sensory branch of the femoral nerve (Fig. 3.6a, b).

It is essential to note that in the structure of the SN it is possible to visualize the medial (tibial division) and lateral (peroneal division) trunks, which are gathered under the same sheath. Approximately, at the level of the union from the middle third to the distal third of the thigh, the sciatic nerve undergoes the process of division to constitute the common peroneal and tibial nerves [2].

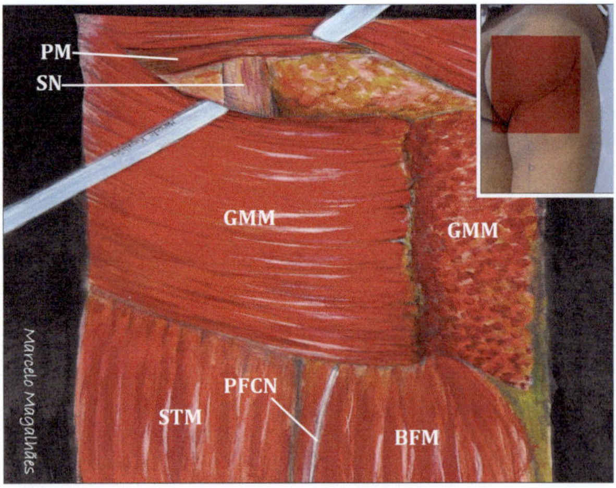

Fig. 3.4 View of the right gluteal region, with exposure of the posterior femoral cutaneous nerve and the sciatic nerve, after opening the fibers of the gluteus maximus muscle. Note the presence of the piriformis muscle over the sciatic nerve. *BFM* = biceps femoris muscle, *GMM* = gluteus maximus muscle, *PFCN* = posterior femoral cutaneous nerve, *PM* = piriformis muscle, *SN* = sciatic nerve, *STM* = semitendinosus muscle

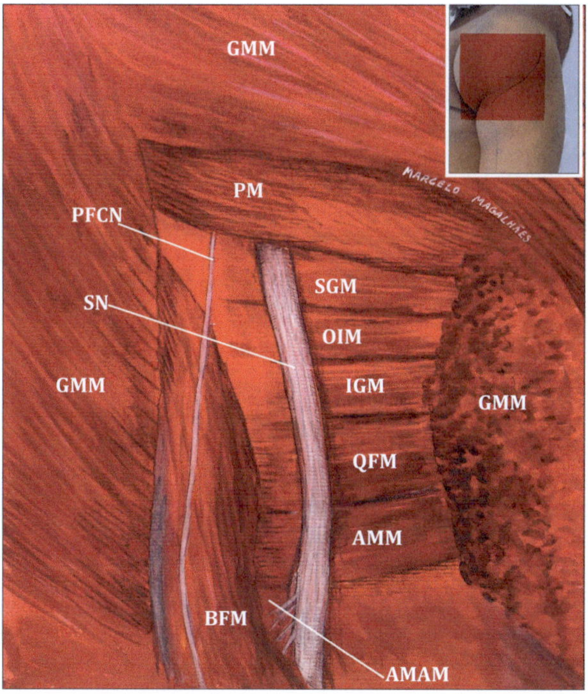

Fig. 3.5 View of the right gluteal region, with exposure of the posterior femoral cutaneous nerve and the sciatic nerve, after sectioning the fibers of the gluteus maximus muscle. Note the presence of the piriformis muscle over the sciatic nerve. *AMAM* = adductor magnus muscle, *AMM* = adductor minimus muscle, *BFM* = biceps femoris muscle, *GMM* = gluteus maximus muscle, *IGM* = inferior gemellus muscle, *OIM* = obturator internus muscle, *PFCN* = posterior femoral cutaneous nerve, *PM* = piriformis muscle, *QFM* = quadratus femoris muscle, *SGM* = superior gemellus muscle, *SN* = sciatic nerve

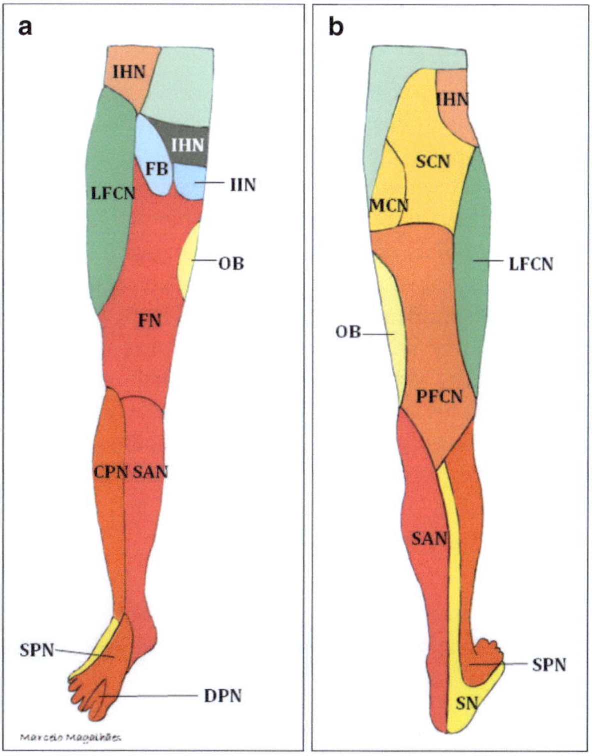

Fig. 3.6 (**a**, **b**) Anterior and posterior view of the sensory territories of the main nerves of the lower limb. *CPN* = common peroneal nerve, *DPN* = deep peroneal nerve, *FB* = femoral branch (genitofemoral nerve), *FN* = femoral nerve, *IHN* = iliohypogastric nerve, *IIN* = ilioinguinal nerve, *LFCN* = lateral femoral cutaneus nerve, *MCN* = medial cluneal nerve, *OB* = obturator nerve, *SAN* = saphenous nerve, *SCN* = superior cluneal nerve, *SPN* = superficial peroneal nerve, *SN* = sural nerve. *The ilioinguinal nerve area also has fibers from the genital branch of the genitofemoral nerve

3.1.1 *Vascular Irrigation of the Sciatic Nerve*

Georgakis et al. (2008) demonstrated that the arterial irrigation of the SN is carried out through sciatic arteries that can appear in a number from one to four [12]. It was observed that in 50% of cases, the sciatic arteries originated from the medial circumflex femoral artery, 39% from the inferior gluteal artery, 7% from the first perforating artery, and 4% from the internal pudendal artery [12]. The average length of these arteries varied greatly according to their origin. When the sciatic artery originated from the superior division of the inferior gluteal artery, it has an average length of 15.8 mm, when it originated from direct branches of the inferior gluteal artery, 35.9 mm and from branches of the first perforating artery, 22.7 mm [12].

Stolarczyk et al. (2000) demonstrated the presence of an intrinsic and extrinsic microvascular system in the SN, which are independent and join through anastomoses [13]. Studies conducted on rat SN showed that removal of the epineurium resulted in a 58% reduction in nerve blood flow. These data suggest that most of the blood nutrition of this nerve in rats originates from the surface of this [13]. Zamir et al. (2012) also corroborated the data from Stolarczyk et al. (2000) through an anatomical study with rat SN, conducted by neuroimaging examination and anatomical dissection [13, 14]. The studies infer that the intrinsic and extrinsic microvascular system of the SN operates bidirectionally, allowing greater resistance to ischemia in case of interruption of arterial nutrition in one of the systems [13, 14].

3.2 Anatomy of the Common Peroneal Nerve

The common peroneal nerve (CPN) is a branch of the SN that originates in the distal third of the posterior compartment of the thigh. The CPN, in turn, presents a lateral trajectory at the level of the knee to reach the lateral portion of the neck of the fibula and penetrate a tunnel constituted by the two heads of the fibularis longus muscle.

Several points of nerve compression occur in the vicinity of the fibula, such as: posterior crural intermuscular septum, anterior crural intermuscular septum, intermuscular septum, and deep tendinous fascia. For satisfactory decompression of the peroneal nerve in compressive syndromes, it is always necessary, if possible, to open all of the aforementioned fasciae and septa.

After the nerve rounds the neck of the fibula, it originates its two most important branches: deep peroneal nerve (DPN) and superficial peroneal nerve (SPN). It is important to mention that the common peroneal nerve also produces a joint branch for the sensory innervation of the lateral part of the knee joint [15] (Figs. 3.7, 3.8, 3.9, 3.10, 3.11, and 3.12).

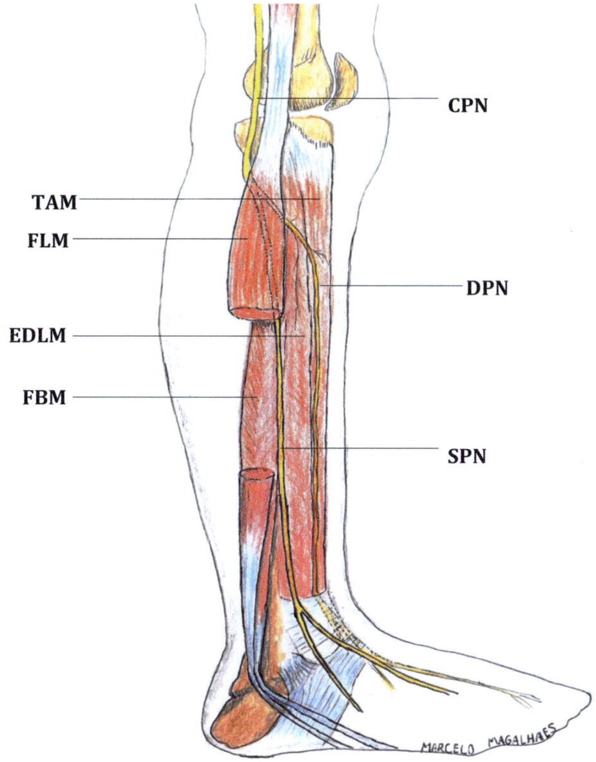

Fig. 3.7 Division of the sciatic nerve into the peroneal nerve. *CPN* = common peroneal nerve, *DPN* = deep peroneal nerve, *EDLM* = extensor digitorum longus muscle, *FBM* = fibularis brevis muscle, *FLM* = fibularis longus muscle, *SPN* = superficial peroneal nerve, *TAM* = tibialis anterior muscle

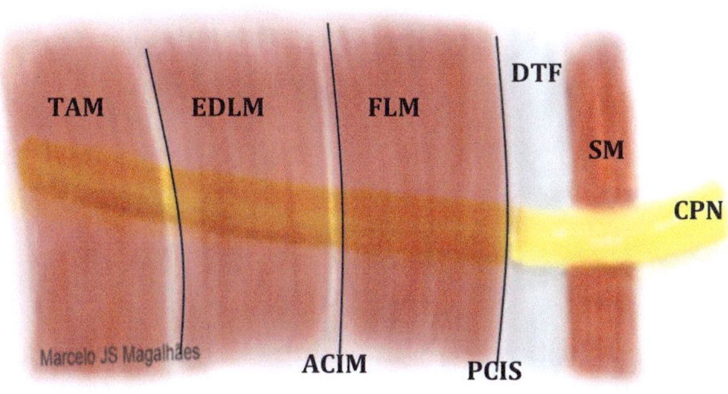

Fig. 3.8 Common peroneal nerve in the left lower limb. *ACIM* = anterior crural intermuscular septum, *CPN* = common peroneal nerve, *DTF* = deep tendinous fascia, *EDLM* = extensor digitorum longus muscle, *FLM* = fibularis longus muscle, *IS* = intermuscular septum, *PCIS* = posterior crural intermuscular septum, *SM* = soleus muscle, *TAM* = tibialis anterior muscle

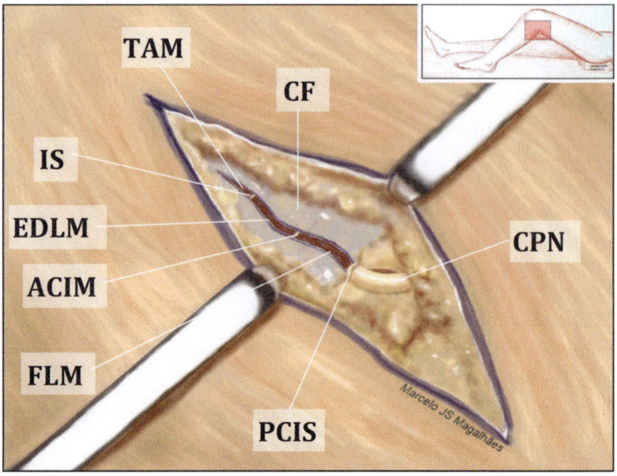

Fig. 3.9 Common peroneal nerve and its course at the level of the neck of the fibula. *ACIM* = anterior crural intermuscular septum, *CF* = crural fascia, *CPN* = common peroneal nerve, *EDLM* = extensor digitorum longus muscle, *FLM* = fibular longus muscle, *IS* = intermuscular septum, *PCIS* = posterior crural intermuscular septum, *TAM* = tibialis anterior muscle

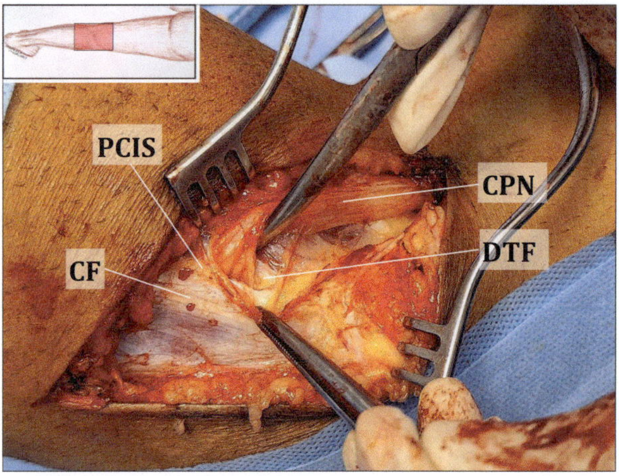

Fig. 3.10 Peroneal nerve in the right lower limb. Patient in prone position. Note that the crural fascia of the leg has not yet been opened for the exposure of the septa. *CF* = crural fascia, *CPN* = common peroneal nerve, *DTF* = deep tendinous fascia, *PCIS* = posterior crural intermuscular septum

3.2.1 Anatomy of the Superficial Peroneal Nerve

The superficial peroneal nerve (SPN), after originating from the common peroneal nerve, presents a trajectory inside the lateral compartment of the leg. In a proximal position, it courses under the fibularis longus muscle and more distally, it positions itself between the fibularis brevis, fibularis longus, and extensor digitorum longus muscles. In the leg, the SPN produces a motor branch for the fibularis longus and fibularis brevis muscles. In the distal third of the leg, in the anterolateral region, the SPN pierces the deep fascia of the leg and produces the nerves: medial dorsal cutaneous and intermediate dorsal cutaneous. The SPN is the responsible for the sensory innervation of the dorsum of the foot, except for a small area of skin located in the first digital space which is performed by the DPN and by a dorsal skin region in the two lateral toes which is performed by the sural nerve [2].

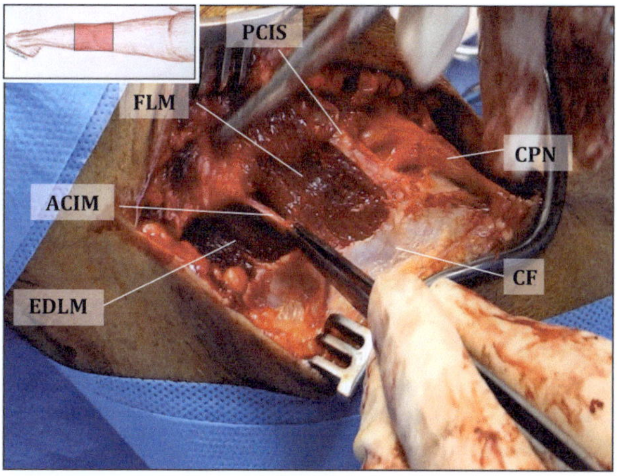

Fig. 3.11 Peroneal nerve in the right lower limb. Patient is in prone position. Note that at this surgical stage, some septa are already exposed. The deep tendinous fascia has been opened and part of the crural fascia has been resected. *ACIM* = anterior crural intermuscular septum, *CF* = crural fascia, *CPN* = common peroneal nerve, *EDLM* = extensor digitorum longus muscle, *FLM* = fibularis longus muscle, *PCIS* = posterior crural intermuscular septum

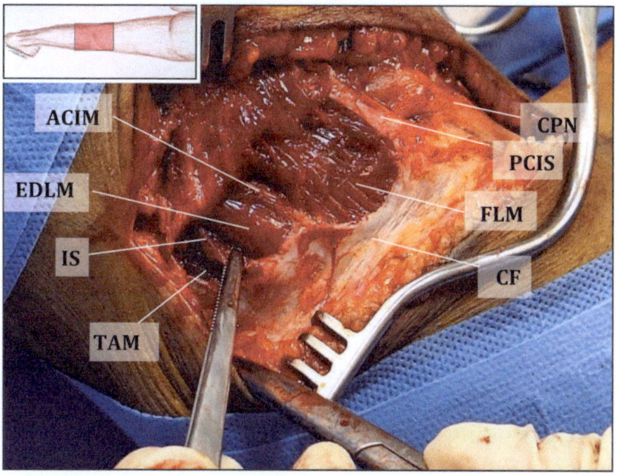

Fig. 3.12 Peroneal nerve in the right lower limb. Patient is in prone position. The opening of the crural fascia of the leg allowed the visualization of the septa. *ACIM* = anterior crural intermuscular septum, *CPN* = common peroneal nerve, *EDLM* = extensor digitorum longus muscle, *IS* = intermuscular septum, *PCIS* = posterior crural intermuscular septum, *FLM* = fibularis longus muscle, *TAM* = tibialis anterior muscle, *CF* = crural fascia

Anatomical studies show that the SPN can be positioned in the lateral compartment of the leg in 57–73% of cases, in the anterior compartment in 8.1–23% and its branches in both compartments between 5% and 26% [17–20]. Tomaszewski et al. (2017) in a meta-analysis showed that the division of the distal branches occurs in a suprafascial plane in 82.7% of cases (Type I), intracompartmental division with superficialization of the branches as distinct entities in 15.6% (Type II), and absence of the intermediate dorsal cutaneous branch in 1.8% (Type III) [21].

3.2.2 *Intraseptal Tunnel of the Superficial Peroneal Nerve*

Valisena et al. (2021) in an anatomical study involving 15 lower limbs showed that the point of emergence of the SPN in the deep fascia of the leg was about 10.37 cm proximal to the lateral malleolus. In ten specimens, it was possible to identify the presence of an intraseptal tunnel, and in eight cases, the SPN left the tunnel as a standard of single trunk, and in two cases, with the pattern of its branches. The average length of the intraseptal tunnel was 2.63 cm (minimum value of 1 cm and maximum of 4 cm) [22].

The tunnel has a fibrous-looking floor, where the ceiling presents a thin wall. The physical characteristics of the ceiling wall of the SPN tunnel are more compatible with those identified in the crural fascia (deep fascia of the leg) [22].

The use of anatomical points for the identification of the SPN can avoid nerve injuries in surgical approaches performed in the anterior and anterolateral compartment of the lower limb. There is an estimate that the anterior surgical approach causes between 7.7% and 16.7% of SPN injury and that in the anterolateral approach 21% [19, 23, 24].

3.2.3 *Anatomy of the Deep Peroneal Nerve*

After the origin of the DPN, it presents a trajectory in the anterior compartment of the leg running deep to the fibularis longus and extensor digitorum longus muscles. In the upper third of the leg, the DPN presents a trajectory between the extensor digitorum longus and the tibialis anterior muscles. At the level of the lower third of the leg, the DPN presents a trajectory inferior to the tendon of the extensor hallucis longus muscle. At this point, it is medial to the anterior tibial artery and has a path between the tendons of the extensor digitorum longus and extensor hallucis longus muscles [25]. There is a distance of 1.3 cm from the ankle, and the nerve divides into lateral and medial branches [25, 26].

It is noted that the bifurcation of the DPN into medial and lateral branches presents anatomical variation described in the literature. In an anatomical study with 36 formalin-fixed lower limbs, it was found that in 31 specimens (86%), the bifurcation occurred within the anterior tarsal tunnel (ATT), in 2 specimens (5.6%), it occurred below and in 3 specimens (8.3%), no division of the nerve into lateral and medial branches was found. In this same study, no division into branches above the ATT was

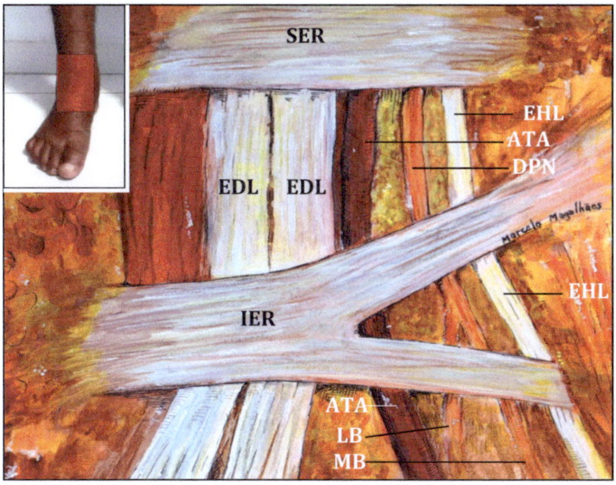

Fig. 3.13 Anterior tarsal tunnel in the right lower limb. *ATA* = anterior tibial artery, *DPN* = deep peroneal nerve, *EDL* = extensor digitorum longus, *EHL* = extensor hallucis longus, *IER* = inferior extensor retinaculum, *LB* = lateral branch, *MB* = medial branch, *SER* = superior extensor retinaculum. Note that the deep peroneal nerve passes under the superior and inferior extensor retinaculum. The tendon of the tibialis anterior muscle lies medial to the tendon of the extensor hallucis longus, deep to the overlying adipose tissue depicted in this region

observed [16]. At the level of the bifurcation, the DPN presents a transverse diameter in formalized specimen of 3.2 mm ± 0.6 mm. The distance between the bifurcation and the first interdigital space is 131.0 mm ± 13.4 mm [16] (Figs. 3.13 and 3.14).

The lateral branch of the DPN innervates the extensor hallucis brevis, extensor digitorum brevis muscles, and the second, third, and fourth metatarsophalangeal joints [27–29].

The medial branch of the DPN presents a trajectory between the tendon of the extensor hallucis longus muscle and the medial edge of the extensor digitorum brevis muscle. After piercing the deep fascia, this medial branch divides into two cutaneous branches for sensory innervation of the first digital space [25, 26].

At the level of the first interdigital space of the foot, an anastomosis was described between the superficial and deep peroneal nerves in 27.8% of the specimens in an anatomical study [16].

It is important to stress that the DPN located cranially to the inferior retinaculum is responsible for the innervation of the tibialis anterior, fibularis tertius, extensor hallucis longus, and extensor digitorum longus muscles. Below this retinaculum, it innervates only the extensor digitorum brevis and extensor hallucis brevis muscles [27–29]. Given these anatomical considerations, a compressive process at the level of the extensor retinaculum can only result in sensory impairment of the first interdigital space and paresis of extensor hallucis brevis and extensor digitorum brevis muscles.

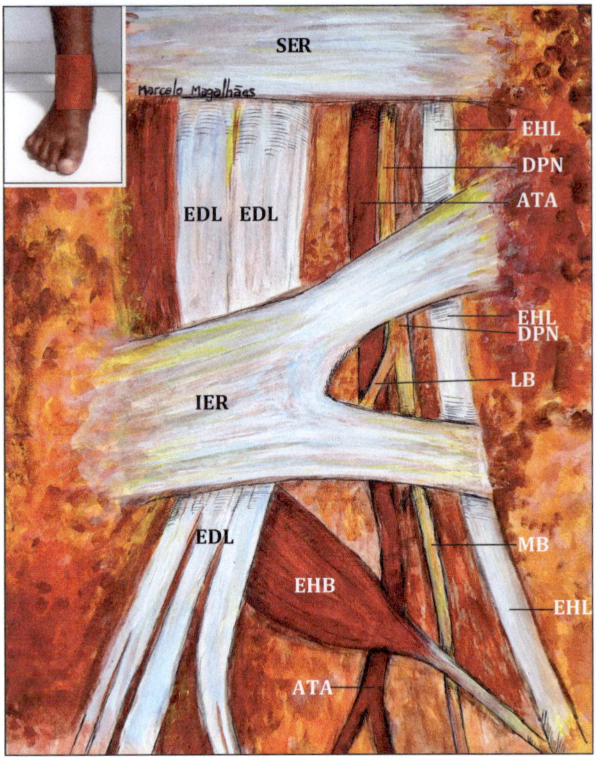

Fig. 3.14 Anterior tarsal tunnel in the right lower limb. *ATA* = anterior tibial artery, *DPN* = deep peroneal nerve, *EDL* = extensor digitorum longus, *EHB* = extensor hallucis brevis, *EHL* = extensor hallucis longus, *IER* = inferior extensor retinaculum, +*LB* = lateral branch, *MB* = medial branch, *SER* = superior extensor retinaculum. Note that distally, the deep peroneal nerve passes under the tendon of the extensor hallucis brevis muscle. The tendon of the tibialis anterior muscle lies medial to the tendon of the extensor hallucis longus, deep to the overlying adipose tissue depicted in this region

3.2.4 Anatomy of the Anterior Tarsal Tunnel

To avoid the "bowstring" effect on the deep peroneal nerve (DPN) at the level of the ankle, the superior and inferior extensor retinaculum acts on the nerve, preventing this phenomenon, given that the nerve follows a trajectory with a curvature close to 90° [25, 26].

The anterior tarsal tunnel (ATT) can be conceptualized as a space of flattened dimensions positioned between the fascia of the navicular and talus bones (ventral) and the inferior extensor retinaculum of the foot [29].

In an anatomical study conducted with 18 formalized cadavers, it was shown that the lateral length of the tarsal tunnel had an extension of about 21.7 ± 4.2 mm and the medial length 55.0 ± 9 mm. The width of the anterior tarsal tunnel, at the level of the lower edge between the tendons of the extensor hallucis longus and extensor digitorum longus muscles, had an extension of 12.6 ± 2.1 mm [22].

The presence of fibrotic bands over the DPN and dorsal artery of the foot, at the level of the ATT is described in 61.1% of studied specimens [22] (Figs. 3.13 and 3.14).

3.3 Anatomy of the Tibial Nerve

The SN is constituted by nerve fibers originating from the spinal nerves L4–S3 that originate the CPN and tibial nerve (TN) at the level of the distal third of the thigh [2] (Figs. 3.15 and 3.16).

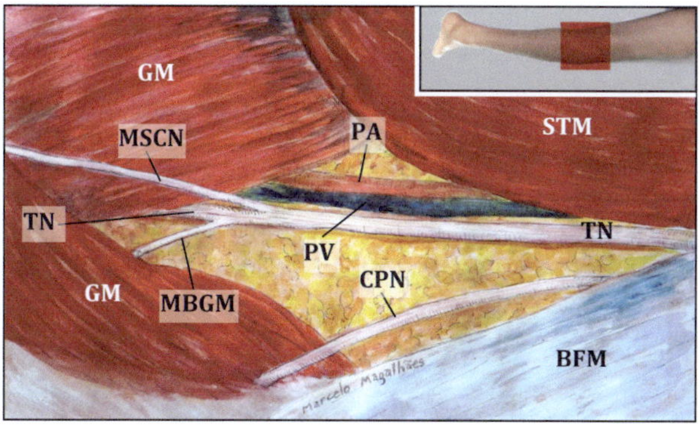

Fig. 3.15 Popliteal fossa of the right lower limb. *BFM* = biceps femoris muscle, *CPN* = common peroneal nerve, *GM* = gastrocnemius muscle, *MBGM* = muscle branch for gastrocnemius muscle, *MSCN* = medial sural cutaneous nerve, *PA* = popliteal artery, *PV* = popliteal vein, *STM* = semitendinosus muscle, *TN* = tibial nerve

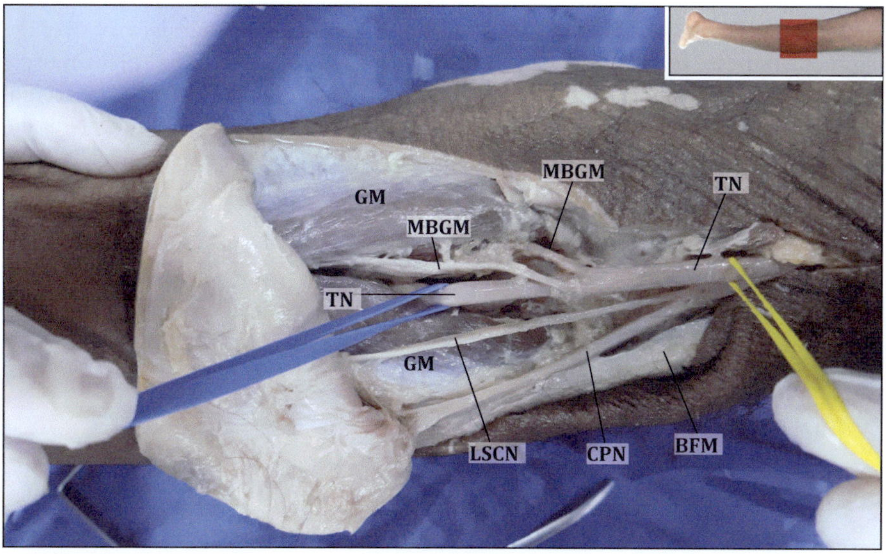

Fig. 3.16 Anatomy of the popliteal fossa in the right lower limb of a formalized specimen. The blue and yellow tapes highlight the tibial nerve in the popliteal fossa. *BFM* = biceps femoris muscle, *CPN* = common peroneal nerve, *GM* = gastrocnemius muscle, *LSCN* = lateral sural cutaneous nerve, *MBGM* = muscle branch for gastrocnemius muscle, *TN* = tibial nerve

The TN is a mixed type nerve that has motor, autonomic, and sensory fibers. In its constitution are nerve fibers of the spinal nerves L4–S3 [2]. It is the nerve responsible for the motility of the following muscles of the lower limb:

- Soleus muscle
- Tibialis posterior muscle
- Gastrocnemius muscle
- Flexor hallucis longus muscle
- Flexor digitorum longus muscle
- Popliteus muscle
- Quadratus plantae muscle
- Adductor hallucis muscle
- Abductor hallucis muscle
- Flexor hallucis brevis muscle
- Flexor digitorum brevis muscle
- First, second, third, and fourth lumbrical muscles
- Abductor digiti minimi muscle
- Flexor digiti minimi muscle
- Interosseous muscle

The sensory fibers of the TN run through the following nerves: medial sural cutaneous, medial plantar branch, lateral plantar branch, and calcaneal branch. It is noted that the sensory territory of the TN corresponds to the lateral portion of the foot, sole, and small portion of skin located distally on the dorsum of the toes, excluding the skin located in the first interdigital space which is done by the DPN.

After the TN passes through the popliteal fossa, it presents a trajectory over the popliteus muscle. It then reaches a deep trajectory in relation to the soleus muscle and superficial in relation to the tibialis posterior muscle. At the level of the medial malleolus, it penetrates the posterior tarsal tunnel (PTT). In general, the TN at the level of this osteofibrous tunnel emits the following branches: calcaneal, medial plantar, and lateral plantar [2] (Figs. 3.15, 3.16, 3.17, 3.18, and 3.19).

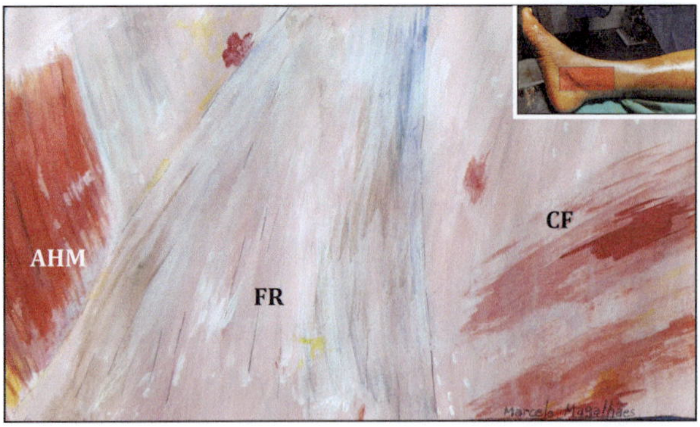

Fig. 3.17 Right ankle with preserved crural fascia and flexor retinaculum. *AHM* = abductor hallucis muscle, *CF* = crural fascia, *FR* = flexor retinaculum

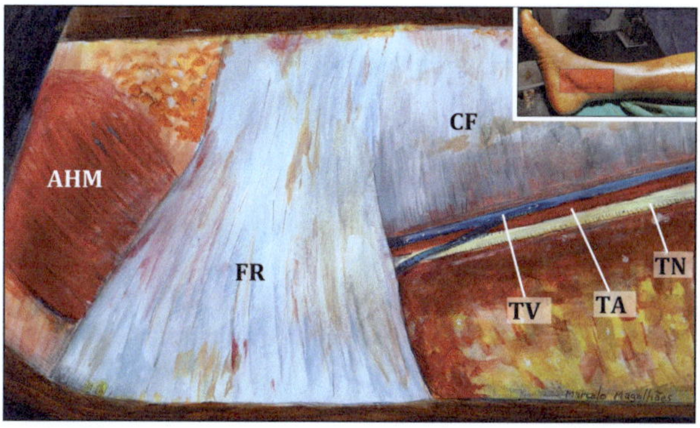

Fig. 3.18 Right ankle after opening the crural fascia. *AHM* = abductor hallucis muscle, *CF* = crural fascia, *FR* = flexor retinaculum, *TA* = tibial artery, *TN* = tibial nerve, *TV* = tibial veins

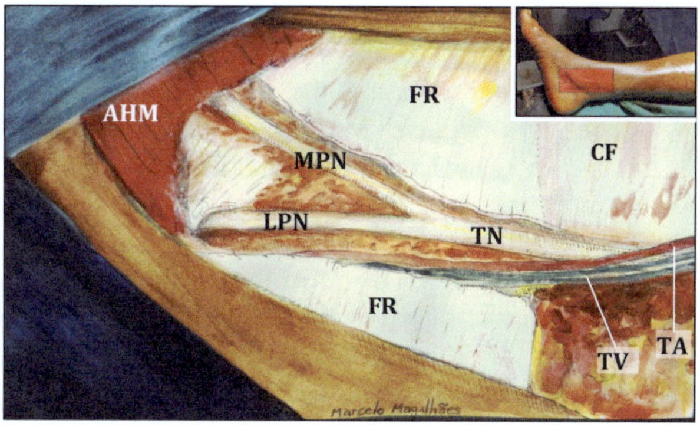

Fig. 3.19 Right ankle after opening the crural fascia and flexor retinaculum. *AHM* = abductor hallucis muscle, *CF* = crural fascia, *FR* = flexor retinaculum, *LPN* = lateral plantar nerve, *MPN* = medial plantar nerve, *TA* = tibial artery, *TN* = tibial nerve, *TV* = tibial veins

Complete proximal injury of the tibial nerve causes the following sensory changes: anesthesia in the plantar region, lateral portion of the foot, and small portion of skin located distally on the dorsum of the toes, excluding the skin located in the first interdigital space, plegia for foot extension, toe flexion, and foot inversion [25].

3.3.1 Anatomy of the Posterior Tarsal Tunnel

The PTT presents as a roof, the flexor retinaculum that attaches to the medial malleolus and calcaneus. Within the tunnel are the tendons of the tibialis posterior, flexor digitorum longus, and flexor hallucis longus muscles, tibial nerve, tibial artery, and tibial veins [2]. The posterior limit of the PTT is the posterior process of the talus, the upper limit, the medial malleolus, and the lateral edge is constituted by the calcaneus and lower edge, the abductor hallucis muscle. The flexor retinaculum is also called lanciniate ligament or internal annular ligament [26] (Figs. 3.17, 3.18, and 3.19).

3.4 Lateral Femoral Cutaneous Nerve

It is a sensory nerve originating from fibers that arise from the posterior division of the spinal nerves L2 and L3 of the lumbar plexus. It has the function of sensory innervation of the anterior and lateral portion of the thigh.

This nerve presents a trajectory that starts inside the pelvis, in the retroperitoneum, and that ends after reaching the lateral region of the thigh [30]. Inside the pelvis, the lateral femoral cutaneous nerve (LFCN) emerges on the lateral edge of the psoas major muscle, with an infero-lateral trajectory over this same muscle. In this path over the psoas major muscle, the LFCN is located between the two layers of the superficial iliac fascia [31, 32]. At a more distal point in the pelvis, this nerve is crossed by the deep circumflex iliac vessels [33]. After crossing the aponeuroticofascial tunnel, also known as the iliopubic tract, this nerve reaches the inguinal ligament [33]. After passing the inguinal ligament, the LFCN leaves the pelvis and reaches the lateral portion of the thigh.

According to Siqueira M.G. et al., the nerve is easily identifiable between 5 and 25 mm medial to the anterior superior iliac spine (ASIS) [2]. Tomaszewski K.A. et al. (2016), in their review in the literature, cite that the nerve is identified 19 mm medial to the ASIS [30]. On the other hand, Grothaus M.C. et al. (2005) describe that this distance varies between 6 and 73 mm [33]. After leaving the inguinal ligament, the LFCN presents a trajectory under the fascia lata that crosses over or through the fibers of the sartorius muscle. After passing the sartorius muscle, it divides into anterior and posterior branches. Both branches pierce the tensor fasciae latae to reach the subcutaneous plane (Figs. 3.20 and 3.21).

3.5 Genitofemoral Nerve

The genitofemoral nerve (GFN) is a predominantly sensory nerve. From a motor point of view, it is responsible only for the motility of the cremaster muscle. It originates from the ventral fibers of the spinal nerves L1 and L2, emerging within the medial edge of the psoas major muscle. This nerve emerges at the intervertebral level L3/L4 to present a trajectory in the fascia of the psoas major muscle. It follows a path that passes posterior to the ureter where it then bifurcates into genital and femoral branches [24] (Fig. 3.21).

The femoral branch of the GFN presents a trajectory lateral to the external iliac artery and posterior to the inguinal ligament. Distally to this ligament, the nerve reaches the tensor fasciae latae muscle, to reach the anterior region of the thigh, where it is responsible for sensory innervation [24].

The genital branch of the GFN presents a trajectory that continues along the psoas major muscle toward the inguinal ring. In males, this branch is responsible for supplying the motor innervation of the cremaster muscle and sensitivity to the spermatic cord, scrotum, and adjacent thigh skin [24, 34–38]. In females, the genital

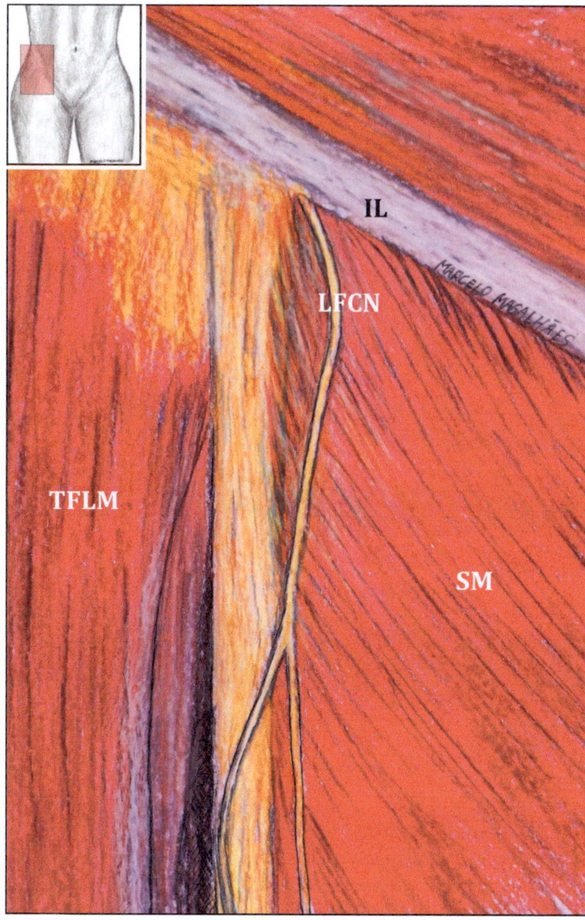

Fig. 3.20 Lateral femoral cutaneous nerve in the right lower limb. *IL* = inguinal ligament, *LFCN* = lateral cutaneous femoral nerve, *SM* = sartorius muscle, *TFLM* = tensor fasciae latae muscle

branch is responsible for the sensory innervation of the pubic region, major labia. Several authors have demonstrated the presence of great anatomical variation of the GFN [24, 39–42].

3.6 Sural Nerve

The sural nerve (SRN) has a purely sensory function and is located in the postero-lateral part of the lower limb. This nerve has important clinical relevance because it serves as a graft for nerve reconstruction procedures. SRN is responsible for the sensory innervation of a small portion of skin on the lateral part of the foot, including the lateral part of the ankle and fifth toe.

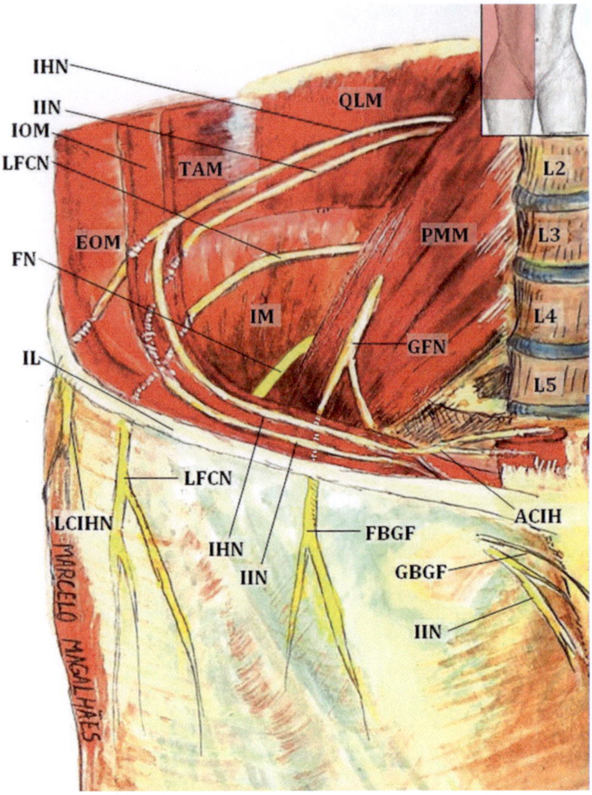

Fig. 3.21 Anatomy of the main nerves of the inguinal region and anterior region of the thigh. *ACIH* = anterior cutaneous branch of iliohypogastric nerve, *FBGF* = femoral branch of genitofemoral nerve, *FN* = femoral nerve, *GBGF* = genital branch of genitofemoral nerve, *GFN* = genitofemoral nerve, *IHN* = iliohypogastric nerve, *IIN* = ilioinguinal nerve, *IL* = inguinal ligament, *IM* = iliacus muscle, *LCIHN* = lateral cutaneous branch of iliohypogastric nerve, *LFCN* = lateral femoral cutaneous nerve, *LSCN* = lateral sural cutaneous nerve, *OEAM* = obliquus externus abdominis muscle, *OIAM* = obliquus internus abdominis muscle, *PMM* = psoas major muscle, *QLM* = quadratus lumborum muscle, *TAM* = transversus abdominis muscle

The SRN commonly originates from the union of a component originating from the tibial nerve (medial sural cutaneous nerve) and a component of the peroneal nerve which can be the lateral sural cutaneous nerve or fibers originating directly from the common peroneal nerve. However, it may be constituted by only the medial component originating from the tibial nerve or the lateral component originating from the common peroneal nerve. Thus, at least five patterns can be identified (Figs. 3.15, 3.16, and 3.22).

In the study by Riedl O. et al. (2013), it was shown that the medial sural cutaneous nerve was the nerve that was present in most of the specimens studied, with the

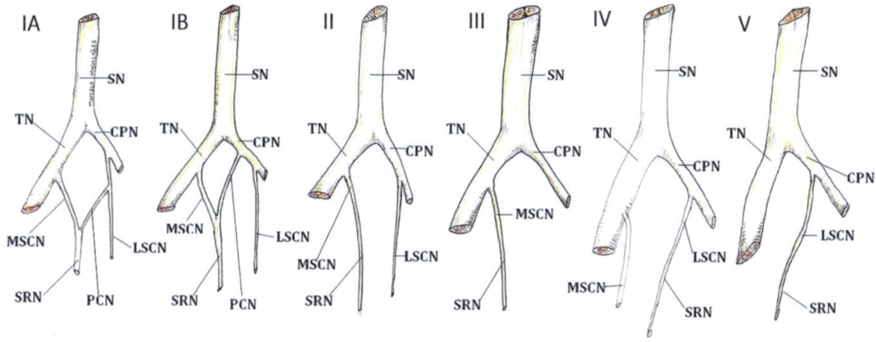

Fig. 3.22 Patterns of sural nerve formation from branches originating from the tibial and peroneal nerves. *CPN* = common peroneal nerve, *LSCN* = lateral sural cutaneous nerve, *MSCN* = medial sural cutaneous nerve, *PCN* = peroneal communicating nerve, *SRN* = sural nerve, *SN* = sciatic nerve, *TN* = tibial nerve

exception of only one case. The medial sural cutaneous nerve almost always originates in the dorsal part of the circumference of the tibial nerve [43–50].

The medial sural cutaneous nerve originates outside the fascia of the leg and its entry point to the subfascial space may contain a fibrous arch that is positioned proximal to the musculotendinous junction of the gastrocnemius muscle [43, 51–55] (Fig. 3.22).

Pattern I = It is the most common pattern with 63% of cases. The SRN is constituted by a medial component originating from the tibial nerve and a lateral component originating from the common peroneal nerve.

Pattern IA = The fibers originating from the lateral sural cutaneous nerve.

Pattern IB = The lateral component originates directly from the common peroneal nerve through a peroneal communicating branch. In pattern IB, the lateral sural cutaneous nerve may or may not be present.

Pattern II = Occurs in 27% of cases. The SRN is constituted only by the medial component originating from the tibial nerve and the lateral sural cutaneous nerve runs independently.

Pattern III = Occurs in 7% of cases. The SRN is constituted only by the medial component originating from the tibial nerve and the lateral sural nerve is absent.

Pattern IV = Occurs in 3% of cases. The SRN is constituted only by the lateral sural cutaneous nerve with the medial sural nerve running independently.

Pattern V = Very rare to be identified. The SRN is constituted only by the lateral sural cutaneous nerve and the medial sural cutaneous nerve is absent.

Regarding the peroneal communicating branch, Huelke D.F. (1957) describes that it originates from the CPN in 42% and in 33% it originates from the lateral sural cutaneous nerve. Riedl O. et al. (2013) reveal that the lateral sural cutaneous nerve typically originates from the CPN in its posteromedial quadrant [24, 43–45, 52, 56–58].

The point of origin of the SRN is always in the proximal half of the leg. Regarding the disposition of the SRN in the fascial plane, it is noted that in 79% of cases, the origin of this nerve is positioned in the subfascial plane. More often, the pinching point of the nerve in the crural fascia corresponds to the meeting of the second and third quarters of the leg [43]. The SRN pierces the crural fascia about 16 cm, proximal to the lateral malleolus, to reach a more lateral position, toward the calcaneal tendon. After piercing the crural fascia, the SRN follows a trajectory close to the small saphenous vein [2].

3.7 Femoral Nerve

The femoral nerve (FN) is the largest branch originating from the lumbar plexus. It originates from the posterior division of the spinal nerves L2, L3, and L4. The FN has both motor and sensory functions in the lower limb.

In the abdomen, the FN, after its formation, follows a path through the psoas major muscle, and more distally, it follows a path between the psoas major and iliacus muscles. Inside the pelvis, the FN is closely related to the external iliac artery, which is positioned anterior and medial to this nerve. More distally, the FN passes under the inguinal ligament and produces a branch for the pectineus muscle and penetrates the femoral triangle [59, 60] (Fig. 3.23).

The femoral triangle is bounded laterally by the sartorius muscle, medially by the adductor longus muscle, and superiorly by the inguinal ligament. The floor of the triangle is made up of the iliopsoas, pectineus, and adductor longus muscles, and its roof is formed by the tensor fasciae latae muscle [61, 62]. On its course, after leaving the inguinal ligament, about 4 cm from it, the FN branches into its anterior and posterior divisions [61].

The anterior division produces four branches, two for the sartorius muscle, one branch that will constitute the medial cutaneous nerve of the thigh, and another branch that will constitute the intermediate cutaneous nerve of the thigh. This muscle assists in the movement of hip flexion [62].

The posterior division produces the longest branch of the FN, which is the saphenous nerve. The saphenous nerve follows a medial course in the thigh and leg, innervating the medial part of the knee and leg, medial malleolus, and medial plantar arch, as well as the medial part of the hallux [62]. This division also produces the branch for the quadriceps femoris muscle (rectus femoris, vastus medialis, vastus intermedius, and vastus lateralis muscles).

The quadriceps femoris muscle acts in the movement of knee extension. The branch that goes to the rectus femoris muscle also has a sensory innervation function of the hip joint. The other branches for the vastus medialis, vastus intermedius, and vastus lateralis muscles also have a sensory component for knee innervation [62].

The rectus femoris muscle in an anatomical study can receive between one and four branches, the most common being the presence of two branches [63].

3.8 Neuroanatomy Obturator Nerve

The obturator nerve (ON) is a mixed nerve that carries sensory and motor fibers. It innervates muscles located in the medial compartment of the thigh and the sensitivity of the skin located on the medial face of the thigh and knee joint. It is constituted by the union of the fibers of the ventral branches of the spinal nerves L2, L3, and L4. Regarding the formation of this nerve, Tshabalala ZN et al. (2022) described a study involving 181 limbs, in which in 80% of the cases, the ON was formed by the spinal nerves L2–L4 and in 20%, by the spinal nerves L3–L4. These authors described that in 1.7% of the cases, the fusion of the fibers of the anterior branches of the spinal nerves occurred outside the psoas major muscle [64] (Fig. 3.23).

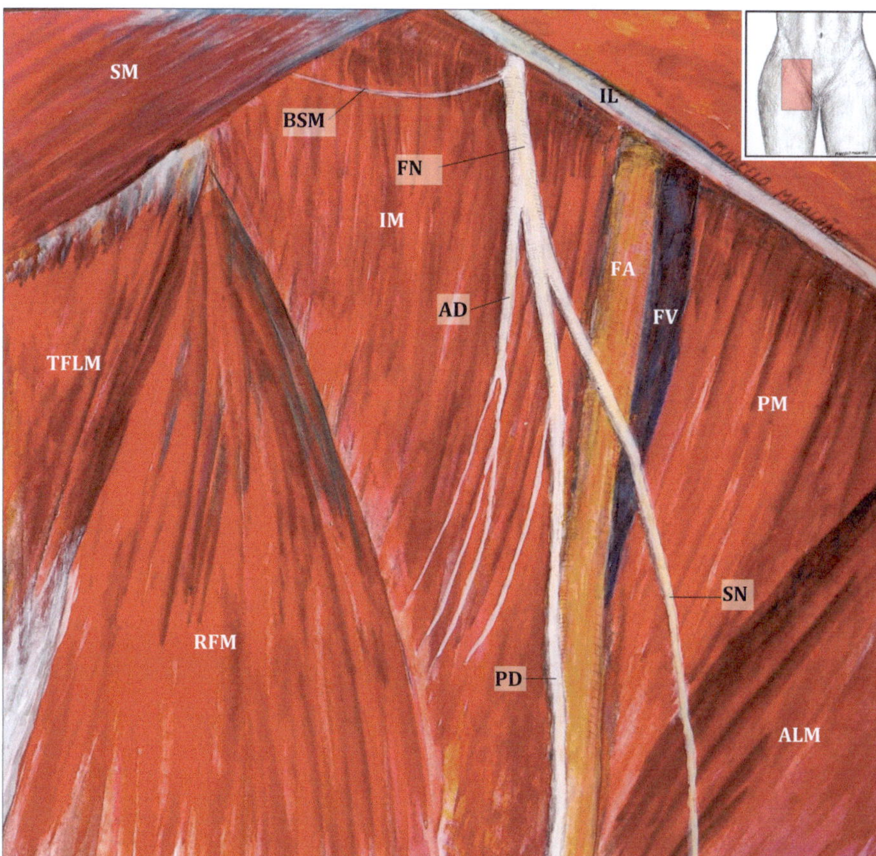

Fig. 3.23 Femoral nerve in right leg. Note that the sartorius muscle was detached and retracted laterally to better expose the femoral nerve and its branches. *AD* = anterior division of femoral nerve, *ALM* = adductor longus muscle, *BSM* = branch for sartorius muscle, *FA* = femoral artery, *FN* = femoral nerve, *FV* = femoral vein, *IL* = inguinal ligament, *IM* = iliacus muscle, *PD* = posterior division of femoral nerve, *PM* = pectineus muscle, *RFM* = rectus femoris muscle, *SM* = sartorius muscle, *SN* = saphenous nerve, *TFLM* = tensor fascia lata muscle

The formation of the trunk of ON occurs inside the psoas major muscle and leaves it at its lateral edge. It penetrates the pelvic region, approximately at the level of the sacroiliac joint. This nerve, associated with the obturator vein and artery, constitutes the neurovascular bundle that penetrates the obturator foramen. Still within the obturator canal, it divides into posterior and anterior branches and a muscular branch.

It is important to mention that the point at the bifurcation of the ON is very variable and can occur both in the intrapelvic cavity, obturator canal, and on the medial face of the thigh [65–70]. Regarding the bifurcation of the ON into its branches, Tshabalala et al. (2022) showed that in 3% of the left side and 1% of the right side it occurred still in the intrapelvic region, in 92% of the cases on the left and 94% on the right the bifurcation occurred inside the obturator canal. And finally, the bifurcation of the ON occurred in 5% of the cases at an extrapelvic point [64]. Tshabalala et al. (2022) also demonstrated that the distance between the ON and the most inferior point of the obturator foramen in females was 44.99 ± 3.42 mm and in males 48.85 ± 3.55 mm [64] (Fig. 3.24).

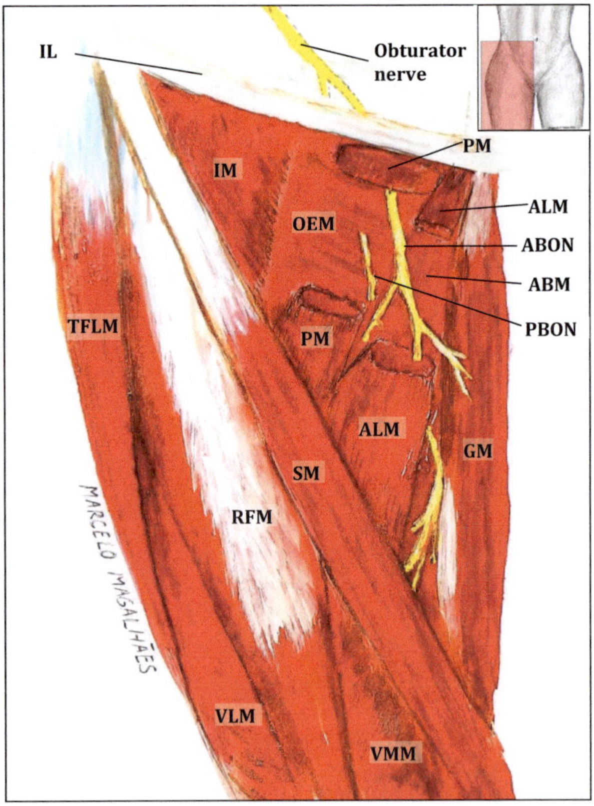

Fig. 3.24 Exposure of the obturator nerve after the resection of the pectineus and adductor longus muscles. *ABM* = adductor brevis muscle, *ABON* = anterior branch of obturator nerve, *ALM* = adductor longus muscle, *GM* = gracilis muscle, *IL* = inguinal ligament, *IM* = iliacus muscle, *OEM* = obturator externus muscle, *PBON* = posterior branch of obturator nerve, *PM* = pectineus muscle, *RFM* = rectus femoris muscle, *SM* = sartorius muscle, *TFLM* = tensor fasciae latae muscle, *VLM* = vastus lateralis muscle, *VMM* = vastus medialis muscle

The anterior branch is responsible for the sensory innervation of the distal 2/3 of the medial face of the thigh. This branch also innervates the adductor brevis, adductor longus, and gracilis muscles [64, 65, 68, 71, 72].

The posterior branch produces the motor fibers for part of the adductor magnus muscle. Regarding anatomical variation of this nerve, the presence of an accessory ON is described by some authors in some anatomical studies. Tshabalala et al. (2022) and Tubbs et al. (2005) [64, 73] did not identify the presence of an accessory ON. However, in the study by Akkaya et al. (2008) [74], the accessory ON was identified in 12.5% of the cases and in the study by Anloague and Huijbregts (2009) in 8.8% [75].

3.9 Neuroanatomy of the Ilioinguinal Nerve

The ilioinguinal nerve (IIN) is a mixed type nerve in which motor and sensory axonal fibers can be identified in its structure. It originates from fibers of the anterior branch of the spinal nerves T12 and L1 [78].

After its formation, this nerve emerges on the lateral edge of the psoas major muscle in a caudal direction, in the subperitoneal plane of the anterior wall of the abdomen, anterior to the quadratus lumborum muscle, until it reaches the anterior superior iliac spine [78, 79]. From this point, the IIN crosses and innervates the transversus abdominis and obliquus internus abdominis muscles. At this point, while following a path parallel to the inguinal ligament, the nerve takes a more superficial course, to cross the superficial inguinal ring in men and the round ligament in women. In women, the IIN is responsible for the sensory innervation of the pubic mound, labia majora, and a small anteromedial part of the thigh, and in men, the skin of the anterior face of the scrotum, root of the penis, and a small part of the anteromedial region of the thigh [76, 77] (Fig. 3.21).

3.10 Final Conclusion

The anatomy of the nerves of the lower limb is of great importance to health professionals who work with patients suffering from neuropathies, especially nerve surgeons. It is noted that the main nerve of the lower limb is the sciatic nerve, which when injured causes severe distal deficits to the knee. At least three osteofibrous tunnels are clinically relevant, the peroneal nerve tunnel at the level of the fibula neck, the posterior tarsal tunnel, and the anterior tarsal tunnel. The most common compressive neuropathies of the lower limb occur in these three.

References

1. Currin SS, Mirjalili SA, Meikle G, Stringer MD. Revisiting the surface anatomy of the sciatic nerve in the gluteal region. Clin Anat. 2015;28(1):144–9. https://doi.org/10.1002/ca.22449. PMID: 25131147.
2. Siqueira MG, Martins RS. Anatomia cirúrgica das vias de acesso aos nervos periféricos. (Portuguese version) ed. São Paulo: Dilivros; 2005.
3. Beaton LE, Anson BJ. The relation of the sciatic nerve and of its subdivisions to the piriformis muscle. Anat Rec. 1937;70:1–5.
4. Atomi AD, Oyinbo CA, Francis DAU, Tabowei UL. Anatomic variation of the sciatic nerve: a study on the prevalence, and bifurcation loci in relation to the piriformis and popliteal fossa. Acta Med Acad. 2022;51(1):52–8. https://doi.org/10.5644/ama2006-124.370. PMID: 35695403; PMCID: PMC9982851.
5. Kanawati AJ. Variations of the sciatic nerve anatomy and blood supply in the gluteal region: a review of the literature. ANZ J Surg. 2014;84(11):816–9. https://doi.org/10.1111/ans.12675. PMID: 24842563.
6. Jankovic D, Peng P, van Zundert A. Brief review: piriformis syndrome: etiology, diagnosis, and management. Can J Anaesth. 2013;60(10):1003–12. https://doi.org/10.1007/s12630-013-0009-5.
7. Pokorny D, Jahoda D, Veigl D, Pinskerova V, Sosna A. Topographic variations of the relationship of the sciatic nerve and the piriformis muscle and its relevance to palsy after total hip arthroplasty. Surg Radiol Anat. 2006;28(1):88–91.
8. Singh AK, Sharma RC. Relationship between the sciatic nerve and piriformis muscle. Neurosci Res Lett. 2011;2(1):26–8.
9. Chiba S. Multiple positional relationships of nerves arising from the sacral plexus to the piriformis muscle in humans [in Japanese]. Kaibogaku Zasshi. 1992;67(6):691–724.
10. Uluutku MH, Kurtoglu Z. Variations of nerves located in deep gluteal region. Okajimas Folia Anat Jpn. 1999;76(5):273–6.
11. Berihu BA, Debeb YG. Anatomical variation in bifurcation and trifurcations of sciatic nerve and its clinical implications: in selected university in Ethiopia. BMC Res Notes. 2015;8:633. https://doi.org/10.1186/s13104-015-1626-6.
12. Georgakis E, Soames R. Arterial supply to the sciatic nerve in the gluteal region. Clin Anat. 2008;21:62–5.
13. Stolarczyk A, Papierski K, Adamczyk G, Siński M, Sawionek L, Przybylski J. Functional studies on sciatic nerve blood flow in respect to its vascular supply and tonic neural activity. J Physiol Pharmacol. 2000;51:483–9.
14. Zamir M, Twynstra J, Vercnocke AJ, et al. Intrinsic microvasculature of the sciatic nerve in the rat. J Peripher Nerv Syst. 2012;17:377–84.
15. Mackinnon SE. Nerve surgery. 1st ed. New York: Thieme; 2014.
16. Ikiz ZAA, Ucerler H, Uygur M. Dimensions of the anterior tarsal tunnel and features of the deep peroneal nerve in relation to clinical application. Surg Radiol Anat. 2007;29(7):527–530. https://doi.org/10.1007/s00276-007-0229-x.
17. Adkison DP, Bosse MJ, Gaccione DR, Gabriel KR. Anatomical variations in the course of the superficial peroneal nerve. J Bone Joint Surg Am. 1991;73(1):112–4.
18. Barrett SL, Dellon AL, Rosson GD, et al. The clinical importance of variations in the surgical anatomy of the superficial peroneal nerve in the mid-third of the lateral leg. J Bone Joint Surg Am. 2006;88(3):174–6.
19. Ducic I, Dellon AL, Graw KS. The clinical importance of variations in the surgical anatomy of the superficial peroneal nerve in the mid-third of the lateral leg. Ann Plast Surg. 2006;56:635–8.
20. Rosson GD, Dellon AL. Superficial peroneal nerve anatomic variability changes surgical technique. Clin Orthop Relat Res. 2005;438:248–52.
21. Tomaszewski KA, Graves MJ, Vikse J, et al. Superficial fibular nerve variations of fascial piercing: a meta-analysis and clinical consideration. Clin Anat. 2017;30(1):120–5.

22. Valisena S, Gamulin A, Hannouche D. The intraseptal course of the superficial peroneal nerve: an anatomic study. Foot Ankle Int. 2021;42(9):1171–8. https://doi.org/10.1177/10711007211002508. PMID: 34151593; PMCID: PMC8446894.
23. Darland AM, Kadakia AR, Zeller JL. Branching patterns of the superficial peroneal nerve: implications for ankle arthroscopy and for anterolateral surgical approaches to the ankle. J Foot Ankle Surg. 2015;54:332–7.
24. Kosinski C. The course, mutual relations and distribution of the cutaneous nerves of the metazonal region of leg and foot. J Anat. 1926;60(pt 3):274–97.
25. Adelman KA, Wilson G, Wolf JA. Anterior tarsal tunnel syndrome. J Foot Surg. 1988;27(4):299–302.
26. Sarrafian S. The anatomy of the foot and ankle. Philadelphia: J.B. Lippincott; 1983.
27. Dellon AL. Deep peroneal nerve entrapment on the dorsum of the foot. Foot Ankle Int. 1990;11(2):73–80.
28. Standring S, editor. Gray's anatomy. 39th ed. London: Churchill Livingstone; 2005. p. 1505.
29. Zongzhao L, Jiansheng Z, Li Z. Anterior tarsal tunnel syndrome. J Bone Joint Surg. 1991;73B(3):470–3.
30. Tomaszewski KA, Popieluszko P, Henry BM, et al. The surgical anatomy of the lateral femoral cutaneous nerve in the inguinal region: a meta-analysis. Hernia. 2016;20:649–57. https://doi.org/10.1007/s10029-016-1493-7.
31. Dias Filho LC, Valença MM, Guimarães Filho FAV, et al. Lateral femoral cutaneous neuralgia: an anatomical insight. Clin Anat. 2003;16:309–16. https://doi.org/10.1002/ca.10106.
32. Martinoli C, Miguel-Perez M, Padua L, Gandolfo N, Zicca A, Tagliafico A. Imaging of neuropathies about the hip. Eur J Radiol. 2013;82:17–26. https://doi.org/10.1016/j.ejrad.2011.04.034.
33. Grothaus MC, Holt M, Mekhail AO, Ebraheim NA, Yeasting RA. Lateral femoral cutaneous nerve: an anatomic study. Clin Orthop Relat Res. 2005;437:164–8. https://doi.org/10.1097/01.blo.0000164526.08610.97.
34. Cesmebasi A, Yadav A, Gielecki J, Tubbs RS, Loukas M. Genitofemoral neuralgia: a review. Clin Anat. 2015;28(1):128–35. https://doi.org/10.1002/ca.22481. Epub 2014 Nov 5. PMID: 25377757.
35. Hollinshead WH. Anatomy for surgeons: Volume 2. The thorax, abdomen and pelvis. New York: Harper & Brothers; 1956. p. 870.
36. Amid PK, Chen DC. Surgical treatment of chronic groin and testicular pain after laparoscopic and open preperitoneal inguinal hernia repair. J Am Coll Surg. 2011;213:531–6.
37. Starling JR, Harms BA. Diagnosis and treatment of genitofemoral and ilioinguinal neuralgia. World J Surg. 1989;13:586–5.
38. Perry CP. Laparoscopic treatment of genitofemoral neuralgia. J Am Assoc Gynecol Laparosc. 1997;4:231–4.
39. Izard G, Gailleton R, Randrianasolo S, Houry R. Treatment of inguinal hernias by McVay's technique. Apropos of 1332 cases. Ann Chir. 1996;50:755–66.
40. Lange JF, Wijsmuller AR, van Geldere D, Simons MP, Swart R, Oomen J, Kleinrensink GJ, Jeekel J, Lange JF. Feasibility study of three-nerve-recognizing Lichtenstein procedure for inguinal hernia. Br J Surg. 2009;96:1210–4.
41. Alfieri S, Rotondi F, Di Giorgio A, Fumagalli U, Salzano A, Di Miceli D, Ridolfini MP, Sgagari A, Doglietto G, Groin Pain Trial Group. Influence of preservation versus division of ilioinguinal, iliohypogastric, and genital nerves during open mesh herniorrhaphy: prospective multicentric study of chronic pain. Ann Surg. 2006;243:553–38.
42. Chen DC, Hiatt JR, Amid PK. Operative management of refractory neuropathic inguinodynia by a laparoscopic retroperitoneal approach. JAMA Surg. 2013;148:962–7.
43. Riedl O, Frey M. Anatomy of the sural nerve. Plast Reconstr Surg. 2013;131(4):802–10. https://doi.org/10.1097/prs.0b013e3182818cd4.
44. Riedl O, Koemuercue F, Marker M, Hoch D, Haas M, Deutinger M. Sural nerve harvesting beyond the popliteal region allows a significant gain of donor nerve graft length. Plast Reconstr Surg. 2008;122:798–805.

45. Coert JH, Dellon AL. Clinical implications of the surgical anatomy of the sural nerve. Plast Reconstr Surg. 1994;94:850–5.
46. Mahakkanukrauh P, Chomsung R. Anatomical variations of the sural nerve. Clin Anat. 2002;15:263–6.
47. Sokolow P. Zur Anatomie des Nervus suralis beim Menschen und Affen. Z Gesamte Anat. 1933;100:194–217.
48. Aktan Ikiz ZA, Uçerler H, Bilge O. The anatomic features of the sural nerve with an emphasis on its clinical importance. Foot Ankle Int. 2005;26:560–7.
49. Mestdagh H, Drizenko A, Maynou C, Demondion X, Monier R. Origin and make up of the human sural nerve. Surg Radiol Anat. 2001;23:307–12.
50. Ortiguela ME, Wood MB, Cahill DR. Anatomy of the sural nerve complex. J Hand Surg Am. 1987;12:1119–23.
51. Romanes GJ. Cunningham's textbook of anatomy. 12th ed. Oxford: Oxford Medical Publications; 1981.
52. Huelke DF. A study of the formation of the sural nerve in adult man. Am J Phys Anthropol. 1957;15:137–47.
53. Sekiya S, Suzuki R, Miyawaki M, Chiba S, Kumaki K. Formation and distribution of the sural nerve based on nerve fascicle and nerve fiber analyses. Anat Sci Int. 2006;81:84–91.
54. Husson JL, Mathieu M, Briand B, Meadeb J, Barumbi O, Masse A. Syndrome of compression of the external saphenous nerve (or the sural nerve) (in French). Acta Orthop Belg. 1989;55:491–7.
55. Andreassi G. Osservazioni intorno all'origine, comportamento e distribuzione dei nervi cutaneo mediale della sura, ramo anastomotico peoniero e cutaneo laterale della sural nell úomo. Ricerche di Morfologia. 1931;11:83–100.
56. Sekiya S, Kumaki K. Sural-tibial nerve communications in humans. Anat Sci Int. 2002;77:140–4.
57. Dolan RW, McAvoy DW, Carr M. Anatomical variations of the sensory nerves to the fibular osteocutaneous flap. Arch Facial Plast Surg. 2000;2:252–5.
58. Sunderland S, Ray LJ. The intraneural topography of the sciatic nerve and its popliteal divisions in man. Brain. 1948;71:242–73.
59. Basinger H, Hogg JP. Anatomy, abdomen and pelvis: femoral triangle. In: StatPearls [Internet]. Treasure Island: StatPearls Publishing; 2023.
60. Clar DT, Bordoni B. Anatomy, abdomen and pelvis: femoral region. In: StatPearls [Internet]. Treasure Island: StatPearls Publishing; 2022.
61. Orebaugh SL. The femoral nerve and its relationship to the lateral circumflex femoral artery. Anesth Analg. 2006;102(6):1859–62.
62. Refai NA, Black AC, Tadi P. Anatomy, bony pelvis and lower limb: thigh femoral nerve. In: StatPearls [Internet]. Treasure Island: StatPearls Publishing; 2024. Available from: https://www.ncbi.nlm.nih.gov/books/NBK556065/.
63. Plante D, Janelle N, Angers-Goulet M, Corbeil P, Takech MA, Belzile EL. Anatomical variants of the rectus femoris motor innervation. J Hip Preserv Surg. 2019;6(2):170–6.
64. Tshabalala ZN, Human-Baron R, van der Walt S, Louw EM, van Schoor AN. The anatomy of the obturator nerve and its branches in a South African cadaver sample. Transl Res Anat. 2022;27:100201.
65. Wasse M. Interadductor approach to obturator nerve blockade for spastic conditions of adductor thigh muscles. Anesthesiol Pain Med. 1993;18(1):13–7.
66. Bradshaw C, McCrory P, Bell S, Brukner P. Obturator nerve entrapment a cause of groin pain in athletes. Am J Sports Med. 1997;25(3):402–8.
67. Vloka JD, Hadić A. Obturator and genitor femoral nerve blocks. Tech Reg Anesth Pain Manag. 1999;3(1):28–32.
68. Ricciardi E, Jakimovska M, Maniglio P, Schimberni M, Frega A, Kobal B, Moscarini M. Laparoscopic injury of the obturator nerve during fertility-sparing procedure for cervical cancer. World J Surg Oncol. 2012;10(1):1–3.

69. Moore KL, Dalley AF, Agur AM. Clinically oriented anatomy. 8th ed. Philadelphia: Wolters Kluwer Health; 2013. p. 555–7.
70. Kumka M. Critical sites of entrapment of the posterior division of the obturator nerve: anatomical considerations. J Can Chiropr Assoc. 2010;54(1):33.
71. Anagnostopoulou S, Kostopanagiotou G, Paraskeuopoulos T, Chantzi C, Lolis E, Saranteas T. Anatomic variations of the obturator nerve in the inguinal region: implications in conventional and ultrasound regional anesthesia techniques. Anesthesiol Pain Med. 2009;34(1):33–9.
72. Tipton JS. Obturator neuropathy. Curr Rev Musculoskelet Med. 2008;1(3–4):234–7.
73. Tubbs RS, Salter EG, Wellons JC III, Blount JP, Oakes WJ. Anatomical landmarks for the lumbar plexus on the posterior abdominal wall. J Neurosurg Spine. 2005;2(3):335–8.
74. Akkaya T, Comert A, Kendir S, Acar H, Gumus H, Tekdemir I, Elhan A. Detailed anatomy of accessory obturator nerve blockade. Minerva Anestesiol. 2008;74(4):119–22.
75. Anloague PA, Huijbregts P. Anatomical variations of the lumbar plexus: a descriptive anatomy study with proposed clinical implications. J Man Manip Ther. 2009;17(4):107E–14E. https://doi.org/10.1179/106698109791352201.
76. Kohan L, McKenna C, Irwin A. Ilioinguinal neuropathy. Curr Pain Headache Rep. 2020;24(1):2. [PubMed: 31960176]
77. Whiteside JL, Barber MD, Walters MD, Falcone T. Anatomy of ilioinguinal and iliohypogastric nerves in relation to trocar placement and low transverse incisions. Am J Obstet Gynecol. 2003;189(6):1574–8; discussion 1578. [PubMed: 14710069].
78. Manolakos K, Zygogiannis K, Manolakos O, Mousa C, Papadimitriou G, Fotoniatas I. Anatomical variations of ilioinguinal nerve: a systematic review of the literature. Surg Neurol Int. 2024;15:225. https://doi.org/10.25259/SNI_232_2024. PMID: 39108371; PMCID: PMC11301818
79. Elsy B, Asiri WHM, Osman LESE, Alghamdi MAS. Origin and branching pattern of the iliohypogastric and ilioinguinal nerves and their exits in relation to the psoas major muscle: a cadaveric study. Anat Cell Biol. 2025;58(1):14–21. https://doi.org/10.5115/acb.24.175. Epub 2025 Jan 10. PMID: 39788734; PMCID: PMC11933812.

Chapter 4
General Aspects of Common Peroneal Nerve Entrapment

4.1 Introduction

The compressive neuropathy of the peroneal nerve (CNPN) is the most common compressive neuropathy of the lower limb and the third most common neuropathy, right after carpal tunnel syndrome and cubital tunnel syndrome. Its clinical importance also lies due to paresis of foot dorsiflexion, leading the patient to develop "foot drop." It is noteworthy that diseases located distant from the peroneal nerve can lead the patient to develop a similar clinical picture, such as disc herniation that compresses the L5 spinal nerve. The medical literature describes different treatment modalities for the management of patients with this compressive syndrome.

Among the oldest known descriptions of CNPN is the work of Sultan C. (1921) on a ganglionic cyst as the cause of CNPN. Brooks DM (1952) described a series of cases of CNPN caused by a ganglionic cyst. In 1966, Noble W. described two case reports in which the peroneal nerve injury was caused by a trauma in which the patient presented ankle inversion resulting in intraneural hemorrhage by the injury of the vasa nervorum. In 1966, White J. also published a case report in which the peroneal nerve injury occurred due to traumatic injury, whose mechanism involved traction of the affected limb. Cobb CA et al. (1974) described two case reports of ganglionic cyst as the etiology of CNPN [1–4].

Few studies describe the incidence of CNPN in the general population. Studies conducted in Egypt revealed that the incidence of this neuropathy is around 19–40/100,000 inhabitants, totaling between 0.6% and 1.2% of all identified neuropathies [5, 6].

The medical literature describes several articles in which CNPN arose as complications of orthopedic procedures. Marciniak et al. (2013) suggest that this mononeuropathy is identified in 2–27% of patients who undergo high osteotomies of the tibia and fibula. Bouche et al. (2013) in their work identified that 0.3–1.3% of patients who underwent knee arthroplasty developed this neuropathy [7, 8].

M. J. S. Magalhães, *Lower Extremity Nerve Entrapments*,
https://doi.org/10.1007/978-3-031-90058-7_4

Patients also with clinical trauma of the knee associated with dislocation can develop CNPN. Moatshe et al. (2017) in a prospective study, involving 303 patients with knee dislocation, observed that CNPN was diagnosed in 16–40% of cases [9].

The objective of this chapter is to conduct a review on the neuropathy of the peroneal nerve, emphasizing the epidemiological aspects, anatomical, symptomatology, and most relevant differential diagnoses.

4.2 Anatomy of the Peroneal Nerve

The common peroneal nerve (CPN) originates from the sciatic nerve, approximately in the distal third of the thigh (Figs. 4.1a, b, 4.2, 4.3, and 4.4).

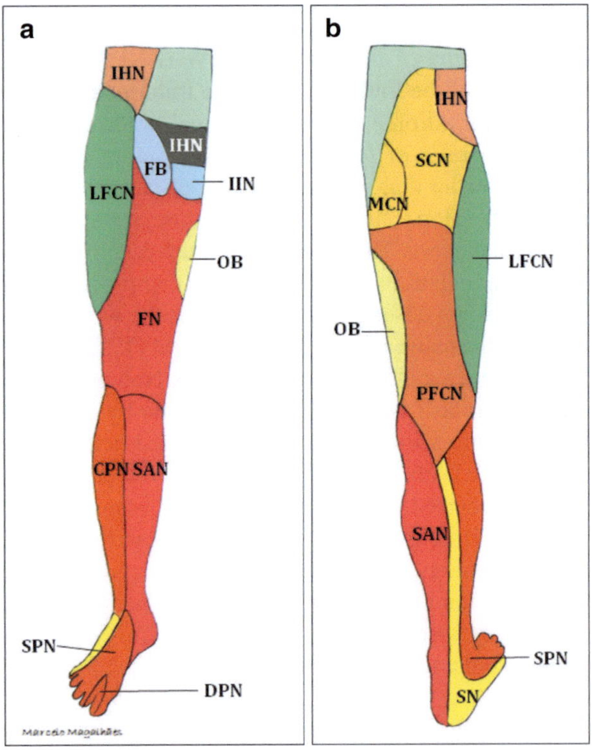

Fig. 4.1 (**a**, **b**) Anterior and posterior view of the sensory territories of the main nerves of the lower limb. Note in dark orange the skin area innervated by the peroneal nerve. *CPN* = common peroneal nerve, *DPN* = deep peroneal nerve, *FB* = femoral branch- genitofemoral nerve, *FN* = femoral nerve, *IHN* = iliohypogastric nerve, *IIN* = ilioinguinal nerve, *LFCN* = lateral femoral cutaneous nerve, *MCN* = medial cluneal nerve, *OB* = obturator nerve, *PFCN* = posterior femoral cutaneous nerve, *SAN* = saphenous nerve, *SCN* = superior cluneal nerve, *SPN* = superficial peroneal nerve, *SN* = sural nerve. *The ilioinguinal nerve area also has fibers from the genital branch of the genitofemoral nerve

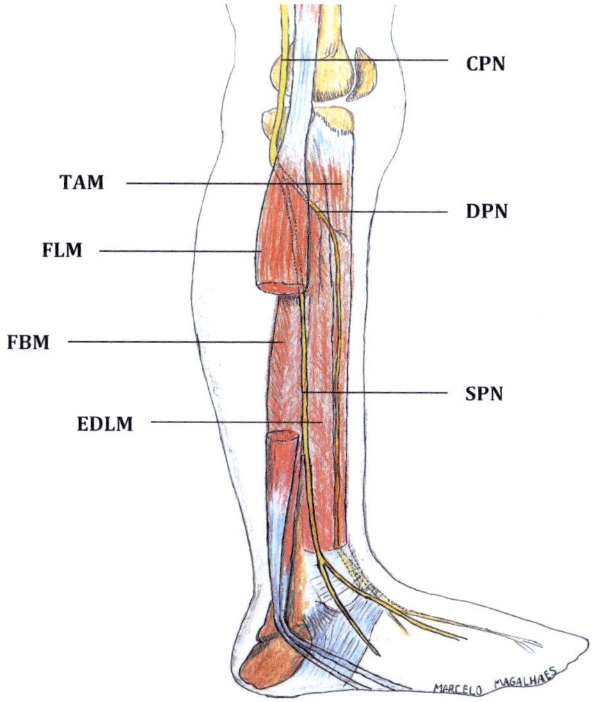

Fig. 4.2 Common peroneal nerve after its formation in the distal third of the thigh and division into superficial and deep peroneal nerve. *EDLM* = extensor digitorum longus muscle, *FBM* = fibularis brevis muscle, *FLM* = fibularis longus muscle (peroneus longus muscle), *TAM* = tibialis anterior muscle, *CPN* = common peroneal nerve, *DPN* = deep peroneal nerve, *SPN* = superficial peroneal nerve

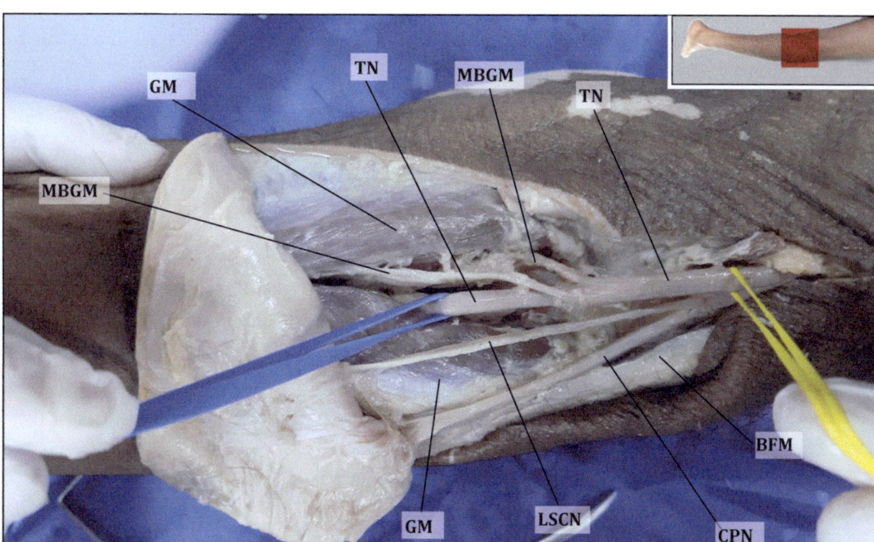

Fig. 4.3 Anatomy of the popliteal fossa in the right posterior fossa of a formalized specimen. Blue and yellow tapes highlight the tibial nerve in the popliteal fossa. *BFM* = biceps femoris muscle, *CPN* = common peroneal nerve, *GM* = gastrocnemius muscle, *LSCN* = lateral sural cutaneous nerve, *MBGM* = muscle branch for gastrocnemius muscle, *PA* = popliteal artery, *PV* = popliteal vein, *STM* = semitendinosus muscle, *TN* = tibial nerve

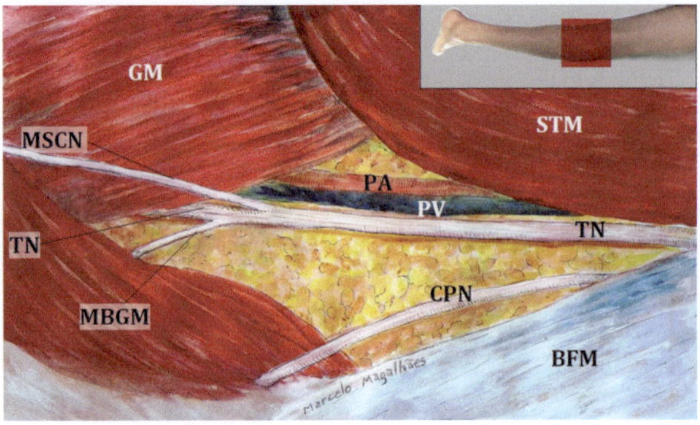

Fig. 4.4 Popliteal fossa of the right lower limb. *CPN* = common peroneal nerve, *FBM* = biceps femoris muscle, *GM* = gastrocnemius muscle, *MBGM* = muscle branch for gastrocnemius muscle, *PA* = popliteal artery, *PV* = popliteal vein, *STM* = semitendinosus muscle, *TN* = tibial nerve

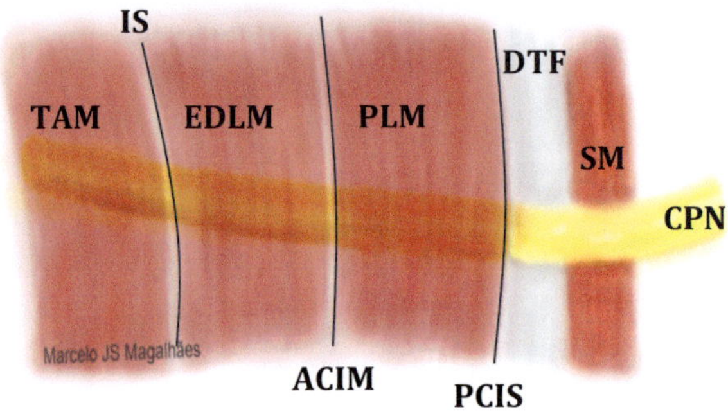

Fig. 4.5 Arrangement of ligaments and septa along the path of the peroneal nerve. *ACIM* = anterior crural intermuscular septum, *CPN* = common peroneal nerve, *DTF* = deep tendinous fascia, *EDLM* = extensor digitorum longus muscle, *IS* = intermuscular septum, *PCIS* = posterior crural intermuscular septum, *PLM* = peroneus longus muscle (fibularis longus muscle), *SM* = soleus muscle, *TAM* = tibialis anterior muscle

After its origin, it follows a trajectory towards the neck of the fibula, to penetrate a tunnel constituted by the two heads of the fibularis longus muscle. A possible point of nerve constriction is present between the posterior edge of the fibularis longus muscle and the lateral edge of the fibula; this septum is called the posterior crural intermuscular septum. A little more distally, another point of compression can occur, in the septum arranged between the fibularis longus muscle and the extensor digitorum longus muscle, which is also known as the anterior crural intermuscular septum (Figs. 4.5, 4.6, 4.7, 4.8, and 4.9).

The anatomical knowledge of the peroneal nerve is fundamental during surgical approach, as the non-release of nerve compression from these anatomical elements can compromise the functional result of the patient.

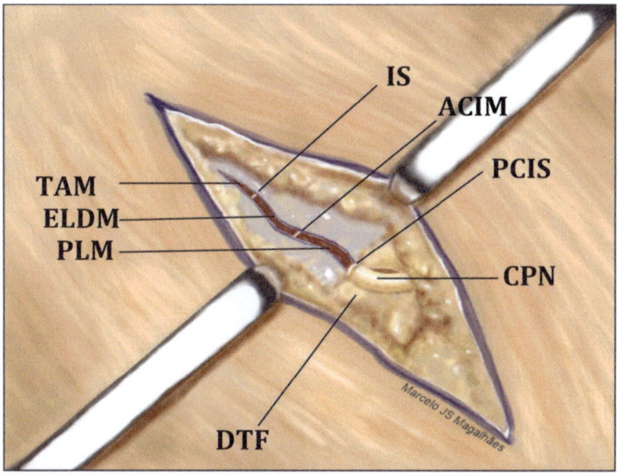

Fig. 4.6 Common peroneal nerve in left lower limb. *ACIM* = anterior crural intermuscular septum, *CPN* = common peroneal nerve, *DTF* = deep tendinous fascia, *EDLM* = extensor digitorum longus muscle, *IS* = intermuscular septum, *PCIS* = posterior crural intermuscular septum, *PLM* = peroneus longus muscle (fibularis longus muscle), *SM* = soleus muscle, *TAM* = tibialis anterior muscle

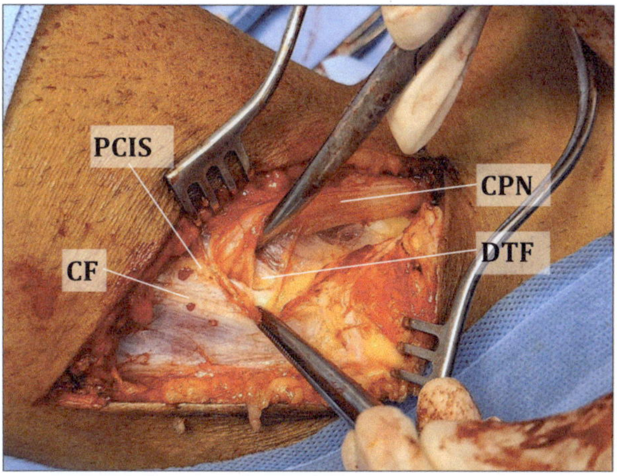

Fig. 4.7 Peroneal nerve in right lower limb. Patient in prone position. *CF* = crural fascia, *CPN* = common peroneal nerve, *DTF* = deep tendinous fascia, *PCIS* = posterior crural intermuscular septum

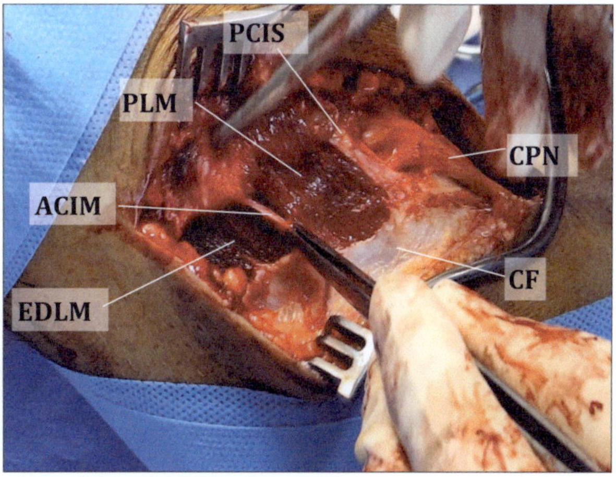

Fig. 4.8 Peroneal nerve in right lower limb. Patient in prone position. *ACIM* = anterior crural intermuscular septum, *CF* = crural fascia, *CPN* = common peroneal nerve, *EDLM* = extensor digitorum longus muscle, *PCIS* = posterior crural intermuscular septum, *PLM* = peroneus longus muscle (fibularis longus muscle)

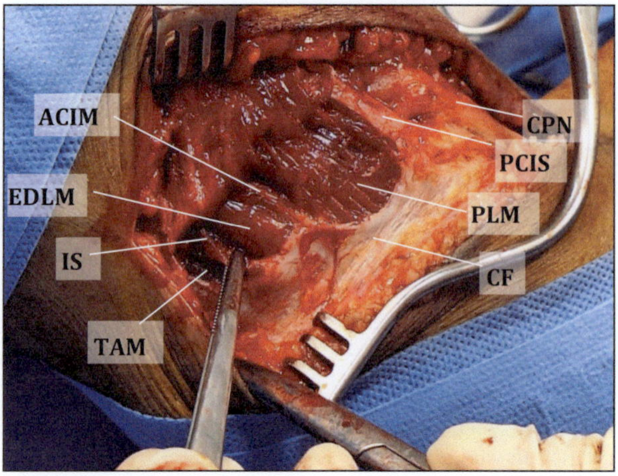

Fig. 4.9 Peroneal nerve in right lower limb. Patient in prone position. *ACIM* = anterior crural intermuscular septum, *CF* = crural fascia, *CPN* = common peroneal nerve, *EDLM* = extensor digitorum longus muscle, *IS* = intermuscular septum, *PCIS* = posterior crural intermuscular septum, *PLM* = peroneus longus muscle (fibularis longus muscle), *TAM* = tibialis anterior muscle

4.2.1 Anatomy of the Superficial Peroneal Nerve

The superficial peroneal nerve (SPN), after originating from the CPN, follows a trajectory inside the lateral compartment of the leg. In a proximal position, it runs under the fibularis longus muscle, and more distally, it positions itself between the fibularis brevis, fibularis longus, and extensor digitorum longus muscles (Fig. 4.2).

In the leg, the SPN produces a motor branch for the fibularis longus muscle and fibularis brevis muscle. These two muscles are responsible for the eversion of the foot. In the distal third of the leg, in the anterolateral region, the SPN perforates the deep fascia of the leg and produces the nerves: medial dorsal cutaneous and intermediate dorsal cutaneous.

The SPN is responsible for the sensory innervation of the dorsum of the foot, except for a small area of skin located in the first digital space which is performed by the deep peroneal nerve and a dorsal skin region in the two lateral toes, which is performed by the sural nerve [10, 11] (Fig. 4.1a, b).

Anatomical studies show that the SPN can position itself in the lateral compartment of the leg between 57% and 73% of cases, in the anterior compartment between 8.1% and 23%, and its branches in both compartments between 5% and 26% [12–14].

Tomaszewski et al. (2017) in a meta-analysis demonstrated that the division of the distal branches of the SPN occurs in a suprafascial plane in 82.7% of cases (Type 1), intracompartmental division, with superficialization of the branches as distinct entities in 15.6% (Type 2), and absence of the intermediate dorsal cutaneous branch in 1.8% (Type 3) [15].

4.2.2 *Intraseptal Tunnel of the Superficial Peroneal Nerve*

Valisena et al. (2021) in an anatomical study involving 15 lower limbs showed that the emergence point of the SPN in the deep fascia of the leg was about 10.37 cm proximal to the lateral malleolus [16].

In 10 specimens, it was possible to identify the presence of an intraseptal tunnel, in 8 cases, the SPN left the tunnel as a single trunk and in 2 cases, with the pattern of its branches. The average length of the intraseptal tunnel was 2.63 cm (minimum value of 1 cm and maximum of 4 cm) [16].

The tunnel has a fibrous-looking floor, where the ceiling presents a thin wall. The physical characteristics of the ceiling wall of the SPN tunnel are more compatible with those identified in the crural fascia (deep fascia of the leg) [16].

The use of anatomical points for the identification of the SPN can avoid its injury in surgical approaches performed in the anterior and anterolateral compartment of the lower limb. There is an estimate that the anterior surgical approach causes between 7.7% and 16.7% of SPN injury and that in anterolateral approach 21% [17–20].

4.2.3 *Anatomy of the Deep Peroneal Nerve*

After the CPN wraps around the neck of the fibula, it originates its three most important branches: deep peroneal nerve (DPN), SPN, and an articular branch for the sensitive innervation of the lateral part of the knee joint [20, 21].

After the origin of the DPN, it presents a trajectory in the anterior compartment of the leg running deep to the fibularis longus muscle and extensor digitorum longus muscle. In the upper third of the leg, the DPN presents a trajectory between the extensor digitorum longus and the tibialis anterior muscles. Already at the level of the lower third of the leg, it presents a trajectory below the tendon of the extensor hallucis longus muscle. At this point, it is lateral to the anterior tibial artery and has a path between the tendons of the extensor digitorum longus and the extensor hallucis longus muscles [22]. There is a distance of 1.3 cm from the ankle, and this nerve divides into lateral and medial branches [20, 21].

It is noted that bifurcation of the DPN into medial and lateral branches presents anatomical variation described. In an anatomical study with 36 lower limbs of formalized specimens, it was found that in 31 (86%) specimens, the bifurcation of the DPN occurred within the anterior tarsal tunnel (ATT), 2 (5.6%) below and in 3 (8.3%) no division of the nerve into lateral and medial branches was found. In this same study, no division into branches above the ATT was observed [16]. At the level of the bifurcation, the DPN presents a transverse diameter, in formalized specimen, of 3.2 ± 0.6 mm. The distance between the bifurcation and the first interdigital space is 131.0 ± 13.4 mm [16] (Figs. 4.10 and 4.11).

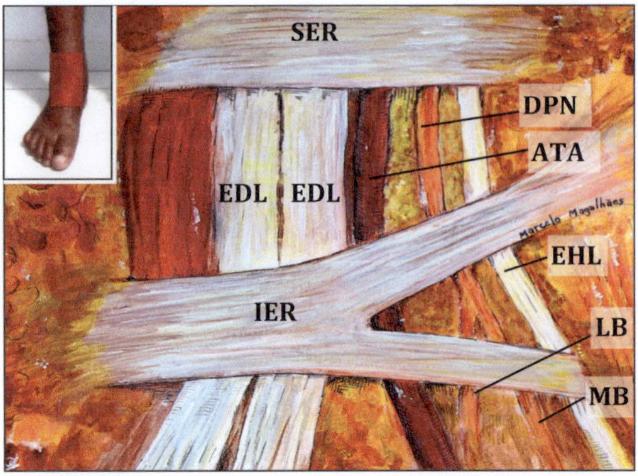

Fig. 4.10 Anterior tarsal tunnel in right lower limb. Note that the deep peroneal nerve is under the superior and inferior extensor retinaculum. *ATA* = anterior tibial artery, *DPN* = deep peroneal nerve, *EDL* = extensor digitorum longus, *EHL* = extensor hallucis longus, *IER* = inferior extensor retinaculum, *LB* = lateral branch, *MB* = medial branch, *SER* = superior extensor retinaculum. The tendon of the tibialis anterior muscle lies medial to the tendon of the extensor hallucis longus, deep to the overlying adipose tissue depicted in this region

The lateral branch of the deep peroneal nerve innervates the extensor hallucis brevis and extensor digitorum brevis muscles and the sensitivity of the second, third, and fourth metatarsophalangeal joints [23–25].

The medial branch of the deep peroneal nerve presents a trajectory between the tendon of the extensor hallucis longus muscle and the medial edge of the extensor digitorum hallucis brevis muscle of the toes. After piercing the deep fascia, this medial branch divides into two cutaneous branches for sensitive innervation of the first digital space [20, 21]. An anatomical study found that at the level of the first interdigital space of the foot, anastomosis between the superficial and deep peroneal nerves occurs in 27.8% of cases [16].

It is important to emphasize that the DPN located cranially to the inferior retinaculum is responsible for the innervation of the muscles: tibialis anterior, fibularis tertius, extensor hallucis longus, and extensor digitorum longus. Below this retinaculum, it only innervates the muscles: extensor digitorum brevis and extensor hallucis brevis [23–25]. For motor function, this nerve is responsible for the dorsiflexion of the foot, extension of the toes, and hallux. Given these anatomical considerations, a compressive process at the level of the extensor retinaculum can only result in sensory impairment of the first interdigital space and paresis of the muscles: extensor digitorum brevis and extensor hallucis brevis.

As the DPN presents a trajectory of almost 90° at the level of the ankle, the bowstring effect on the nerve is avoided by the action of the superior and inferior extensor retinaculum [20, 21].

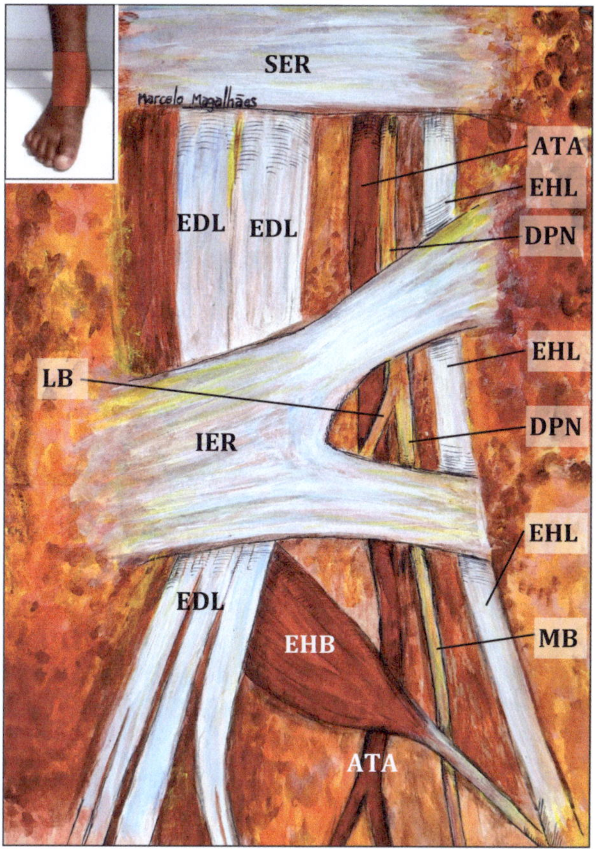

Fig. 4.11 Anterior tarsal tunnel in right lower limb. *ATA* = anterior tibial artery, *DPN* = deep peroneal nerve, *EDL* = extensor digitorum longus, *EHB* = extensor hallucis brevis, *EHL* = extensor hallucis longus, *IER* = inferior extensor retinaculum, *LB* = lateral branch, *MB* = medial branch, *SER* = superior extensor retinaculum. *Note that distally the deep peroneal nerve passes under the tendon of the extensor hallucis brevis muscle. The tendon of the tibialis anterior muscle lies medial to the tendon of the extensor hallucis longus, deep to the overlying adipose tissue depicted in this region

4.2.4 Anterior Tarsal Tunnel

The anterior tarsal tunnel can be conceptualized as a space of flattened dimensions positioned between the fascia of the navicular and talus bones (ventral) and the inferior extensor retinaculum of the foot [25]. In an anatomical study conducted with 18 formalized cadavers, it was shown that the lateral length of the tarsal tunnel is around 21.7 ± 4.2 mm and the medial length 55.0 ± 9 mm. The width of the anterior tarsal tunnel at the level of the lower edge between the tendons of the extensor hallucis longus and extensor digitorum longus muscles presents the extension of 12.6 ± 2.1 mm [16]. The presence of fibrotic bands over the deep peroneal nerve and dorsal artery of the foot, at the level of the anterior tarsal tunnel, is described in 61.1% of studied specimens [16] (Figs. 4.10 and 4.11).

4.3 Risk Factors for CNPN

The CNPN presents several risk factors for its onset, from traumas in the knee region to infectious diseases. It is essential to note that to remember that a fraction of patients identified with this diagnosis, despite undergoing extensive propaedeutic, do not have any identifiable risk factor [26].

Among the group of metabolic diseases, diabetes mellitus (DM) stands out as a risk factor for CNPN [27]. Another metabolic disease associated with this mononeuropathy is hypothyroidism [28]. Yasuoka et al. (1993) described the case report of a 65-year-old male patient with hypothyroidism, who presented impairment of the DPN. Physical examination revealed the presence of pre-tibial edema. Two months after starting treatment with levothyroxine, the neurological symptoms disappeared [29].

Several case reports describe rheumatic diseases such as systemic lupus erythematosus, dermatopolymyositis as a risk factor for peroneal neuropathy [30–32]. Hussein A. (1987) described the case report of a 9-year-old female patient with clinical symptoms of peroneal and radial nerve paralysis. After months of treatment with methylprednisolone and physiotherapy, she showed partial improvement of peroneal nerve paralysis and complete recovery of the radial nerve [32].

Among nerve tumors, schwannoma stands out; when located within the osteofibrous tunnel through which the peroneal nerve passes, they may cause nerve compression [33]. Rafai et al. (2006) described the case report involving a 70-year-old female patient with peroneal nerve schwannoma that triggered the clinical picture of neuropathy [33].

Weight loss is also described as a risk factor for CNPN. Cruz et al. (2000) described a study involving 150 patients, in which 20% of the participants, who lost an average of 10.9 kg, presented this neuropathy [34]. Local trauma of the peroneal nerve has also been described as a risk factor for this neuropathy. In this group, fibula fracture and knee dislocation can be identified [7].

CNPN has also been described after orthopedic procedures such as knee arthroplasty and tibial osteotomies, given the proximity of the nerve in surgical approaches [35].

Among the group of cystic lesions is the ganglion cyst in which post-surgical recurrences are frequent [7].

The habit of crossing the legs and remaining in a squatting position has already been described as a risk factor for this neuropathy [26]. The use of rigid immobilization of the lower limb, such as plaster, or decubitus in which the patient's leg remains in contact with hard surfaces, also increases the risk for the patient to develop CNPN [36].

4.4 Differential Diagnosis of CNPN

Different diseases that compromise nerves of the lower limb and spine can mimic the symptoms of CNPN.

Sciatica that compromises the L5 spinal nerve presents symptomatology similar to CNPN. A detail in the physical examination can assist in the process of identifying the etiology; in the radiculopathy of the L5 spinal nerve, the patient may have paresis for foot inversion, which is performed by the posterior tibial muscle whose innervation is performed by the tibial nerve [37].

4.5 Physical Examination of the Patient with CNPN

The physical examination of the patient suspected of CNPN should include inspection of the lower limb, deep myotendinous reflexes of the calcaneus and knee, sensitivity test, strength tests, and Tinel's test at the level of the fibula neck.

Rarely, on physical examination, will there be identified atrophy of the muscles contained in the anterior and lateral compartment of the leg. When the patient has some expansive lesion in the region of the osteofibrous tunnel, at the level of the fibula neck, some bulging in the skin can be visualized during inspection.

The motor strength test for foot inversion should be performed to assess the involvement of the posterior tibial muscle whose innervation is performed by the tibial nerve (fibers originating from the L5 spinal nerve). The motor strength evaluation for plantar flexion should be performed. The plantar flexion movement is performed by the gastrocnemius and soleus muscles, both innervated by the tibial nerve [38]. The main motor sign of CNPN is the presence of foot drop, leading the patient to develop a steppage gait (Fig. 4.12a, b).

Percussion of the peroneal nerve at the level of the fibula neck (Tinel's Sign) can promote radiation of pain to the distal sensory territory in the anterolateral region of the leg and dorsum of the foot. The calcaneal and patellar myotendinous reflexes are not altered by CNPN. The calcaneal reflex depends on the integrity of the S1 spinal nerve and the patellar reflex on the L3 and L4 spinal nerves [39].

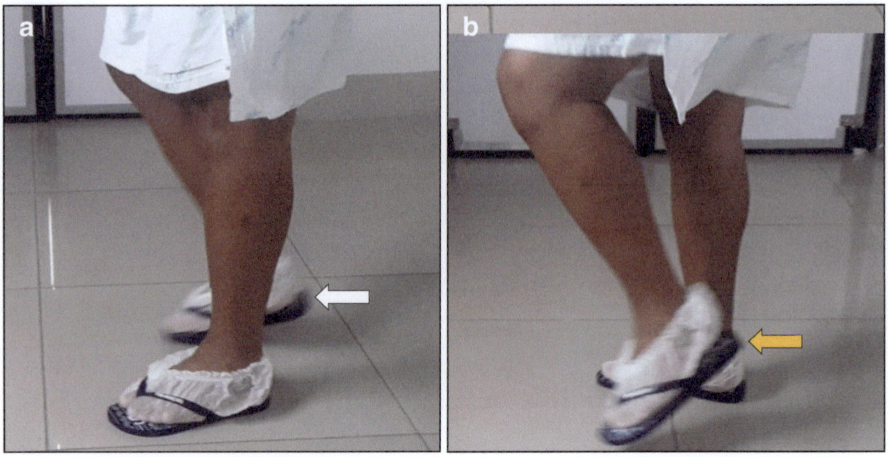

Fig. 4.12 (**a**, **b**) Evaluation of the gait of a patient with foot drop due to injury to the left peroneal nerve. The white arrow reveals that the right foot lifts a few centimeters off the ground to move, however, the left foot, during walking, lifts several centimeters off the ground to compensate for the loss of foot dorsiflexion (yellow arrow).

4.6 Conclusions

CNPN is the most common mononeuropathy of the lower limb with multiple risk factors and etiologies. Anatomical knowledge, the collection of the patient's clinical history, as well as the performance of his neurological examination promotes greater chances of the correct diagnosis.

References

1. Sultan C. Ganglion der nervenscheide des nervus peroneus. Zentralbl Chir. 1921;48:963–5.
2. Brooks DM. Nerve compression by simple ganglia: a review of thirteen collected cases. J Bone Joint Surg Br. 1952;34-B:391–400.
3. Cobb CA, Moiel RH. Ganglion of the peroneal nerve: report of two cases. J Neurosurg. 1974;41:255–9.
4. Noble W. Peroneal palsy due to hematoma in the common peroneal nerve sheath after distal torsional fractures and inversion ankle sprains. J Bone Joint Surg Am. 1966;48-A:1484–95.
5. Khedr EM, Fawi G, Allah Abbas MA, El-Fetoh NA, Zaki AF, Gamea A. Prevalence of common types of compression neuropathies in Qena Governorate/Egypt: a population-based survey. Neuroepidemiology. 2016;46(4):253–60.
6. Kandil MR, Darwish ES, Khedr EM, Sabry MM, Abdulah MA. A community-based epidemiological study of peripheral neuropathies in Assiut, Egypt. Neurol Res. 2012;34(10):960–6.
7. Marciniak C. Fibular (peroneal) neuropathy: Electrodiagnostic features and clinical correlates. Phys Med Rehabil Clin N Am. 2013;24(1):79–89. https://doi.org/10.1016/j.pmr.2012.08.016.
8. Bouche P. Compression and entrapment neuropathies. In: Handbook of clinical neurology, vol. 115. Elsevier B.V.; 2013. p. 311–66. https://doi.org/10.1016/B978-0-444-52902-2.00019-9.

9. Moatshe G, Dornan GJ, Løken S, Ludvigsen TC, Laprade RF, Engebretsen L. Demographics and injuries associated with knee dislocation: a prospective review of 303 patients. Orthop J Sports Med. 2017;5(5):2325967117706521. https://doi.org/10.1177/2325967117706521.
10. Georgakis E, Soames R. Arterial supply to the sciatic nerve in the gluteal region. Clin Anat. 2008;21:62–5.
11. Poirier P. Traité d'anatomie humaine. Paris: Masson; 1896.
12. Adkison DP, Bosse MJ, Gaccione DR, Gabriel KR. Anatomical variations in the course of the superficial peroneal nerve. J Bone Joint Surg Am. 1991;73(1):112–4.
13. Ducic I, Dellon AL, Graw KS. The clinical importance of variations in the surgical anatomy of the superficial peroneal nerve in the mid-third of the lateral leg. Ann Plast Surg. 2006;56:635–8.
14. Rosson GD, Dellon AL. Superficial peroneal nerve anatomic variability changes surgical technique. Clin Orthop Relat Res. 2005;438:248–52.
15. Tomaszewski KA, Graves MJ, Vikse J, et al. Superficial fibular nerve variations of fascial piercing: a meta-analysis and clinical consideration. Clin Anat. 2017;30(1):120–5.
16. Valisena S, Gamulin A, Hannouche D. The intraseptal course of the superficial peroneal nerve: an anatomic study. Foot Ankle Int. 2021;42(9):1171–8. https://doi.org/10.1177/10711007211002508.
17. Darland AM, Kadakia AR, Zeller JL. Branching patterns of the superficial peroneal nerve: implications for ankle arthroscopy and for anterolateral surgical approaches to the ankle. J Foot Ankle Surg. 2015;54:332–7.
18. Rasulić L, Savić A, Vitošević F, Samardžić M, Živković B, Mićović M, Baščarević V, Puzović V, Joksimović B, Novakovic N, Lepić M, Mandić-Rajčević S. Iatrogenic peripheral nerve injuries-surgical treatment and outcome: 10 years' experience. World Neurosurg. 2017;103:841–851.e6. https://doi.org/10.1016/j.wneu.2017.04.099. Epub 2017 Apr 24. PMID: 28450236.
19. Kosinski C. The course, mutual relations and distribution of the cutaneous nerves of the metazonal region of leg and foot. J Anat. 1926;60(pt 3):274–97.
20. Adelman KA, Wilson G, Wolf JA. Anterior tarsal tunnel syndrome. J Foot Surg. 1988;27(4):299–302.
21. Sarrafian S. The anatomy of the foot and ankle. Philadelphia: J.B. Lippincott; 1983.
22. Kanawati AJ. Variations of the sciatic nerve anatomy and blood supply in the gluteal region: a review of the literature. ANZ J Surg. 2014;84(11):816–9. https://doi.org/10.1111/ans.12675.
23. Dellon AL. Deep peroneal nerve entrapment on the dorsum of the foot. Foot Ankle Int. 1990;11(2):73–80.
24. Standring S, editor. Gray's anatomy. 39th ed. Spain: Churchill Livingstone; 2005. p. 1505.
25. Zongzhao L, Jiansheng Z, Li Z. Anterior tarsal tunnel syndrome. J Bone Joint Surg Br. 1991;73-B(3):470–3.
26. Fortier LM, Markel M, Thomas BG, Sherman WF, Thomas BH, Kaye AD. An update on peroneal nerve entrapment and neuropathy. Orthop Rev (Pavia). 2021;13(2):24937. https://doi.org/10.52965/001c.24937.
27. Anderson JC. Common fibular nerve compression: anatomy, symptoms, clinical evaluation, and surgical decompression. Clin Podiatr Med Surg. 2016;33(2):283–91. https://doi.org/10.1016/j.cpm.2015.12.005.
28. Dellon AL. The Dellon approach to neurolysis in the neuropathy patient with chronic nerve compression. Handchir Mikrochir Plast Chir. 2008;40(6):351–60. https://doi.org/10.1055/s-2008-1039216.
29. Yasuoka T, Yokota T, Tsukagoshi H. Deep peroneal nerve palsy associated with hypothyroidism. No To Shinkei. 1993;45(6):563–6. Japanese.
30. Huynh C, Ho SL, Fong KY, Cheung RT, Mok CC, Lau CS. Peripheral neuropathy in systemic lupus erythematosus. J Clin Neurophysiol. 1999;16(2):164–8. https://doi.org/10.1097/00004691-199903000-00010.
31. Florica B, Aghdassi E, Su J, Gladman DD, Urowitz MB, Fortin PR. Peripheral neuropathy in patients with systemic lupus erythematosus. Semin Arthritis Rheum. 2011;41(2):203–11. https://doi.org/10.1016/j.semarthrit.2011.04.001.

32. Hussein A. Juvenile dermatomyositis with respiratory failure and peripheral nerve paralyses: a case report. Klin Padiatr. 1987;199(6):447–8. https://doi.org/10.1055/s-2008-1026837.
33. Rafai MA, El Otmani H, Rafai M, et al. Syndrome de paralysie péronière révélant un schwannome du sciatique poplité externe au col du péroné. Rev Neurol (Paris). 2006;162(8–9):866–8. https://doi.org/10.1016/s0035-3787(06)75092-5. French.
34. Cruz-Martinez A, Arpa J, Palau F. Peroneal neuropathy after weight loss. J Peripher Nerv Syst. 2000;5(2):101–5. https://doi.org/10.1046/j.1529-8027.2000.00007.x.
35. Carender CN, Bedard NA, An Q, Brown TS. Common peroneal nerve injury and recovery after total knee arthroplasty: a systematic review. Arthroplast Today. 2020;6(4):662–7. https://doi.org/10.1016/j.artd.2020.07.017.
36. Bowley MP, Doughty CT. Entrapment neuropathies of the lower extremity. Med Clin North Am. 2019;103(2):371–82. https://doi.org/10.1016/j.mcna.2018.10.013.
37. Carolus AE, Becker M, Cuny J, et al. The interdisciplinary management of foot drop. Dtsch Arztebl Int. 2019;116(20):347–54. https://doi.org/10.3238/arztebl.2019.0347.
38. Masakado Y, Kawakami M, Suzuki K, et al. Clinical neurophysiology in the diagnosis of peroneal nerve palsy. Keio J Med. 2008;57(2):84–9. https://doi.org/10.2302/kjm.57.84.
39. Ginanneschi F, Mondelli M, Piu P, Rossi A. Pathophysiology of knee jerk reflex abnormalities in L5 root injury. Funct Neurol. 2015;30(3):187–91. https://doi.org/10.11138/fneur/2015.30.3.187.

Chapter 5
Complementary Exams in Common Peroneal Nerve Entrapment

5.1 Introduction

The compressive neuropathy of the peroneal nerve (CNPN) is the most common compressive neuropathy of the lower limb and the third most common neuropathy, right after carpal tunnel syndrome and cubital tunnel syndrome. Its clinical importance also lies in the paresis of foot dorsiflexion, leading the patient to develop "foot drop." It is noteworthy that diseases located far from the peroneal nerve (PN), such as a disc herniation compressing the L5 spinal nerve, can lead the patient to develop a clinical syndrome similar to that identified in CNPN. Different diseases and clinical situations increase the chances of the patient developing this type of compressive neuropathy, such as diabetes mellitus, hypothyroidism, collagen diseases, local traumas, calcifications and cysts, and tumors [1–5].

Among the oldest descriptions of CNPN is the work of Sultan C. (1921) that associates this neuropathy with the presence of a ganglion cyst. Brooks D.M. (1952) described a series of cases of this mononeuropathy caused by the ganglion cyst. In 1966, Noble W. described two case reports in which the peroneal nerve injury was caused by a local trauma in which the patient presented ankle inversion resulting in intraneural hemorrhage from the injury of the vasa nervorum. Also in 1966, White J. described the PN injury by trauma, whose mechanism involved traction of the affected limb and Cobb C.A. et al. (1974) described two case reports of CNPN, also associated with the ganglion cyst [6–10].

Few studies describe the incidence of CNPN in the general population. Studies conducted in Egypt revealed that the incidence of this neuropathy is around 19–40/100,000 inhabitants, totaling between 0.6% and 1.2% of all neuropathies [11, 12].

M. J. S. Magalhães, *Lower Extremity Nerve Entrapments*,
https://doi.org/10.1007/978-3-031-90058-7_5

CNPN can arise as complications of orthopedic procedures. Marciniak et al. (2013) identified this neuropathy in 2–27% of patients who underwent high tibial/fibular osteotomies [13]. Bouche et al. (2013) identified that 0.3–1.3% of patients who underwent knee arthroplasty developed CNPN [14].

Patients also with a clinical picture of knee trauma, such as dislocation, can develop CNPN. Moatshe et al. (2017) in a prospective study involving 303 patients observed that CNPN was diagnosed in 16–40% of cases [15].

The aim of this chapter is to review the neuropathy of the PN from the point of view of its complementary exams and physical examination.

5.2 Clinical Diagnosis of the Patient with CNPN

The physical examination of the patient suspected of CNPN should include inspection of the lower limb, deep myotendinous reflexes of the calcaneus and knee, sensitivity test, strength tests, and semiological maneuvers such as the Tinel test at the level of the fibula neck and Lasègue maneuver.

Rarely, on physical examination, atrophy of the muscles contained in the anterior and lateral compartment of the leg will be identified. When the patient has some expansive lesion, in the region of the osteofibrous tunnel at the level of the fibula neck, it may be possible to visualize bulging in the skin during inspection of the limb [2, 3].

The motor strength test for foot inversion should be performed since the posterior tibial muscle is innervated by the tibial nerve (fibers originating from the L5 spinal nerve). Test for motor strength for plantar flexion should also be performed. The plantar flexion movement is performed by the gastrocnemius and soleus muscles, both innervated by the tibial nerve [16]. It is important to remember that CNPN does not cause paresis for foot inversion; however, L5 radiculopathy does. The main motor sign of CNPN is the presence of foot drop, leading the patient to develop a steppage gait.

Percussion of the PN at the level of the fibula neck (Tinel's Sign) can promote radiation of pain to the distal sensory territory in the anterolateral region of the leg and dorsum of the foot, in patients with CNPN.

The calcaneal and patellar myotendinous reflexes are not altered by CNPN. The calcaneal reflex depends on the integrity of the S1 spinal nerve and the patellar reflex on the L3 and L4 spinal nerves [17].

The Lasègue sign should be performed, as its presence may be associated with radiculopathy involving lumbosacral spinal nerves. L5 radiculopathy is an important differential diagnosis for CNPN.

Anesthetic block of the PN may be useful to assess whether the symptoms presented by the patient really result from a neuropathy of this nerve. It is also important to mention that infiltration should be performed with the aid of US, with the aim of avoiding iatrogenic nerve injury [18].

5.3 Ultrasonography of the Peroneal Nerve

US is a relevant tool in the evaluation of the nerve. This exam has the advantage of being a low-cost and easily accessible procedure. The US can reveal the presence of fibrosis and thickening of the nerve. Some relevant differential diagnoses can be identified through this procedure, such as tumors and cystic lesions. Comparing nerves between the affected and healthy limb can be useful [19].

As occurs in other neuropathies, the US can assist in the process of identifying CNPN. There is some evidence that the increase in hypoechoic areas within the nerve suggests an early phase of compressive neuropathy [20].

Another aspect evaluated by the US is the area of the nerve's cross-section. In general, studies calculate this at the point where the cross-sectional area of the nerve presents its largest diameter, generally at the level of the fibula head or above the fibula head. Bignotti et al. (2017) mention that the cross-sectional area of the nerve with a value greater than 12 mm^2 has a sensitivity of 90% and specificity of 92% for the diagnosis of CNPN [19]. Bucklan et al. (2019) cite that the ratio between the cross-sectional area of the nerve at the level of the fibula head and popliteal fossa with a cut-off score of 1.25 could indicate CNPN. This ratio presents sensitivity between 51% and 71%. Despite these aforementioned data, there is no consensus on the most appropriate value for the cross-sectional area of the PN, as a parameter for the diagnosis of neuropathy [20] (Fig. 5.1).

Bignotti et al. (2017) also cite that the loss of fascicular echotexture may be associated with PN neuropathy [19].

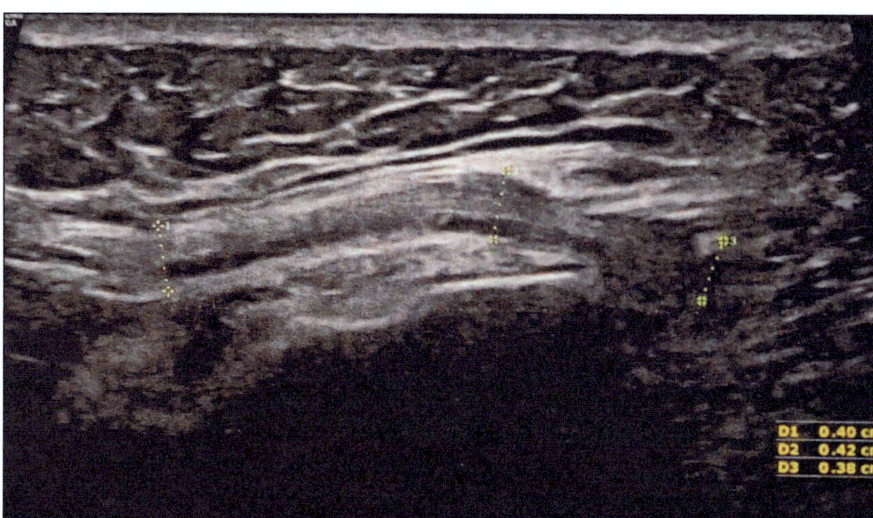

Fig. 5.1 Ultrasound of the lower limb at the level of the peroneal nerve tunnel revealing nerve thickening. The patient has a previous diagnosis of compressive neuropathy of the peroneal nerve

5.4 Electroneuromyography of the Lower Limbs

Electroneuromyography (ENM) of the lower limbs is a test of great value in the evaluation of patients suspected of CNPN. It is a test that allows the evaluation of amplitude and conduction speed. Among these two evaluations, amplitude seems to be more sensitive for the detection of dysfunction of the compromised nerve [21, 22]. It is important to remember that even with the presence of few functioning axons, there is maintenance of conduction speed; however, with any reduction in the number of functioning axons, there is a reduction in amplitude [22].

At least four patterns of CNPN can be identified by ENM [21].

Type 1- Conduction failure (partial or complete). It is the most commonly identified pattern, in about 60% of cases. Usually associated with tumors, traction injury, or compression.
Type 2- Conduction block (partial or complete). Identified in about 25% of cases. Usually results from focal demyelination secondary to traction or compression.
Type 3- Mixed injury pattern, due to axonal loss and conduction block.
Type 4- Axonal loss pattern due to L5 radiculopathy.

ENM is a test of great value in the investigation of the patient with clinical picture of "foot drop." Through this test, it is possible to identify radiculopathies resulting from lumbar disc herniations, lumbosacral plexopathy, mononeuropathies, polyneuropathies, myopathies, and multiple mononeuropathies. ENM also reveals the point of injury, as well as the severity and prognosis.

Commonly, most of the neuropathies identified are of the axonal type. In axonal involvement of a nerve, a reduction in amplitude in the waves of the compound muscle action potential (CMAP) is expected, however, with preservation of nerve conduction speed or minimal impairment of these [23].

The CMAP can be compared to the unaffected lower limb, and this percentage of the unaffected side corresponds to the present axonal loss. It is considered that the comparison between the CMAP between the symptomatic and asymptomatic limb or standard normal value is the best tool to evaluate axonal loss.

In Fig. 5.2, the CMAP waves of the tibial nerve present normal amplitude; however, in Fig. 5.3, it is possible to identify a typical flattening of axonal type nerve lesions in the PN. It is important to note that in axonal lesions, there is a technical difficulty to perform the topography of the point of involvement since there is a decrease in motor responses in the studied nerve as a whole [23].

Neuropathy with the block pattern is observed when there is a significant reduction in the amplitude of the CMAP in proximal stimuli, however, without an increase in its duration [23]. This type of alteration can be identified in the exams of patients with compressive neuropathies. Figure 5.4 shows a reduction in the amplitude of the

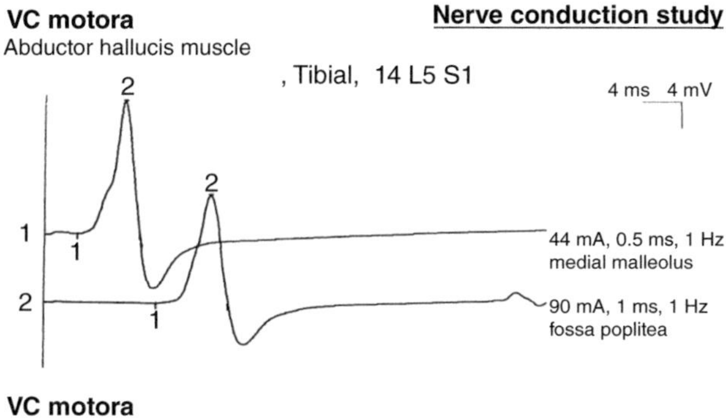

Latência residual e PDF

Lat. res. ms	Norm. LR, ms	Desv. LR., %	Indice lat. term.	Fator Prox.-dist.
3,02	2,0	**+50,9**	0,05	

Fig. 5.2 Electroneuromyography of the lower limbs. Examination of a patient with preserved tibial nerve motor conduction from the evaluation of the abductor hallucis muscle

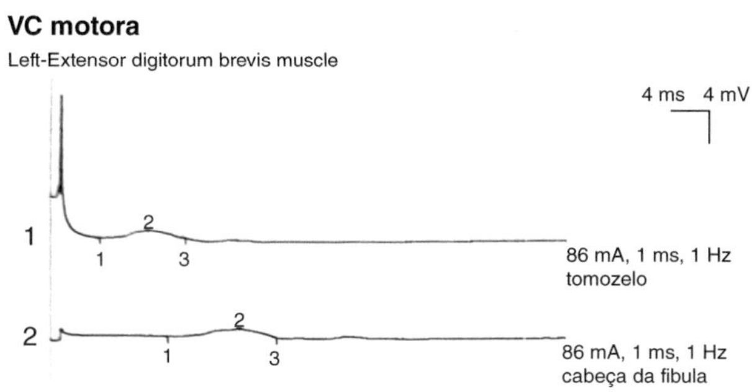

Latência residual e PDF

Lat. res. ms	Norm. LR, ms	Desv. LR., %	Indice lat. term.	Fator Prox.-dist.
3,14	2,0	**+57,1**	0,325	

Fig. 5.3 Electroneuromyography of the lower limbs. The motor conduction of the extensor digitorum brevis muscle showed axonal type lesion from the evaluation. Note the flattening of the wave

PN CMAP in the popliteal fossa. In this specific case, the patient had a diagnosis of PN compressive syndrome.

The medical literature reveals a large number of articles that comment on the reduction of CMAP through the fibula head. Several articles cite that the diagnosis of CNPN would be when the drop in CMAP was >20% [24, 25], others >50% [26–29].

Marciniak C. (2013) reveals that the specificity for the diagnosis of CNPN is 99% when the conduction block is identified at the level of the knee [13].

In demyelinating type lesions, there is a greater temporal dispersion of the CMAP and conduction speed lower than the limit of normality [23]. In demyelination of the PN, it presents focal slowing or conduction block through the neck of the fibula.

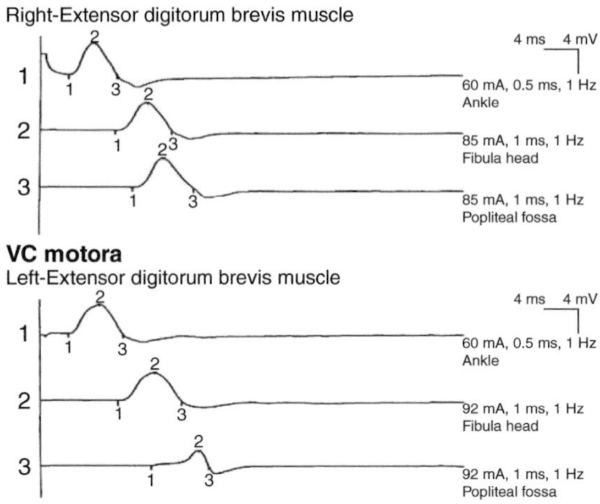

Neuro-EMG-Micro-2M

Latência residual e PDF

Lat. res. ms	Norm. LR, ms	Desv. LR., %	Indice lat. term.	Fator Prox.-dist.
1,97	2,0	**(N)**	0,4	0,961

Latência residual e PDF

Lat. res. ms	Norm. LR, ms	Desv. LR., %	Indice lat. term.	Fator Prox.-dist.
1,84	2,0	**(N)**	0,427	0,52

Fig. 5.4 Electroneuromyography of the lower limbs of a patient with a clinical picture of foot drop resulting from common peroneal neuropathy in the left lower limb. The upper graph reveals motor neuroconduction with compound muscle action potentials (CMAPs) of the left deep peroneal nerve with reduced amplitude and speeds in the popliteal fossa, proximal to the compression point which is at the head of the fibula (conduction block). The upper graph reveals compound muscle action potentials (CMAPs) of the right deep peroneal nerve with preserved amplitudes and speeds

The studies that evaluate the reduction of the conduction speed of the motor nerve were more consistent. A conduction speed <40 m/s was considered a pathological sign in some articles [27, 28], and in others <44 m/s [25, 27, 28].

Some studies evaluated the prognostic power of ENM in the recovery of patients with CNPN. It was observed that the presence of motor block may suggest a better prognosis [27, 29, 30]. Marciniak (2013), on the other hand, cites that the maintenance of a residual CMAP in the exam signals as a predictor of good prognosis [13]. Another author revealed that the presence of CMAP in the tibialis anterior and extensor digitorum brevis muscles is associated with an 81% recovery rate of foot dorsiflexion (motor strength ≥4) within 3 months [31].

The evaluation of the sensory nerve action potential (SNAP) performed in the sensory territory of the PN when it presents reduced amplitude suggests that there is axonal impairment of the nerve. This impairment can be quantified by comparing the amplitude and latency of the response obtained from the SNAP between the affected and healthy limb.

Electromyography can display fibrillation potentials and waves with a positive shape, which may be associated with axonal loss; however, this correlation is poor [32] (Fig. 5.5).

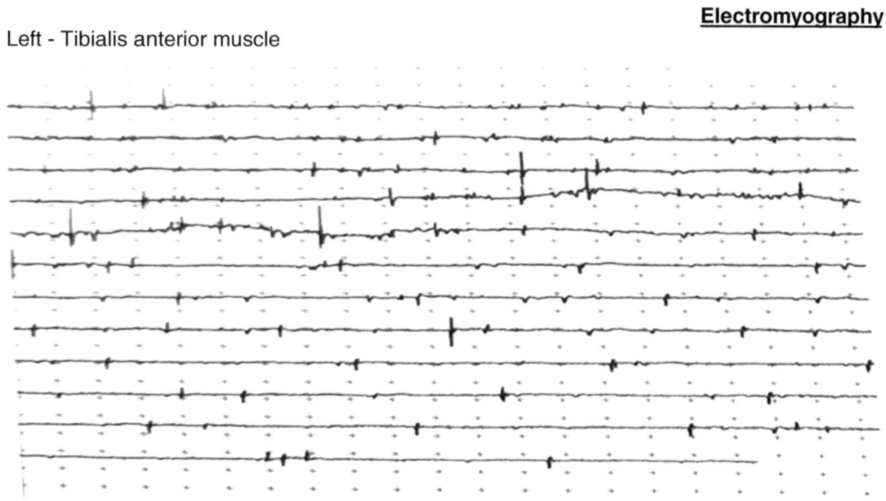

Fig. 5.5 Electromyography of the lower limbs of a patient with a clinical picture of common peroneal nerve neuropathy in the left lower limb. EMG (rest): presence of sharp waves and fibrillations in the left tibialis anterior muscle

5.5 Radiography

Knee radiography is relevant because it allows the identification of fractures, bone tumors, calcifications, as well as deformities present in the knee [3, 4, 33].

Hazmy W. (2001) described a case report of CNPN secondary to a proximal fibula osteochondroma, in an 11-year-old child. After surgical resection, there was control of symptoms [33]. Leveille et al. (2023) also described a case report of a 1 year old child, with CNPN resulting from osteochondroma that only after 8 months of surgical resection showed motor recovery [3].

Angelini et al. (2019) described the case report of a 68-year-old male patient, with clinical picture of CNPN resulting from calcified myonecrosis at the level of the tibia. The calcification arose as a result of tibia fracture that occurred 40 years ago. The radiography revealed extensive soft tissue calcification of the anterior and posterior compartment of the leg. The patient underwent biopsy that evolved with infection that was treated for long period of antibiotic therapy. The patient was asymptomatic after 2 years from the initial approach [4].

5.6 Magnetic Resonance

Magnetic resonance imaging (MRI) is an important complementary exam, especially for the exclusion of secondary causes of CNPN, such as peripheral nerve tumors, extra and intraneural ganglion cysts [5]. The denervation of the muscles in neuropathy is an indirect sign of nerve involvement that can be identified in this type of complementary exam, as is identified in Fig. 5.6.

Panwar et al. (2017) published a series of cases in which 245 patients with peripheral neuropathies underwent MRI for investigation of etiology. The authors identified 45 cystic lesions among these patients, 13 of which were intraneural ganglion cysts, with 7 of these affecting the common peroneal nerve (CPN). Among the other lesions identified were paralabral cysts, extraneural ganglion cysts, and abscesses due to Hansen's disease [5].

Regarding the specific findings of CNPN, Bignotti et al. (2017) revealed that the T2 sequence in the MRI exam can present hyperintensity or increase in the diameter of the nerve [19]. Such changes have sensitivity of 87.5% and specificity of 85%. Bendszus et al. (2003) revealed that using MRI in T1 and TIRM (turbo inversion recovery magnitude sequences) sequences, it is possible to identify pattern of muscle denervation that confers sensitivity and specificity of 100% in the detection of CNPN [34].

Lee et al. (2012) revealed that MRI is capable of detecting regional muscle edema (specificity of 93%, sensitivity of 62%), muscle atrophy (specificity 100%, sensitivity 31%), and fatty infiltration in the muscle (specificity 93%, sensitivity 62%) [35].

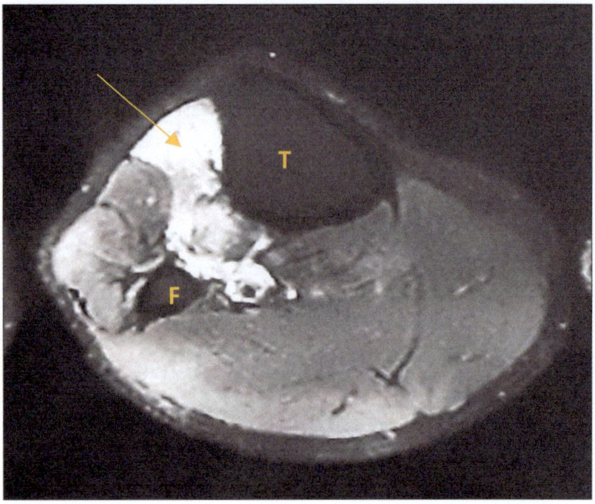

Fig. 5.6 Magnetic resonance imaging of the right leg of a patient with a picture of compressive neuropathy of the right peroneal nerve. The yellow arrow points to the muscle of the anterior compartment of the leg with a hyperintense appearance due to denervation. T = tibia, F = fibula

5.7 Computed Tomography

Computed tomography (CT) assists in the process of identification of diseases that may be underlying the CNPN such as, ganglion cysts, knee arthritis, tumors, fractures, and calcifications [4, 36].

5.8 Conclusions

The diagnosis of CNPN can be made through the patient's clinical picture; however, complementary exams play relevant role in the identification of differential diagnoses and secondary causes of this neuropathy. Among the complementary exams, electroneuromyography stands out.

References

1. Corriveau M, Lescher JD, Hanna AS. Peroneal nerve decompression. Neurosurg Focus. 2018;44(VideoSuppl 1):V6. https://doi.org/10.3171/2018.1.FocusVid.17575. PMID: 29291292.
2. Hazmy W. Peroneal nerve palsy secondary to proximal fibular osteochondroma: a case report. Med J Malaysia. 2001;56(Suppl C):89–90. PMID: 11814260.
3. Leveille CF, Zhu XM, Chen J, Burrow SR, Wang Y, Tarnopolsky M, Barkho JO. Pediatric peroneal nerve palsy secondary to fibular osteochondroma. J Am Acad Orthop Surg Glob Res Rev. 2023;7(10):00123. https://doi.org/10.5435/JAAOSGlobal-D-23-00123.
4. Angelini A, Mavrogenis AF, Pagliarini E, Trovarelli G, Fanelli GN, Cappellesso R, Ruggieri P. Calcific myonecrosis of the leg: a rare entity. Medicina (Kaunas). 2019;55(9):542. https://doi.org/10.3390/medicina55090542.
5. Panwar J, Mathew A, Thomas BP. Cystic lesions of peripheral nerves: are we missing the diagnosis of the intraneural ganglion cyst? World J Radiol. 2017;9(5):230–44. https://doi.org/10.4329/wjr.v9.i5.230.
6. Sultan C. Ganglion der Nervenscheide des Nervus peroneus. Zentralbl Chir. 1921;48:963–5.
7. Brooks DM. Nerve compression by simple ganglia: a review of thirteen collected cases. J Bone Joint Surg Br. 1952;34-B:391–400.
8. Cobb CA, Moiel RH. Ganglion of the peroneal nerve: report of two cases. J Neurosurg. 1974;41:255–9.
9. Noble W. Peroneal palsy due to hematoma in the common peroneal nerve sheath after distal torsional fractures and inversion ankle sprains. J Bone Joint Surg Am. 1966;48-A:1484–95.
10. White J. The results of traction injuries to the common peroneal nerve. J Bone Joint Surg Br. 1968;50-B:346–50.
11. Khedr EM, Fawi G, Allah Abbas MA, El-Fetoh NA, Zaki AF, Gamea A. Prevalence of common types of compression neuropathies in Qena Governorate, Egypt: a population-based survey. Neuroepidemiology. 2016;46(4):253–60.

12. Kandil MR, Darwish ES, Khedr EM, Sabry MM, Abdulah MA. A community-based epidemiological study of peripheral neuropathies in Assiut, Egypt. Neurol Res. 2012;34(10):960–6.
13. Marciniak C. Fibular (peroneal) neuropathy: electrodiagnostic features and clinical correlates. Phys Med Rehabil Clin N Am. 2013;24(1):121–37.
14. Bouche P. Compression and entrapment neuropathies. In: Handbook of clinical neurology, vol. 115. Elsevier B.V.; 2013. p. 311–66. https://doi.org/10.1016/B978-0-444-52902-2.00019-9.
15. Moatshe G, Dornan GJ, Løken S, Ludvigsen TC, Laprade RF, Engebretsen L. Demographics and injuries associated with knee dislocation: a prospective review of 303 patients. Orthop J Sport Med. 2017;5(5):2325967117706521. https://doi.org/10.1177/2325967117706521.
16. Davis TJ, Schon LC. Branches of the tibial nerve: anatomic variations. Foot Ankle Int. 1995;16(1):21–9. https://doi.org/10.1177/107110079501600105. PMID: 7697149.
17. Ginanneschi F, Mondelli M, Piu P, Rossi A. Pathophysiology of knee jerk reflex abnormalities in L5 root injury. Funct Neurol. 2015;30(3):187–91. https://doi.org/10.11138/fneur/2015.30.3.187.
18. Nirenberg MS. A simple test to assist with the diagnosis of common fibular nerve entrapment and predict outcomes of surgical decompression. Acta Neurochir. 2020;162(6):1439–44. https://doi.org/10.1007/s00701-020-04344-3.
19. Bignotti B, Assini A, Signori A, Martinoli C, Tagliafico A. Ultrasound versus MRI in common fibular neuropathy. Muscle Nerve. 2017;55(6):849–57. https://doi.org/10.1002/mus.25418.
20. Oosterbos C, Decramer T, Rummens S, Weyns F, Dubuisson A, Ceuppens J, Schuind S, Groen J, van Loon J, Rasulic L, Lemmens R, Theys T. Evidence in peroneal nerve entrapment: a scoping review. Eur J Neurol. 2022;29(2):665–79. https://doi.org/10.1111/ene.15145.
21. Bucklan JN, Morren JA, Shook SJ. Ultrasound in the diagnosis and management of fibular mononeuropathy. Muscle Nerve. 2019;60(5):544–8.
22. Pickett JB. Localizing peroneal nerve lesions to the knee by motor conduction studies. Arch Neurol. 1984;41:192–5.
23. Gondin FAA, Freitas MRG, Pereira RC. Neuropatias periféricas. 1ª ed. São Paulo: Ominifarma; 2020.
24. Bayrak İK, Oytun Bayrak A, Türker H, Akpinar ÇK, Bolat N. Diagnostic value of ultrasonography in peroneal neuropathy. Turk J Med Sci. 2018;48(6):1115–20.
25. Kwon HK, Kim L, Park YK. Compound nerve action potential of common peroneal nerve and sural nerve action potential in common peroneal neuropathy. J Korean Med Sci. 2008;23(1):117–21.
26. Aprile I, Caliandro P, La Torre G, et al. Multicenter study of peroneal mononeuropathy: clinical, neurophysiologic, and quality of life assessment. J Peripher Nerv Syst. 2005;10(3):259–68.
27. Nageeb RS, Mohamed WS, Nageeb GS, Desoky EA, Azmy TM. Role of superficial peroneal sensory potential and high-resolution ultrasonography in confirmation of common peroneal mononeuropathy at the fibular neck. Egypt J Neurol Psychiatry Neurosurg. 2019;55(1):1–8.
28. Kang PB, Preston DC, Raynor EM. Involvement of superficial peroneal sensory nerve in common peroneal neuropathy. Muscle Nerve. 2005;31(6):725–9.
29. Tsukamoto H, Granata G, Coraci D, Paolasso I, Padua L. Ultrasound and neurophysiological correlation in common fibular nerve conduction block at fibular head. Clin Neurophysiol. 2014;125(7):1491–5.
30. Bsteh G, Löscher WN, Gruber H, Seppi K, Wanschitz JV. Prognosis and prognostic factors in non-traumatic acute-onset compressive mononeuropathies: radial and peroneal mononeuropathies. J Peripher Nerv Syst. 2013;18:981.
31. Derr JJ, Micklesen PJ, Robinson LR. Predicting recovery after fibular nerve injury: which electrodiagnostic features are most useful? Am J Phys Med Rehabil. 2009;88(7):547–53.
32. Gilchrist JM, Sachs GM. Electrodiagnostic studies in the management and prognosis of neuromuscular disorders. Muscle Nerve. 2004;29:165–90.
33. Hazmy W. Peroneal nerve palsy secondary to proximal fibular osteochondroma-A case report. Med J Malaysia. 2001;56 Suppl C:89–90. PMID: 11814260.

34. Bendszus M, Wessig C, Reiners K, Bartsch AJ, Solymosi L, Koltzenberg M. MR imaging in the differential diagnosis of neurogenic foot drop. AJNR Am J Neuroradiol. 2003;24(7):1283–9.
35. Lee PP, Chalian M, Bizzell C, et al. Magnetic resonance neurography of common peroneal (fibular) neuropathy. J Comput Assist Tomogr. 2012;36(4):455–61.
36. Masakado Y, Kawakami M, Suzuki K, Abe L, Ota T, Kimura A. Clinical neurophysiology in the diagnosis of peroneal nerve palsy. Keio J Med. 2008;57(2):84–9. https://doi.org/10.2302/kjm.57.84. PMID: 18677088.

Chapter 6
Management of Common Peroneal Nerve Entrapment

6.1 Introduction

The compressive neuropathy of the peroneal nerve (CNPN) is the most common compressive neuropathy of the lower limb and the third most common mononeuropathy of the limbs, right after carpal tunnel syndrome, and cubital tunnel syndrome. As addressed in other chapters, the compression point of the peroneal nerve (PN) is most commonly identified at the level of the fibula neck, due to its peculiar anatomical characteristics.

The clinical importance of CNPN also occurs due to the paresis of foot dorsiflexion due to the involvement of the tibialis anterior muscle, leading the patient to develop "foot drop."

It is relevant to remember that diseases present at distant points of the PN can lead the patient to develop a clinical picture similar to CNPN, such as a herniated disc compressing the L5 spinal nerve. The medical literature describes different treatment modalities for the management of patients with this compressive syndrome that can be performed through medications, physiotherapies, minimally invasive techniques, and surgical procedures.

Regarding the historical aspects of this disease, among the oldest known descriptions of CNPN is the work of Sultan C. (1921) on a ganglionic cyst as the cause of CNPN. Brooks D.M. (1952) described a series of cases of CNPN also caused by a ganglionic cyst. In 1966, Noble W. described two case reports in which the PN injury was caused by trauma resulting from ankle inversion, resulting in intraneural hemorrhage due to injury to the vasa nervorum. In 1966, White J. also published a case report in that the PN injury occurred due to traumatic injury, the mechanism of which involved traction of the affected limb. Cobb et al. (1974) described two case reports of ganglion cyst as the etiology of CNPN [1–4].

Supplementary Information The online version contains supplementary material available at https://doi.org/10.1007/978-3-031-90058-7_6.

M. J. S. Magalhães, *Lower Extremity Nerve Entrapments*,
https://doi.org/10.1007/978-3-031-90058-7_6

Few studies describe the incidence of CNPN in the general population. Data collected from the population of Egypt revealed that the incidence of this neuropathy is around 19–40/100,000 inhabitants, totaling between 0.6% and 1.2% of all identified neuropathies [5, 6].

The medical literature describes several articles in which CNPN can arise as a result of orthopedic procedures. Marciniak et al. (2013) suggest that this mononeuropathy is identified in 2–27% of patients who underwent high tibial osteotomies [7]. Bouche et al. (2013) in their work identified that between 0.3% and 1.3% of patients who underwent knee arthroplasty developed this neuropathy [8].

Patients with clinical trauma of the knee associated with dislocation may also develop CNPN. Moatshe et al. (2017) in a prospective study, involving 303 patients, observed that CNPN was diagnosed in 16–40% of cases [9].

The aim of this chapter is to conduct a review on the neuropathy of the peroneal nerve, emphasizing conservative and surgical treatment of patients.

6.2 Conservative Treatment

Patients with CNPN can benefit from motor physiotherapy, especially in the presence of paresis for the dorsiflexion of the foot. This treatment modality consists of stretching, strengthening, proprioception, and balance exercises [10]. The use of ice and bandaging "taping" is also described in medical literature as adjuvant treatment modalities for these patients [10].

Those who have paresis for dorsiflexion of the foot should use ankle-foot orthosis (AFO) that promotes ankle immobilization at 90° to prevent shortening of the Achilles tendon [10]. These orthoses promote lateral and medial stability of the ankle during walking, in the support phase which assists the patient. Some orthoses are constructed from carbon fibers that provide greater resistance and lightness to their structures (Fig. 6.1).

Comorbidities that are potentially associated with CNPN, such as vitamin deficiencies, collagen diseases, and metabolic diseases, should also be treated. It is important for the patient to avoid crossing the leg and/or perform activity in which the body position may result in direct compression of the peroneal nerve at the level of the fibula neck [11–15].

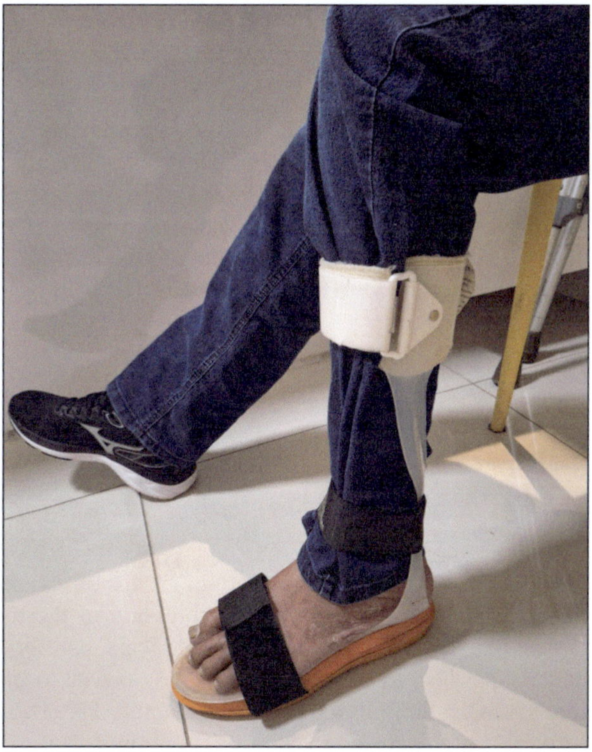

Fig. 6.1 Ankle-foot orthosis (AFO) used by a patient with a foot-drop condition

6.3 Minimally Invasive Techniques

6.3.1 Peroneal Nerve Stimulation as Treatment for CNPN

The use of peripheral nerve stimulation as a form of treatment for CNPN is described in the literature. In a case report, Oswald et al. (2019) revealed significant pain control in patients with neuropathic pain resulting from this neuropathy. Neurostimulation was able to reduce the pain scale score from 9.0 to 2.3. In principle, this is an innovative treatment modality that requires publications involving a larger number of patients and follow-up time for better definition of its role in the treatment of patients with CNPN [16].

6.3.2 *Treatment of Peroneal Neuropathy Through Ultrasound-Guided Pulsed Radiofrequency*

The use of ultrasound-guided pulsed radiofrequency as a form of treatment for a patient with terminal branch neuropathy of the superficial peroneal nerve is reported in the literature. Silva et al. (2023) described the case report of a male patient, handball player, 34 years old, who developed clinical symptoms of superficial peroneal nerve neuropathy after an ankle sprain episode. After treatment with this modality, the patient continued to have good control of pain symptoms, even after 2 years of follow-up [17].

6.4 Surgical Treatment

6.4.1 *Indication of Surgical Treatment for CNPN*

There is clinical evidence that certain groups of patients may benefit from surgical treatment, which consists of decompression of the tunnel through which the PN passes [17, 18]. Patients with a significant paresis of foot dorsiflexion should undergo surgical treatment without delay, as well as those who present pain refractory to medications after a period of 3 months [17, 18]. Among other indications for surgical treatment, one can cite the rapid neurological deterioration of the patient [17].

However, the most appropriate time to perform decompression surgery in patients with only sensory symptoms is not yet clearly established.

6.4.2 *Surgical Decompression of the Common Peroneal Nerve and Superficial and Deep Branches*

The patient can remain in two positions for the decompression of the PN tunnel, in prone position, with the lower limbs extended or in supine position, with the lower limb to be operated on with knee flexion at a 90° angle. In the second position, a cushion should be placed between the legs to prevent movement of the limb during the procedure. To facilitate the correct positioning of the limb in flexion, it can be fixed to the surgical table with some type of tape or use the foot support (Fig. 6.2).

It is interesting to previously ask the patient about the presence of allergies to the types of tapes most commonly available in the hospital environment, such as adhesive tape and micropore. Trimming should be performed, when necessary, moments before performing limb antisepsis.

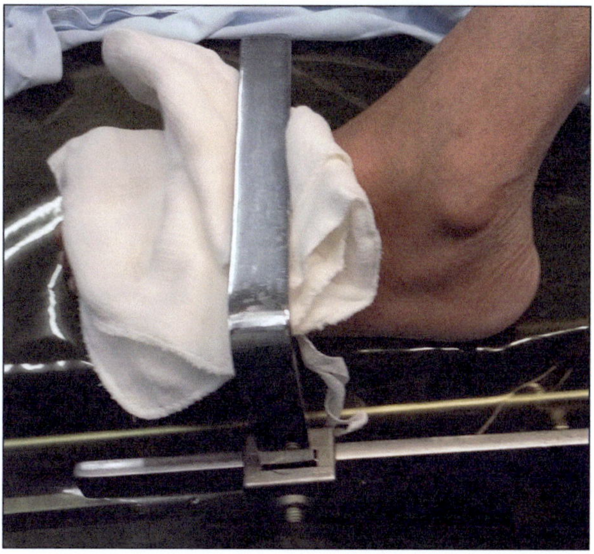

Fig. 6.2 Foot support during positioning in dorsal decubitus with knee flexion for surgical treatment. Patient with a lesion of the common peroneal nerve

When opting for the prone position, a cushion should be placed under the anterior superior iliac spine and on the ankle, with the aim of promoting a slight flexion of the hip and knee.

Anesthesia should be of the general type and without the use of muscle blockers.

Surgical marking is essential to avoid wasting time during surgery and better approach to perform nerve decompression. The surgical marking of the incision must necessarily pass at the level of the neck of the fibula which is identified by manual palpation, after the patient is properly positioned. The patient who has thicker subcutaneous tissue is more prone to a less reliable marking.

Anesthetic infiltration should be careful, as the common peroneal nerve (CPN) has an oblique trajectory in the neck of the fibula and very close to the skin surface.

An approximately 7 cm incision in the skin should be careful. Once the thigh and leg fascia is identified, an incision should be made for the recognition of the common peroneal nerve, in the proximal part of the incision (Figs. 6.3, 6.4, 6.5, 6.6, 6.7, 6.8, and 6.9; Video 6.1).

After visualizing the common peroneal nerve, the identification and opening of the crural fascia, positioned over the fibularis longus, extensor digitorum longus, and tibialis anterior muscles, should be performed. The deep tendinous fascia positioned under the PN should then be sectioned. The next step is the opening of the posterior and anterior intermuscular crural septum. Finally, the intermuscular septum should also be sectioned with the aim of a complete decompression of the nerve.

During the process of opening ligaments and fascias, unnecessary manipulation of the CPN and its deep and superficial branches should be avoided. Once the articular branch is identified, it should be preserved.

During synthesis, it is not necessary to close the fascia and ligaments already sectioned.

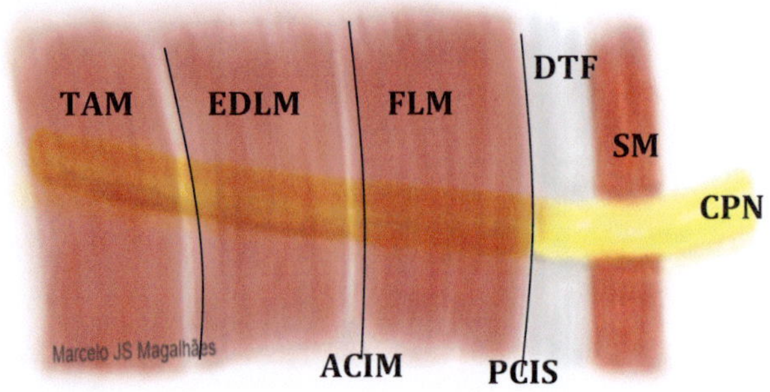

Fig. 6.3 Common peroneal nerve in the left lower limb. *ACIM* = anterior crural intermuscular septum, *CPN* = common peroneal nerve, *DTF* = deep tendinous fascia, *EDLM* = extensor digitorum longus muscle, *FLM* = fibularis longus muscle, *IS* = intermuscular septum, *PCIS* = posterior crural intermuscular septum, *SM* = soleus muscle, *TAM* = tibialis anterior muscle

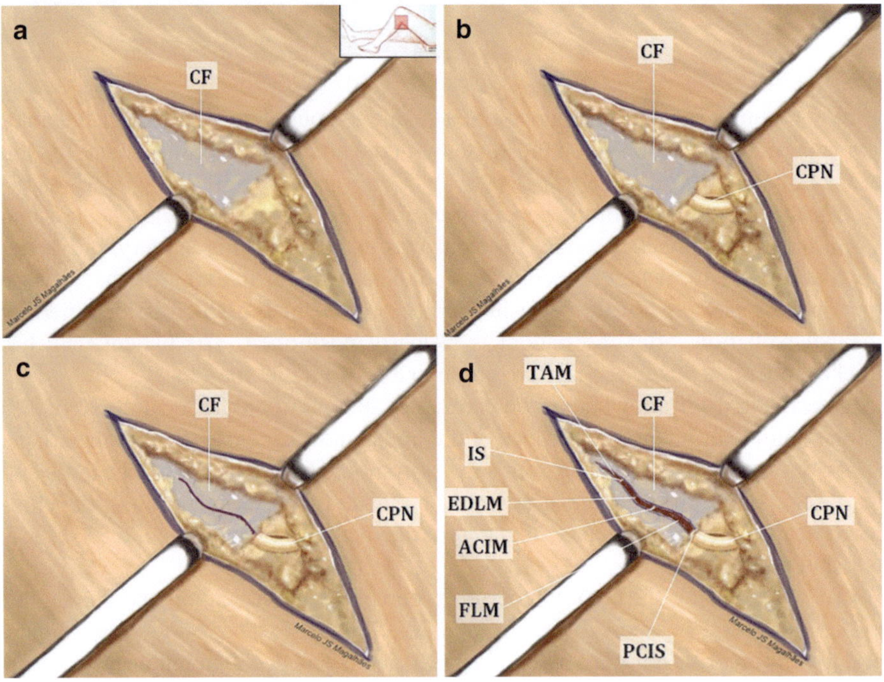

Fig. 6.4 (**a–d**) Common peroneal nerve in the left lower limb. First 4 steps to the exposure of the main septa of the peroneal nerve tunnel. (**a**) Exposure of the crural fascia of the leg. (**b**) Exposure of the common peroneal nerve. (**c**) Opening of the crural fascia of the leg to visualize the underlying musculature. (**d**) Exposure of the main septa of the peroneal nerve tunnel. *ACIM* = anterior crural intermuscular septum, *CF* = crural fascia, *CPN* = common peroneal nerve, *EDLM* = extensor digitorum longus muscle, *FLM* = fibularis longus muscle, *IS* = intermuscular septum, *PCIS* = posterior crural intermuscular septum, *TAM* = tibialis anterior muscle

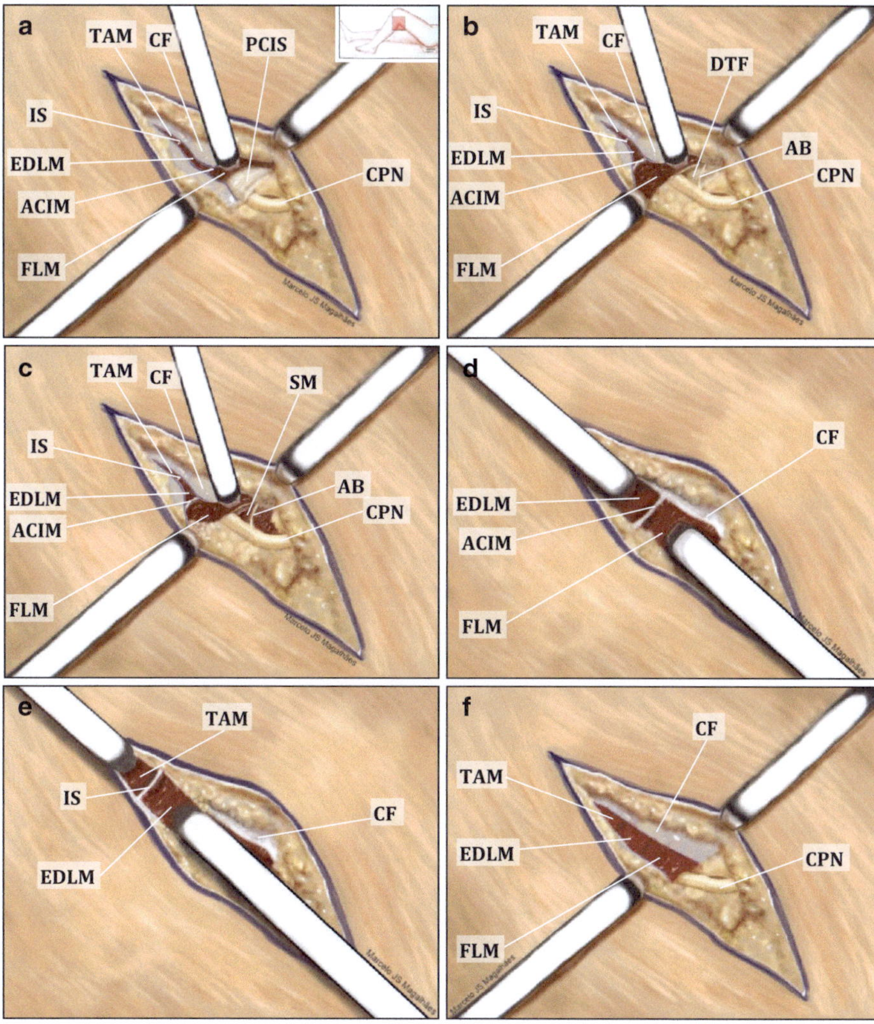

Fig. 6.5 (**a–f**) Common peroneal nerve in the left lower limb. Opening of the main septa of the peroneal nerve tunnel. (**a**) Exposure of the posterior crural intermuscular septum. (**b**) Opening of the posterior crural intermuscular septum with exposure of the articular branch and better exposure of the common peroneal nerve and exposure of the deep tendinous fascia. (**c**) Opening of the deep tendinous fascia. (**d**) Exposure of the anterior crural intermuscular septum for its opening. (**e**) Exposure of the intermuscular septum for its opening. (**f**) Surgical bed after the opening of all septa. *AB* = articular branch, *ACIM* = anterior crural intermuscular septum, *CF* = crural fascia, *CPN* = common peroneal nerve, *DTF* = deep tendinous fascia, *EDLM* = extensor digitorum longus muscle, *FLM* = fibularis longus muscle, *IS* = intermuscular septum, *PCIS* = posterior crural intermuscular septum, *SM* = soleus muscle, *TAM* = tibialis anterior muscle

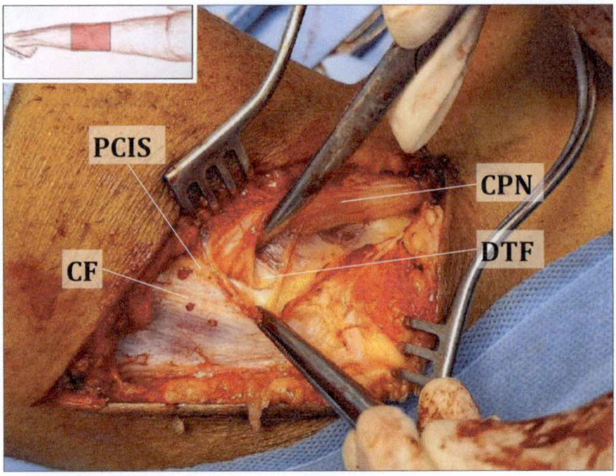

Fig. 6.6 Peroneal nerve in the right lower limb. Patient in prone position. Note that the crural fascia of the leg has not yet been opened for the exposure of the septa. *CF* = crural fascia, *CPN* = common peroneal nerve, *DTF* = deep tendinous fascia, *PCIS* = posterior crural intermuscular septum

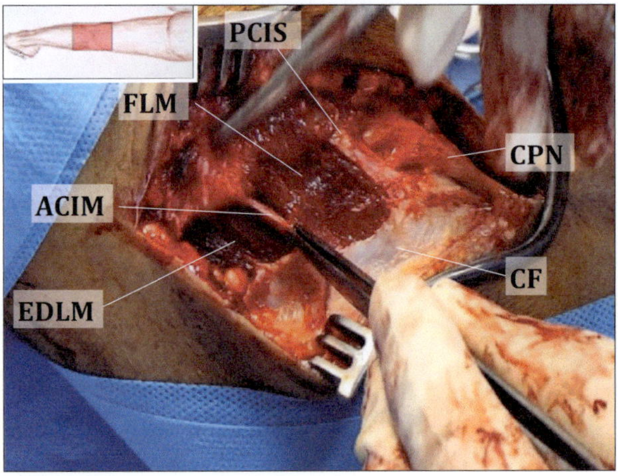

Fig. 6.7 Peroneal nerve in the right lower limb. Patient in prone position. Note that at this surgical stage some septa are already exposed. The deep tendinous fascia has been opened and part of the crural fascia has been resected. *ACIM* = anterior crural intermuscular septum, *CF* = crural fascia, *CPN* = common peroneal nerve, *EDLM* = extensor digitorum longus muscle, *FLM* = fibularis longus muscle, *PCIS* = posterior crural intermuscular septum

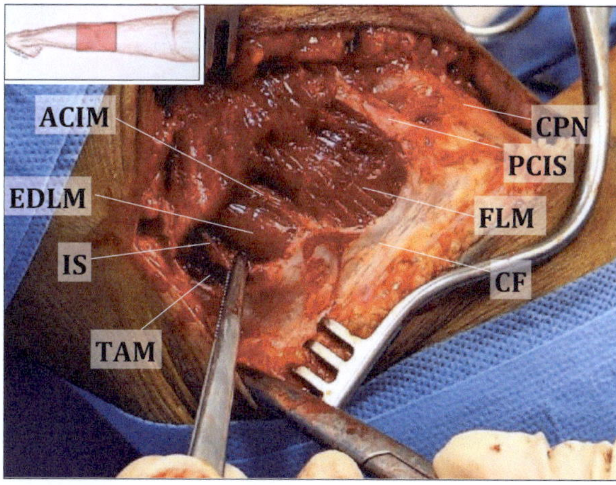

Fig. 6.8 Peroneal nerve in the right lower limb. Patient in prone position. The opening of the crural fascia of the leg allowed the visualization of the septa. *ACIM* = anterior crural intermuscular septum, *CF* = crural fascia, *CPN* = common peroneal nerve, *EDLM* = extensor digitorum longus muscle, *FLM* = fibularis longus muscle, *IS* = intermuscular septum, *PCIS* = posterior crural intermuscular septum, *TAM* = tibialis anterior muscle

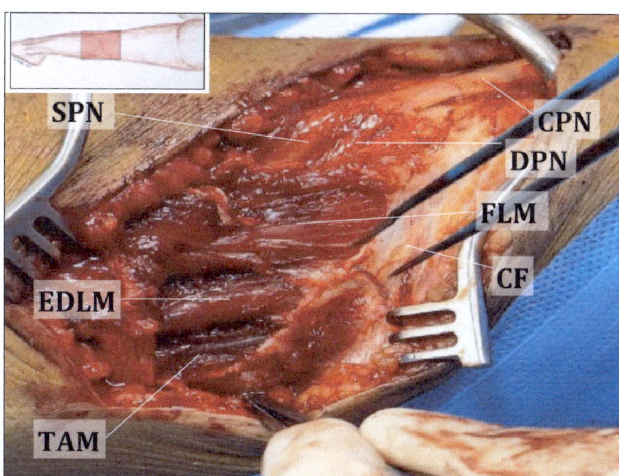

Fig. 6.9 Peroneal nerve in the right lower limb. Patient in prone position. Note that all fasciae and ligaments have been sectioned for the decompression of the peroneal nerve. *CF* = crural fascia, *CPN* = common peroneal nerve, *DPN* - Deep peroneal nerve, *EDLM* = extensor digitorum longus muscle, *FLM* = fibularis longus muscle, *SPN* - Superficial peroneal nerve, *TAM* = tibialis anterior muscle

If necessary, the PN can also be decompressed in its proximal portion, through skin retraction that facilitates the visualization of this nerve.

6.4.3 *Complications Resulting from Surgical Decompression as Treatment for CNPN*

Patients with CNPN may present with paresis for dorsiflexion of the foot (dropped foot) and tendon shortening of the calcaneus, which gives the patient the equinovarus foot. Not infrequently, it is necessary to perform calcaneus tendon lengthening to give these patients' ankles a more physiological angle. The lengthening procedure, in general, is performed when necessary, concomitantly in patients undergoing myotendinous transfer of the tibialis posterior muscle for the treatment of dropped foot deformity (Figs. 6.10 and 6.11a, b; Video 6.2)

6.4.4 *Results of Surgical Decompression of the Peroneal Nerve*

In a systematic review on the outcomes of treatments for patients with different types of PN injury, Mackay M.J. et al. (2022) revealed that among 42 articles identified, neurolysis was responsible for a result ≥M3 (British Medical Research Council) in 81.4% of cases [19].

6.4.5 *Complications of Surgical Decompression of the Peroneal Nerve*

In a systematic review involving 39 studies, totaling 368 patients, who underwent surgical decompression of the CPN for the treatment of this neuropathy, Chow et al. (2021) revealed that the main complications identified were infection 0.52% ($N = 2$), dehiscence 0.27% ($N = 1$), hematoma 0.54% ($N = 2$), hemorrhage 0.27% ($N = 1$), recurrence of PN paralysis 0.27% ($N = 1$), and death from sepsis 0.27% ($N = 1$) [20].

6.4.6 *Surgical Failure of PN Decompression*

Some patients with a dropped foot due to paresis of the peroneal nerve may persist with motor deficit, despite having undergone surgical treatment with adequate decompressive technique.

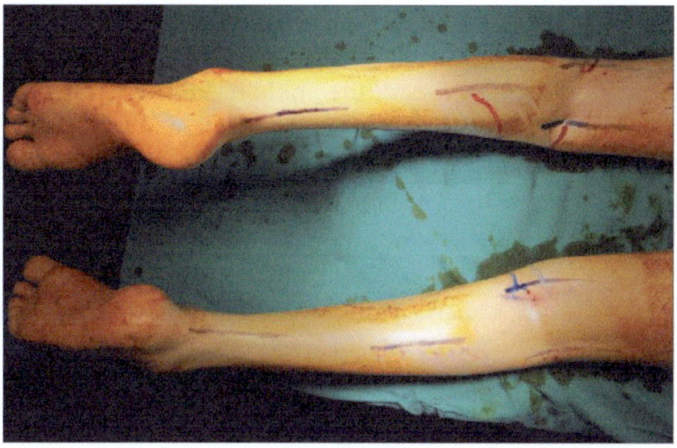

Fig. 6.10 Tendon shortening secondary to paralysis of the peroneal nerve. Male patient, victim of severe cranioencephalic trauma, with a long period of intensive treatment in a hospital environment. The patient developed bilateral peroneal neuropathy and subsequent tendon shortening of the dorsiflexor muscles of the foot and flexor of the knee bilaterally. Note the presence of the feet in equinovarus position and reduction of knee extension. The markings indicate the incisions used for surgical lengthening of various tendons

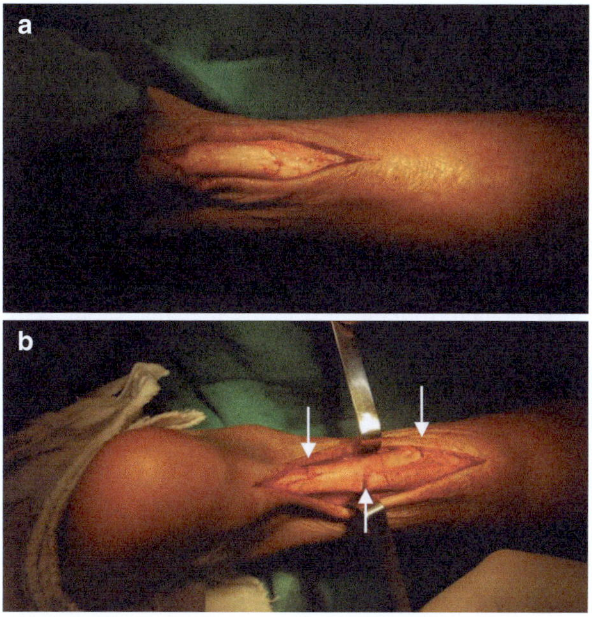

Fig. 6.11 (**a**) Achilles tendon lengthening technique. Note the linear incision on the back of the leg. (**b**) Achilles tendon lengthening technique. The white arrows indicate the 3 incisions made with a scalpel. Note that the incisions are alternated and never cross the midline

Among the options available for the correction of steppage gait are ankle arthrodesis and myotendinous transfer of the tibialis posterior muscle to the tendon of the tibialis anterior muscle. Arthrodesis of the ankle has the disadvantage of creating a rigid joint. On the other hand, in the myotendinous transfer, the dorsiflexion movement is restored at the expense of the sacrifice of the tendon of the tibialis posterior muscle, which is sutured to the tendon of the tibialis anterior (responsible for the dorsiflexion of the foot). In this case, the patient loses the inversion movement of the foot, despite maintaining the extension movement of the foot. It is important to note that for the myotendinous transfer technique of the tibialis posterior, the patient must demonstrate foot inversion on physical examination (Video 6.3).

Patients with a long period of paresis of the dorsiflexion of the foot and/or inability to properly rehabilitate with physiotherapy may have shortening of the Achilles tendon, consequently presenting the foot in plantar extension position. Therefore, some patients will need tendon stretching, as already mentioned. After surgery, the patient should remain for about 6 weeks with the foot immobilized in an orthopedic boot [21].

6.5 Nerve Transfer as a Treatment Modality for Peroneal Nerve Injury

The transfer of motor fibers from the tibial nerve to the deep peroneal nerve has been described in several works in the medical literature. The results in general in the published articles were not encouraging from the point of view of restoring the dorsiflexor function of the foot. Flores et al. (2013) in a series of cases presented unsatisfactory results in terms of recovery of foot dorsiflexion [22]. In a case report published by Ratanshi et al. (2017), a patient with intraneural ganglion cyst, whose symptoms were characterized by pain and dropped foot, was treated by connecting the articular branch of the peroneal nerve, decompression, and transfer of a motor nerve branch from the flexor muscle hallucis longus to the motor branch of the tibialis anterior muscle. The patient evolved with pain control and recovery of the motor of foot dorsiflexion [23] (Figs. 6.12 and 6.13).

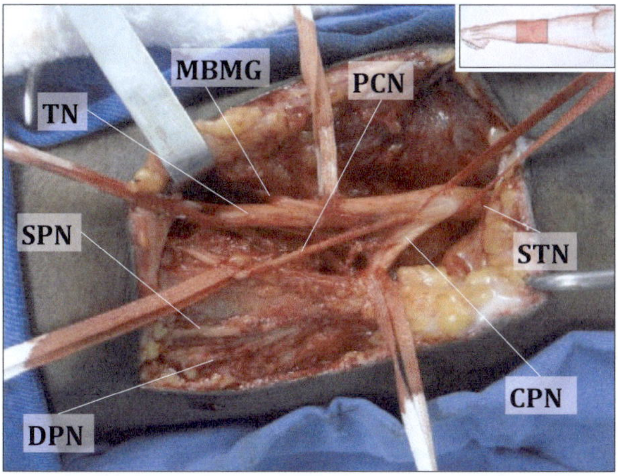

Fig. 6.12 Surgical access in the right popliteal fossa area with extension to the fibular region, for the transfer of the medial motor branch of the gastrocnemius to the deep peroneal nerve. *CPN* = common peroneal nerve, *DPN* = deep peroneal nerve, *MBMG* = motor branch for medial gastrocnemius muscle, *PCN* = peroneal communicating nerve, *SPN* = superficial peroneal nerve, *STN* = sciatic nerve, *TN* = tibial nerve

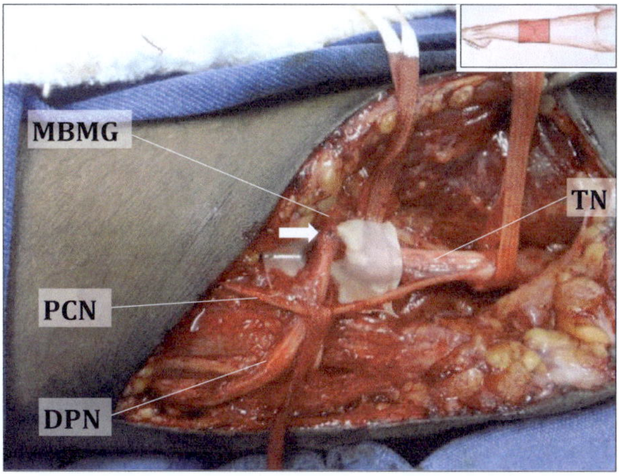

Fig. 6.13 Surgical access in the right popliteal fossa area with extension to the fibular region. The white arrow points to the neurotization between the medial gastrocnemius motor branch and the deep peroneal nerve. *DPN* = deep peroneal nerve, *PCN* = peroneal communicating nerve, *MBMG* = motor branch for medial gastrocnemius muscle, *TN* = tibial nerve

6.6 Conclusions

The management of patients with CNPN through decompressive surgery of the PN presents high success rates and low complication index. In addition to conservative treatment, minimally invasive modalities of managing patients with this compressive neuropathy need more studies that present a larger number of patients with longer follow-up time for better evaluation of the results.

References

1. Sultan C. Ganglion der nervenscheide des nervus peroneus. Zentralbl Chir. 1921;48:963–5.
2. Brooks DM. Nerve compression by simple ganglia: a review of thirteen collected cases. J Bone Joint Surg Br. 1952;34-B:391–400.
3. Cobb CA, Moiel RH. Ganglion of the peroneal nerve. Report of two cases. J Neurosurg. 1974;41:255–9.
4. Noble W. Peroneal palsy due to hematoma in the common peroneal nerve sheath after distal torsional fractures and inversion ankle sprains. J Bone Joint Surg Am. 1966;48-A:1484–95.
5. Khedr EM, Fawi G, Allah Abbas MA, El-Fetoh NA, Zaki AF, Gamea A. Prevalence of common types of compression neuropathies in Qena Governorate/Egypt: a population-based survey. Neuroepidemiology. 2016;46(4):253–60.
6. Kandil MR, Darwish ES, Khedr EM, Sabry MM, Abdulah MA. A community-based epidemiological study of peripheral neuropathies in Assiut, Egypt. Neurol Res. 2012;34(10):960–6.
7. Marciniak C. Fibular (peroneal) neuropathy. Electrodiagnostic features and clinical correlates. Phys Med Rehabil Clin N Am. 2013;24:121. https://doi.org/10.1016/j.pmr.2012.08.016.
8. Bouche P. Compression and entrapment neuropathies. In: Handbook of clinical neurology, vol. 115. Elsevier B.V.; 2013. p. 311–66. https://doi.org/10.1016/B978-0-444-52902-2.00019-9.
9. Moatshe G, Dornan GJ, Løken S, Ludvigsen TC, Laprade RF, Engebretsen L. Demographics and injuries associated with knee dislocation: a prospective review of 303 patients. Orthop J Sport Med. 2017;5(5):2325967117706521. https://doi.org/10.1177/2325967117706521.
10. Lezak B, Massel DH, Varacallo M. Peroneal nerve injury. [Updated 2024 Feb 25]. In: StatPearls [Internet]. Treasure Island: StatPearls Publishing; 2024. Available from: https://www.ncbi.nlm.nih.gov/books/NBK549859/.
11. Fortier LM, Markel M, Thomas BG, Sherman WF, Thomas BH, Kaye AD. An update on peroneal nerve entrapment and neuropathy. Orthop Rev (Pavia). 2021;13(2):24937. https://doi.org/10.52965/001c.24937.9.
12. Anderson JC. Common fibular nerve compression anatomy, symptoms, clinical evaluation, and surgical decompression. Clin Podiatr Med Surg. 2016;33(2):283–91. https://doi.org/10.1016/j.cpm.2015.12.0058.
13. Dellon AL. The Dellon approach to neurolysis in the neuropathy patient with chronic nerve compression. Handchir Mikrochir Plast Chir. 2008;40(6):351–60. https://doi.org/10.1055/s-2008-1039216.
14. Yasuoka T, Yokota T, Tsukagoshi H. Deep peroneal nerve palsy associated with hypothyroidism. No To Shinkei. 1993;45(6):563–6. Japanese.
15. Bowley MP, Doughty CT. Entrapment neuropathies of the lower extremity. Med Clin North Am. 2019;103(2):371–82. https://doi.org/10.1016/j.mcna.2018.10.013.
16. Oswald J, Shahi A, Chakravarthy KV. Prospective case series on the use of peripheral nerve stimulation for focal mononeuropathy treatment. Pain Manag. 2019;9:551–8. https://doi.org/10.2217/pmt-2019-0028.

17. Martins da Silva R, Pereira A, Branco R, Carvalho JL. Ultrasound-guided pulsed radiofrequency treatment for superficial peroneal nerve entrapment in a professional handball player. Cureus. 2023;15(7):e42043. https://doi.org/10.7759/cureus.42043. PMID: 37593284; PMCID: PMC10427882.
18. Poage C, Roth C, Scott B. Peroneal nerve palsy: evaluation and management. J Am Acad Orthop Surg. 2016;24(1):1–10. https://doi.org/10.5435/JAAOS-D-14-00420. PMID: 26700629.
19. Mackay MJ, Ayres JM, Harmon IP, Tarakemeh A, Brubacher J, Vopat BG. Traumatic peroneal nerve injuries: a systematic review. JBJS Rev. 2022;10(1):e20. https://doi.org/10.2106/JBJS.RVW.20.00256.
20. Chow AL, Levidy MF, Luthringer M, Vasoya D, Ignatiuk A. A clinical outcomes after neurolysis for the treatment of peroneal nerve palsy: a systematic review and meta-analysis. Ann Plast Surg. 2021;87(3):316–23. https://doi.org/10.1097/SAP.0000000000002833. PMID: 34397520.
21. Park JS, Casale MI. Posterior tibial tendon transfer for common peroneal nerve injury. Clin Sports Med. 2020;39(4):819–28. https://doi.org/10.1016/j.csm.2020.07.003. Epub 2020 Aug 14. PMID: 32892969.
22. Flores LP, Martins RS, Siqueira MG. Clinical results of transferring a motor branch of the tibial nerve to the deep peroneal nerve for treatment of foot drop. Neurosurgery. 2013;73(4):609–16.
23. Ratanshi L, Clark TA, Giuffre JL. Immediate nerve transfer for the treatment of peroneal nerve palsy secondary to an intraneural ganglion: case report and review. Plast Surg (Oakv). 2017;25(1):5458.

Chapter 7
Tendon Transfer for Treatment of Sequela of Nerve Injury in Lower Limbs

7.1 Introduction

Among the possible complications of compressive neuropathy and traumatic injury to the peroneal nerve is paresis for foot dorsiflexion, also known as "drop foot." Patients with sciatic nerve injuries may also present drop foot with or without preserved function of the tibial component.

It is noted that some patients even after the correct management of injuries to the peroneal or sciatic nerve course with this deficit that leads to steppage gait. Over time, different techniques have been developed with the aim of solving or mitigating this old motor deficit in this group of patients. Among the surgical options, described in the literature for these patients, are ankle arthrodesis and myotendinous transfers.

The core of the myotendinous transfer techniques is based on the principle of performing tenodesis of a tendon with preserved function in a tendon without motor function. In general, the motor deficit resulting from the sacrifice of the functioning tendon should not promote a more severe motor deficit than that already present. It is desirable that the tendons involved in this surgical procedure have a similar caliber.

The techniques of myotendinous transfer for the correction of drop foot have undergone adaptations over time. Despite the initial description having been made in the twentieth century, it is still performed today with satisfactory results, especially due to the speed with which dorsiflexion is obtained, unlike nerve reconstruction techniques, where the first results appear only months after the procedure. An advantage of this treatment modality is the possibility of performing it late after the onset of motor symptoms. Thus, patients, even years after the initial manifestation of the motor nerve injury, can still benefit from this surgery.

Supplementary Information The online version contains supplementary material available at https://doi.org/10.1007/978-3-031-90058-7_7.

M. J. S. Magalhães, *Lower Extremity Nerve Entrapments*,
https://doi.org/10.1007/978-3-031-90058-7_7

Other myotendinous transfer techniques have been described for the treatment for patients with femoral or tibial nerve injuries.

The myotendinous transfer of the tibialis anterior tendon with or without the fibularis longus tendon to the calcaneus, for example, is used to prevent deformity resulting from paresis of the gastrocnemius and soleus muscles. Another example is the myotendinous transfer of the biceps femoris and semitendinosus tendons to the patella, which is performed for the treatment of the paralyzed quadriceps muscle [1].

The history of the myotendinous transfer technique of the tibialis posterior muscle (TPM) for treatment of patients with foot drop begins with Ober (1933), who described the circumtibial technique [2]. A few years later, in 1937, Mayer described the surgical technique in which the route of the TPM tendon is performed through the interosseous membrane. This author, however, credited this new technique to Putti [3]. Carayon et al. (1967) described a dual technique, in which the TPM tendon has route through the interosseous membrane to undergo tenodesis with the tibialis anterior tendon and tenodesis of flexor digitorum longus (FDL) tendon to the extensor digitorum longus (EDL) and extensor hallucis longus (EHL) tendons [4]. Srinivasan et al. (1968) described a technique in which the TPM tendon is split into two strips. In this way, the medial tendon strip performs tenodesis with the EHL tendon and the lateral strip, with the EDL and fibularis tertius tendons [5]. Other techniques have been described in recent decades, such as that of Riordan, also known as the Bridle procedure, described by McCall et al. (1991) [6], and the modified Bridle technique, described by Rodriguez (1992) [7].

According to a systematic review conducted by Stevoska et al. (2023) on myotendinous transfer, it was revealed that paralysis of the common peroneal nerve was the most identified etiology, with 89% (33/37 studies) of cases, of these, 20 were due to trauma and 11 due to Hansen's disease. In 8% (3/37 studies), it was not possible to identify a cause [8].

Stevoska et al. (2023) also revealed that the types of tendon fixation most used in myotendinous transfer were tendon-tendon 67% (28 out of 42 studies) and tendon to bone 33% (14 out of 42 studies) [8].

The lengthening of the calcaneal tendon as a measure to improve the surgical results of myotendinous transposition was identified in 67% of the patients in this study (737 out of 1227 feet) [8].

The aim of this chapter is to describe the main myotendinous transfer techniques available to restore dorsiflexion movement in patients with foot drop.

7.2 Indication of Myotendinous Transfer for Correction of Foot Drop

Patients who have had foot drop for more than 12 months, with little chance of motor recovery, are the ideal candidates for the myotendinous transfer technique [1, 8, 9].

This indication also extends, especially, to patients with old traumatic nerve injuries where conservative treatment or nerve reconstruction surgery no longer applies and when satisfactory results have not been obtained with conservative and surgical management of compressive neuropathy [10].

7.3 General Aspects of Myotendinous Transfer for Foot Drop

The first step before indicating myotendinous transfer is to perform a neurological evaluation of the patient's lower limb, with the aim of identifying which muscles are paretic. In this way, the examiner evaluates the movements of inversion and eversion of the foot and dorsiflexion and extension of the foot/toes. To perform the TPM myotendinous transfer, the inversion movement of the foot must be preserved [9] (Video 7.1).

The next step is to assess the existence of calcaneal tendon shortening. The prior identification of this problem allows the surgeon to better plan for the lengthening of this tendon unit at the same surgical time as the myotendinous transposition. If the patient has passive mobility that allows, without great effort, the dorsiflexion of the foot, tendon lengthening will not be necessary.

The use of ankle foot orthesis (AFO) associated with regular physiotherapy protects the patient, suffering from peroneal nerve injury, from developing calcaneal tendon shortening [9]. Fritschi et al. (1971) suggest that in specific cases, where patients present an isolated lesion of the deep component of the peroneal nerve and with preservation of the eversion movement of the foot, the posterior tibial myotendinous transfer is not indicated, as it would cause an imbalance between the inverting and everting forces of the foot [17]. In these cases, according to these same authors, the most indicated tendon for transfer would be the fibularis longus [11, 17].

7.4 Surgical Lengthening of the Calcaneal Tendon

Patients with peroneal nerve neuropathy may present calcaneal tendon shortening which gives the patient an equine foot. Not infrequently, it is necessary to perform lengthening of this tendon to give the ankle a more physiological angle.

The indication for surgical lengthening of this tendon occurs when the patient's ankle joint does not allow passive dorsiflexion movement. There are different techniques described such as the "Z" lengthening technique and Hoke, which will be described in the following two topics.

7.4.1 *Hoke Technique for Surgical Lengthening of the Calcaneal Tendon*

Hoke first described in 1931 the technique of triple hemisection of the calcaneal tendon [12]. In 1979, Bleck described this same technique in an open surgical approach [13], and Hoefnagels et al. (2007) mention percutaneous approach for this surgery [14].

With the patient in the prone position and the patient's foot in maximum dorsiflexion, the Achilles tendon is identified and its anatomical boundaries are marked by palpation.

A marking proximal to the insertion is made from the medial edge to the midline of the tendon. The intermediate marking is made an inch cranial to the first marking, and the incision is made in the tendon from its midline to its lateral edge. A third incision is made an inch cranial to the second incision. This last one starts from the midline of the tendon and goes towards its medial edge.

In children, the length of the distal phalanx of the thumb can be used as a measure. The incision can be made percutaneously or open depending on the surgeon's experience. After making the incisions, forced dorsiflexion of the foot should be performed (Figs. 7.1a, b; Video 7.2).

Among the complications of this technique are tendon rupture after its elongation, injury to the sural and tibial nerves, injury to the tendon of the flexor hallucis longus muscle, and wound dehiscence [14].

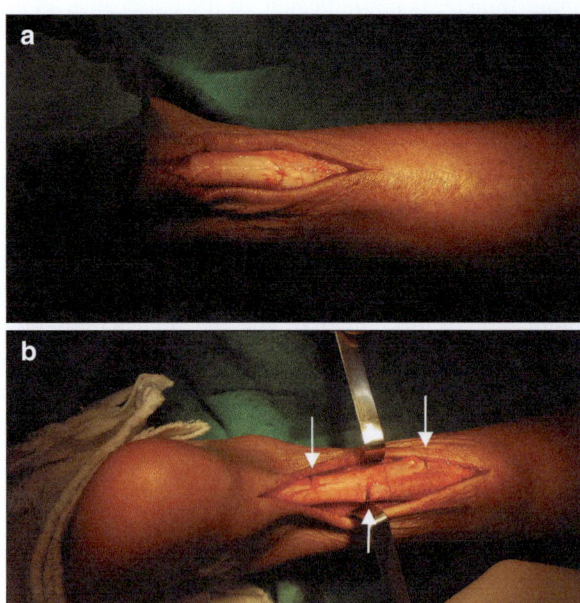

Fig. 7.1 (**a**) Hoke's technique for Achilles tendon lengthening. Note the linear surgical incision exposing the back of the tendon. (**b**) Achilles tendon lengthening technique. The white arrows indicate the 3 incisions made with a scalpel. Note that the incisions are alternated and never cross the midline of the tendon

7.4.2 "Z" Lengthening Technique of the Achilles Tendon

It is a technique indicated for the treatment of clubfoot and hemiplegic spasticity. It is also used for the correction of tendon shortening secondary to peroneal nerve injury.

A linear incision in the skin at the level of the medial edge of the Achilles tendon is made. Then, the skin is reflected and the posterior face of the Achilles tendon is visualized. The opening of the loose tissue that covers the tendon is only made in its midline, with the aim of maintaining the vascularization of the local structures. The tendon is incised longitudinally in its midline until it is completely separated into two units. Then, a lateral hemisection is made in the lateral bundle, at a proximal point, and another distal hemisection is made in the medial bundle.

To perform this technique, an adequate distance between the medial and lateral incisions must be maintained so that the final contact area for the tenodesis is not too short, after performing the dorsiflexion of the foot.

After the incisions are made, the foot should be subjected to dorsiflexion, until it reaches a neutral position. After this maneuver, the tenodesis is performed, preferably with non-braided surgical sutures.

As a complication, the patient may develop weakness of the triceps surae muscle, local infection, and surgical wound dehiscence [15].

7.5 Circumtibial Technique of Myotendinous Transfer of the Tibialis Posterior

Before starting the procedure, it is relevant to check the availability of the rigid short leg brace used in the immediate postoperative period.

Before anesthesia induction, the patient should be examined one more time to verify the function of the tibialis posterior muscle through voluntary inversion of the foot. At this moment, the insertion point of this tendon can be marked on the skin.

The patient should be placed in the supine position, with the limb to be subjected to the procedure positioned in extension, with a small cushion under the knee. After the limb is sterilized, the skin incisions should be marked.

The first incision refers to the insertion point of the tibialis posterior muscle tendon, on the medial side of the foot, the second incision a little above the medial malleolus, and the third incision on the dorsum of the foot (Fig. 7.2).

An incision of approximately 4 cm is made on the medial part of the foot between the medial malleolus and the first cuneiform bone. After making the first incision, the tendon of the tibialis posterior muscle is located. Once identified, it can be pulled to perform foot inversion. It should be ensured that all the tendon fibers have been cut, otherwise, the tendon will not be able to be pulled through the second incision. Before cutting the tendon, a braided suture can be passed through its end to pull it after it is cut. This will facilitate its removal through the second incision.

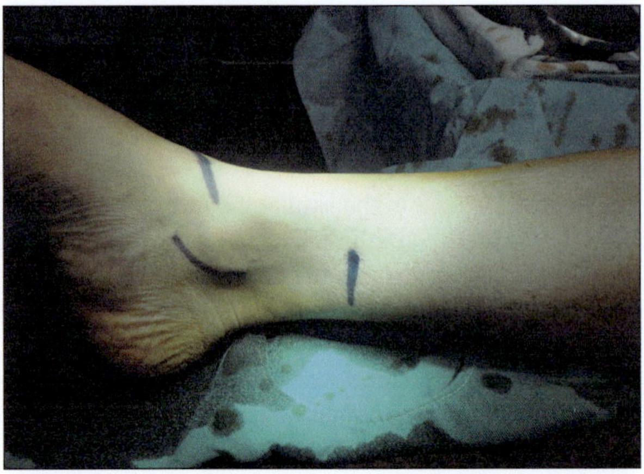

Fig. 7.2 Myotendinous transfer technique via the circumtibial route. Marking of the surgical incisions on the right foot

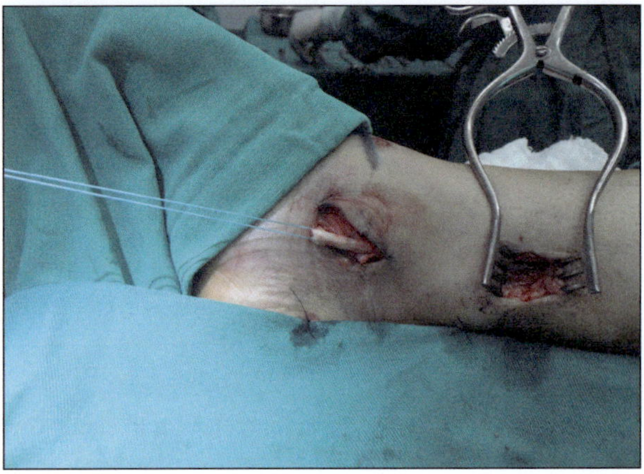

Fig. 7.3 Myotendinous transfer technique via the circumtibial route. Note in the first incision on the medial side of the foot, the tendon of the posterior tibial muscle already detached from the bone and with surgical thread sutured at its end

After making the incision located above the medial malleolus, surgical technologist should perform traction movements of the tendon using the suture previously passed at the distal end of the tendon. Simultaneously, through digital palpation, the surgeon locates the tendon, detecting its movement in a deep plane, inside the second incision (Fig. 7.3).

Once located, the tendon is pulled until it is removed through the second incision. If you did not completely cut the tendon's insertion in the first incision, it will not be possible to remove it (Fig. 7.4).

After making the third incision, it is necessary to identify the tendons of the tibialis anterior (TA), extensor digitorum longus (EDL), and extensor hallucis longus (EHL) muscles (Fig. 7.5).

The tendon of the tibialis posterior muscle should be transferred to the third incision through the subcutaneous plane (circumtibial route), which can be performed with the help of a hemostatic clamp attached to the suture attached to the end of the tendon (Fig. 7.6).

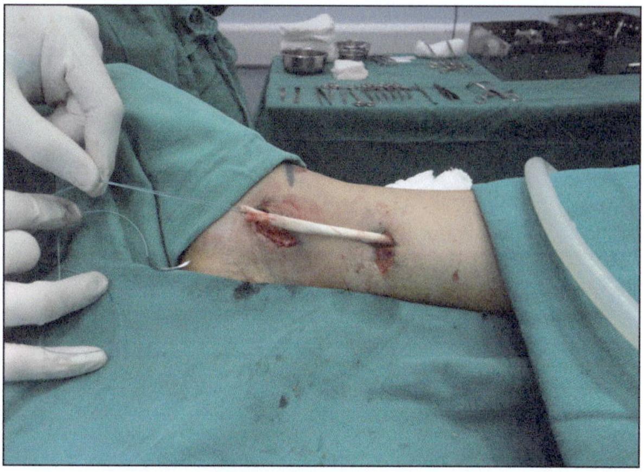

Fig. 7.4 Myotendinous transfer technique via the circumtibial route. Note in the second incision on the medial side of the leg, the tendon of the tibialis posterior muscle pulled and removed from the first incision

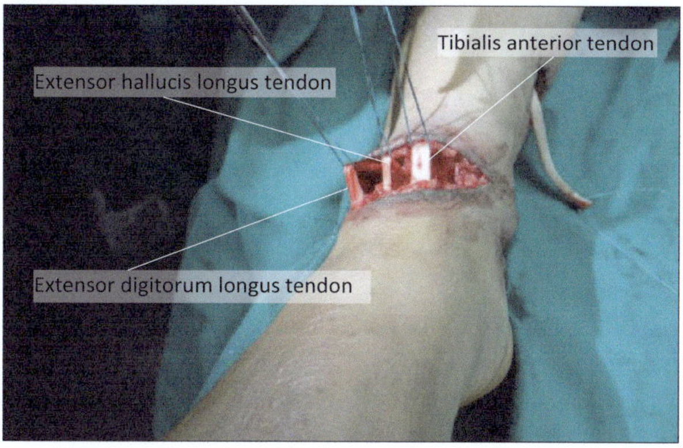

Fig. 7.5 Myotendinous transfer technique via the circumtibial route. Dorsal incision of the foot revealing the tendons of the tibialis anterior, extensor hallucis longus, and extensor digitorum longus muscles

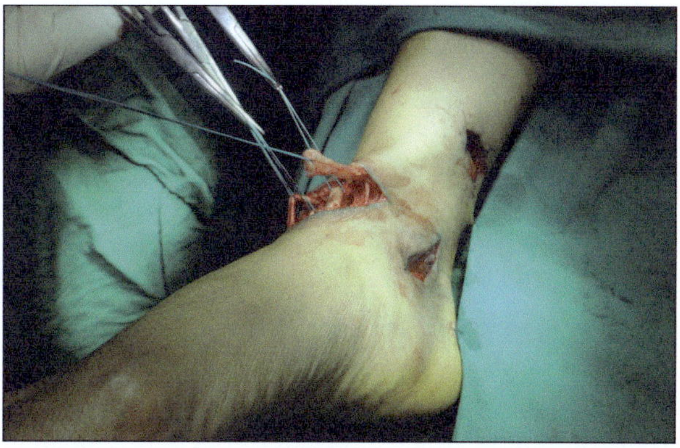

Fig. 7.6 Myotendinous transfer technique via the circumtibial route. Note in the third incision located on the dorsum of the foot, the tendon of tibialis posterior muscle pulled and removed from the second incision. Also note the tendons of the extensor retinaculum already identified and pulled by a surgical thread

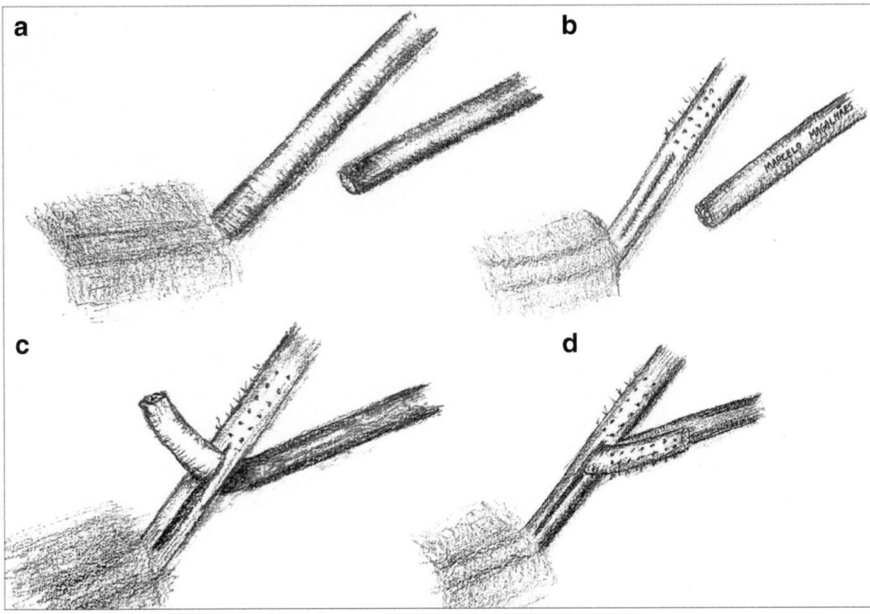

Fig. 7.7 Myotendinous transfer technique via the circumtibial route. Steps (**a**–**d**) illustrate the step-by-step process for tenodesis of the posterior tibial tendon to the anterior tibial tendon. (Author's personal technique)

When the tip of the tendon of the tibialis posterior muscle is already located in the third incision, this will be sutured to the tendon of the tibialis anterior muscle. The tenodesis process should be performed with the foot under forced dorsiflexion performed by the surgical assistant. Braided surgical suture increases the chances of local infection and therefore should be avoided (Fig. 7.7).

After suturing the three incisions, the limb should be immobilized in the orthosis still inside the operating room. The patient should avoid stepping on the ground for a period of 6 weeks. For this, a crutch can be used. The non-use of a boot immobilizer and/or rest from walking may compromise the functional result of the surgery (Video 7.3).

7.6 Myotendinous Transposition of the Tibialis Posterior via Interosseous Membrane

The patient should be positioned in dorsal decubitus, with the limb to be submitted to the procedure arranged in extension, with a small cushion under the knee. After asepsis of the limb, the skin incisions should be marked.

An incision of approximately 4 cm is made on the medial part of the foot, between the medial malleolus and the first cuneiform bone. For better identification of the tendon, when traction is performed on it, it is possible to observe the inversion movement of the foot [16]. After correct identification of the tibialis posterior tendon, it is detached from its bone insertion. It is important that all tendon fibers are completely severed from their bone insertion, otherwise, the tendon cannot be removed by the second incision during traction [16].

A braided surgical suture can be temporarily used at the tip of the already disinserted tendon, with the aim of assisting in the process of its removal through the second incision.

The second incision of 4 cm is made on the medial and distal part of the leg, approximately 3 cm above the medial malleolus. From this incision, the tibialis posterior tendon is removed by manual traction [16]. While the surgical assistant pulls the tendon through the surgical suture attached to its end, the surgeon identifies the tendon inside the second surgical incision by digital palpation.

The third incision of approximately 7 cm longitudinal is made distally, in the distal third of the leg, above the cruciform ligament of the ankle [16]. The next step is to identify the tibial artery and vein, deep peroneal nerve, TA muscle tendon, and ELH muscle tendon to perform traction of these elements laterally [16]. Once the interosseous membrane is visualized, an incision is made to create a quadrangular window in its extension [16]. The TPM tendon is passed with the help of surgical instruments (Ober tendon passer or a hemostatic clamp) through the interosseous membrane until it reaches the third incision [16].

The last incision is made on the dorsum of the foot, centered on the second metatarsal. The TPM tendon is passed through the extensor retinaculum and anchored on the dorsum of the foot, on the second metatarsal using a bone tunnel. It is important to note that the foot should be in dorsiflexion during the anchoring of the tendon [16].

7.7 Myotendinous Transfer of the Fibularis Longus for Treatment of Drop Foot

The patient should be positioned in dorsal decubitus, with the limb to be submitted to the procedure, placed in extension, with a small cushion under the knee. After asepsis of the limb, the skin incisions should be marked.

The first oblique-shaped incision is made on the lateral face of the foot, starting at the level of the fifth metatarsal and extending to 1 cm caudal to the lateral malleolus. Through this incision, it will be possible to identify the tendons of the fibularis brevis (FBM) and fibularis longus (FLM) muscles [9]. For correct identification of the tendons, the surgeon can pull them. In the presence of foot eversion movement, recognition of these tendinous structures is confirmed.

A second incision is made on the anterolateral face of the leg, about 5 cm above the lateral malleolus. In this incision, the FLM tendon is identified and pulled until its exit. After this step, the FLM tendon is distally divided into two ends, which are tunneled in the subcutaneous plane to the incisions that will be made on the dorsum of the foot.

One end will undergo tenodesis with the ELH muscle tendon and the other simultaneously with the EDL muscle tendon and fibularis tertius (FT) [17]. The foot, toes should remain in forced dorsiflexion during tenodesis.

It is advisable that the suture be performed with non-absorbable thread and preferably, non-braided thread, with the aim of reducing the incidence of infectious process. After the end of the surgery, the patient should remain with a foot immobilizer orthosis in dorsiflexion for a period of 6 weeks [9].

7.8 Postoperative Care in Myotendinous Transfer

Park et al. (2020) recommend that in the immediate postoperative period, the foot be immobilized in maximum dorsiflexion with the aid of a rigid orthosis for a period of 6 weeks. The stitches should be removed around 2 weeks. From the sixth week, the patient is allowed to start walking, even with the use of the orthosis and also passive physiotherapy. At 3 months, the use of the AFO is advised to keep a night orthosis that maintains the dorsiflexion of the ankle for another 3 months. At 6 months, all movement restrictions are removed, and at 9 months, the patient is cleared for sports activities. However, the patient should be advised that returning to sports activities is not a goal of the surgery [18].

7.9 Surgical Outcomes

According to a systematic review conducted by Stevoska et al. (2023), it was revealed that 94% (205 out of 219) of patients who underwent myotendinous transfer were satisfied with the treatment [8]. Another interesting point in this systematic review was the fact that the different tendon fixation techniques or even the choice of myotendinous transfer used did not affect the score obtained on the available outcome assessment scales [8].

7.10 Differences Between Techniques That Use Circumtibial and Interosseous Routes

It is noted that the circumtibial technique described by Ober (1933) usually results in an ankle with a greater range of motion compared to the interosseous technique, but with a higher degree of foot inversion [2, 11].

7.11 Complications of Myotendinous Transfer

Some measures can be taken to avoid complications resulting from myotendinous transfer for the treatment of foot drop.

Advise the patient to start physiotherapy and use the AFO before the procedure. These guidelines can maintain the range of motion of the ankle joint preserved. Maintaining ankle mobility can spare the patient from a surgical stretching of the Achilles tendon.

The use of braided surgical suture for tenodesis may increase the risk of infection. If the patient has a wound infection, in the presence of the use of this type of surgical suture, a new surgical approach may be necessary to remove the sutures near the surgical wound.

The use of a short rigid boot can reduce the chances of losing the dorsiflexion angle obtained during the surgical procedure. The immobilizing boot made of plaster does not have the same physical resistance as the rigid boot made of metal and plastic polymers, and not infrequently, it can suffer a fracture at the heel angle during the long postoperative rest period.

The patient's rest in the postoperative period is essential. Physical effort on the operated limb can lead to rupture of the tenodesis and promote the failure of the procedure (Figs. 7.8 and 7.9).

Before performing the procedure, it is essential to check if the patient has a limitation of passive dorsiflexion movement of the foot due to shortening of the Achilles tendon. In this case, if the surgical stretching of the tendon is not performed, the final result of the myotendinous transfer may be compromised.

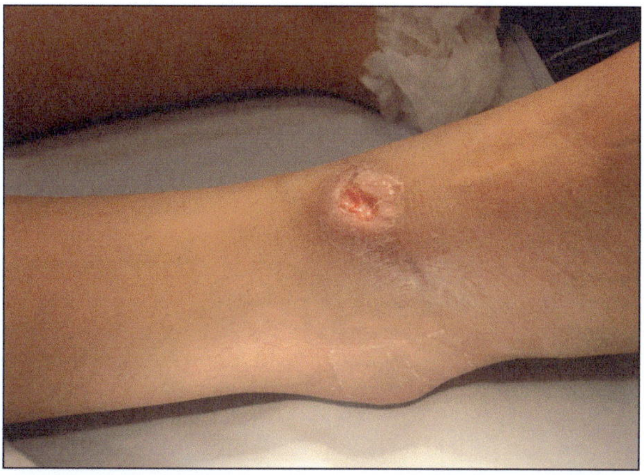

Fig. 7.8 Wound dehiscence on the dorsum of the right foot in a patient who underwent myotendinous transfer for the treatment of foot drop

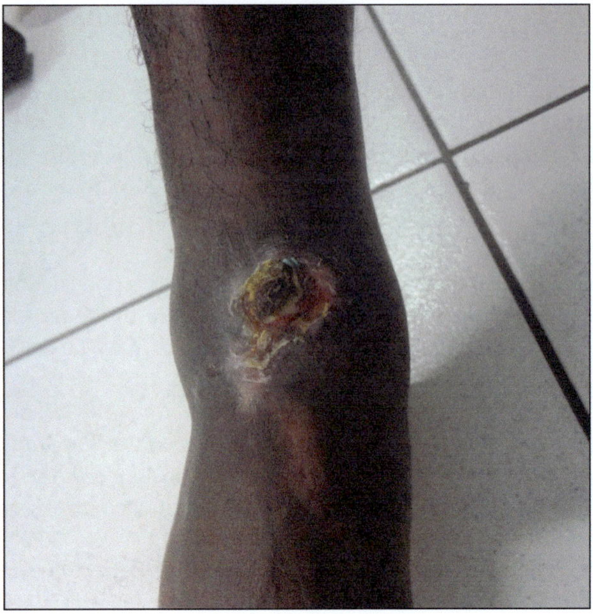

Fig. 7.9 Dehiscence and infection in incision on the dorsum of the right foot in a patient who underwent myotendinous transfer for the treatment of foot drop. Note the presence of exposed surgical suture in the surgical wound

7.12 Conclusion

The techniques of myotendinous transfer for the correction of foot drop have undergone adaptations over time. Despite its description many decades ago, it is still performed today with satisfactory results. This treatment modality presents a quick recovery of the dorsiflexion movement of the foot, unlike the techniques of nerve reconstruction, where the first results appear months after the surgical treatment performed. This technique also has the advantage of being able to be performed late, even years after the nerve injury.

References

1. Wiesseman G. Tendon transfers for peripheral nerve injuries of the lower extremity. Orthop Clin North Am. 1981;12(2):459–67.
2. Ober FR. Tendon transplantation in the lower extremity. N Engl J Med. 1933;209:52–9.
3. Mayer L. The physiological method of tendon transplantation in the treatment of paralytic drop-foot. J Bone Joint Surg. 1937;19:389–94.
4. Carayon A, Bourrel P, Bourges M, Touze M. Dual transfer of the posterior tibial and flexor digitorum longus tendons for drop foot. J Bone Joint Surg Am. 1967;49:144–8.
5. Srinivasan H, Mukherjee SM, Subramaniam RA. Two-tailed transfer of tibialis posterior for correction of drop-foot in leprosy. J Bone Joint Surg Br. 1968;50:623–8. https://doi.org/10.1302/0301-620X.50B3.623.
6. McCall RE, Frederick HA, McCluskey GM, Riordan DC. The Bridle procedure: a new treatment for equinus and equinovarus deformities in children. J Pediatr Orthop. 1991;11:83–9.

7. Rodriguez RP. The Bridle procedure in the treatment of paralysis of the foot. Foot Ankle Int. 1992;13:63–9. https://doi.org/10.1177/107110079201300203.
8. Stevoska S, Pisecky L, Stadler C, et al. Tendon transfer in foot drop: a systematic review. Arch Orthop Trauma Surg. 2023;143:773–84. https://doi.org/10.1007/s00402-021-04162-x.
9. Krishnamurthy S, Ibrahim M, Surgery P, et al. Tendon transfers in foot drop. Indian J Plast Surg. 2019;52:100–8. https://doi.org/10.1055/s-0039-1688105.
10. Ricnard A. Surgical management of neuritis. Kathmandu: Ekta Books; 2004.
11. Soares D. Tibialis posterior transfer for the correction of foot drop in leprosy. Long-term outcome. J Bone Joint Surg Br. 1996;78:61–2.
12. Hoke M. An operation for the correction of extremely relaxed flat feet. J Bone Joint Surg. 1931;13(4):773–83.
13. Bleck EE. Orthopaedic management of cerebral palsy. Philadelphia: WB Saunders; 1979.
14. Hoefnagels EM, Waites MD, Belkoff SM, Swierstra BA. Percutaneous Achilles tendon lengthening: a cadaver-based study of failure of the triple hemisection technique. Acta Orthop. 2007;78(6):808–12.
15. Turco VJ. Surgical correction of the resistant club foot. One-stage posteromedial release with internal fixation: a preliminary report. J Bone Joint Surg Am. 1971;53(3):477–97.
16. Gould JS. Anterior transfer of the posterior tibial tendon through the interosseous membrane. In: Musculoskeletal key [Internet]. [cited 2023 Sep 14]. Available from: https://musculoskeletalkey.com/28-anterior-transfer-of-the-posterior-tibial-tendon-through-the-interosseous-membrane/.
17. Fritschi EP. Reconstructive surgery in leprosy. Bristol: Wright; 1971.
18. Park JS, Casale MJ. Posterior tibial tendon transfer for common peroneal nerve injury. Clin Sports Med. 2020;39(4):819–28. https://doi.org/10.1016/j.csm.2020.07.003.

Chapter 8
Anterior Tarsal Syndrome

8.1 Introduction

The anterior tarsal tunnel syndrome or deep peroneal nerve entrapment (DPNE) is defined as a chronic compressive neuropathy when this nerve structure follows the path within the inferior extensor retinaculum, at the level of the ankle [1, 2].

The anterior tarsal tunnel syndrome is a rare entity when compared to other neuropathies present in the lower limb, such as the compressive syndrome of the common peroneal nerve and posterior tarsal tunnel syndrome [1]. It is estimated that this mononeuropathy is present in 5% of patients with complaints of numbness in the feet [3, 4].

The first description of this compressive syndrome was made by authors Kopell and Thompson in 1963. In 1968, Marinacci named this syndrome and established its electrophysiological diagnosis [4, 5].

Patients with this mononeuropathy usually have symptoms of pain, paresthesias, hypoesthesia, foot weakness, and more rarely, paresis for toe extension [6].

Symptoms tend to occur in the space located between the first and second toes of the foot (first interdigital space), since the deep peroneal nerve is responsible for the sensory innervation of this skin territory [7].

The objective of this chapter is to describe the anatomy of the deep peroneal nerve, the clinical changes of DPNE, complementary exams, conservative/classical surgical, and neuroendoscopic treatment.

Supplementary Information The online version contains supplementary material available at https://doi.org/10.1007/978-3-031-90058-7_8.

M. J. S. Magalhães, *Lower Extremity Nerve Entrapments*,
https://doi.org/10.1007/978-3-031-90058-7_8

8.2 Anatomy

8.2.1 *Anatomy of the Deep Peroneal Nerve*

The common peroneal nerve (CPN) is a branch of the sciatic nerve that originates in the distal third of the posterior compartment of the thigh. The CPN, in turn, has a lateral trajectory at the knee level to contour the lateral portion of the fibular neck and reach the anterior compartment of the leg. After the CPN contours the fibular neck, it originates its two most important branches: deep peroneal nerve (DPN) and superficial peroneal nerve (SPN) [5, 6]. It is important to mention that CPN also produces an articular branch for the sensitive innervation of the lateral part of the knee joint.

After the origin of the DPN, it presents a trajectory in the anterior compartment of the leg running deeply to the fibularis longus and extensor digitorum longus muscles.

In the upper third of the leg, it presents a trajectory between the extensor digitorum longus and tibialis anterior muscles.

At the level of the lower third of the leg, it presents a trajectory below the tendon of the extensor hallucis longus muscle. At this point, it is medial to the anterior tibial artery and has a course between the tendons of the extensor digitorum longus and extensor hallucis longus muscles [1].

It is noted that the bifurcation of the DPN into medial and lateral branches presents anatomical variation described. In an anatomical study with 36 lower limbs, it was found that in 31 (86%) specimens, the bifurcation occurred within the anterior tarsal tunnel, 2 (5.6%) below and 3 (8.3%) no division of the nerve into lateral and medial branches was found. In the same study, no division of the DPN into branches above this osteofibrous tunnel was observed [7]. At the level of the bifurcation, the DPN presents a transverse diameter in formalized specimen of 3.2 ± 0.6 mm. The distance between the bifurcation and the first interdigital space is 131.0 ± 13.4 mm [7] (Figs. 8.1, 8.2, 8.3, and 8.4).

The lateral branch of the DPN innervates the extensor hallucis brevis, extensor digitorum brevis muscles, and the sensitivity of the second, third, and fourth metacarpophalangeal joints [8–10]. The medial branch of the DPN presents a trajectory between the tendon of extensor hallucis longus muscle and the medial edge of the extensor digitorum brevis muscle. After piercing the deep fascia, this medial branch divides into two cutaneous branches for sensitive innervation of the first interdigital space [5, 6]. Aktan et al (2007) show that at the level of the first interdigital space of the foot, an anastomosis between the superficial and deep peroneal nerves is described in 27.8% in anatomical study [7].

The proximal part of the DPN to the inferior retinaculum is responsible for the innervation of the tibialis anterior, fibularis tertius, extensor hallucis longus, and extensor digitorum longus muscles. Below this retinaculum, this nerve only innervates the extensor hallucis brevis and extensor digitorum brevis [8–10]. Given these anatomical considerations, a compressive process at the level of the extensor

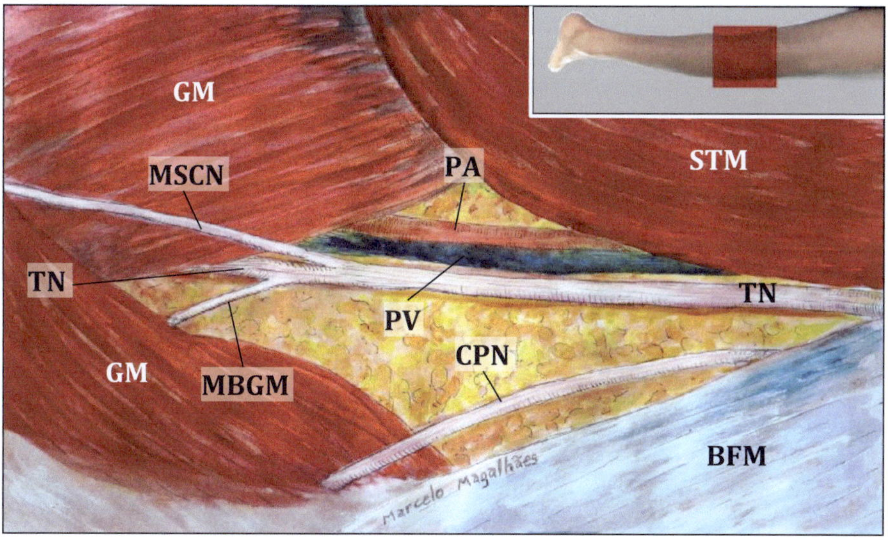

Fig. 8.1 Popliteal fossa of the right lower limb. *BFM* = biceps femoris muscle, *CPN* = common peroneal nerve, *GM* = gastrocnemius muscle, *MBGM* = muscle branch for gastrocnemius muscle, *MSCN* = medial sural cutaneous nerve, *PA* = popliteal artery, *PV* = popliteal vein, *STM* = semitendinosus muscle, *TN* = tibial nerve

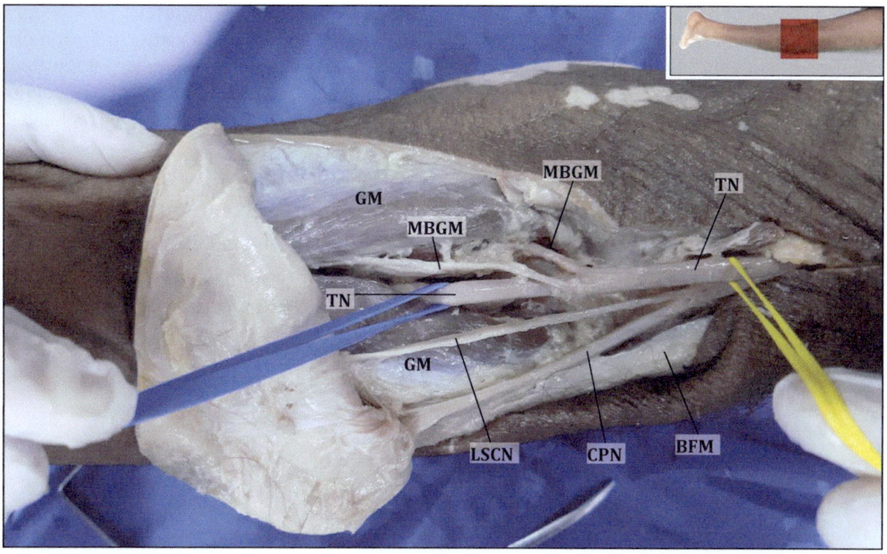

Fig. 8.2 Anatomy of the popliteal fossa in the right lower limb of a formalized specimen. The blue and yellow tapes highlight the tibial nerve in the popliteal fossa. *BFM* = biceps femoris muscle, *CPN* = common peroneal nerve, *GM* = gastrocnemius muscle, *LSCN* = lateral sural cutaneous nerve, *MBGM* = muscle branch for gastrocnemius muscle, *TN* = tibial nerve

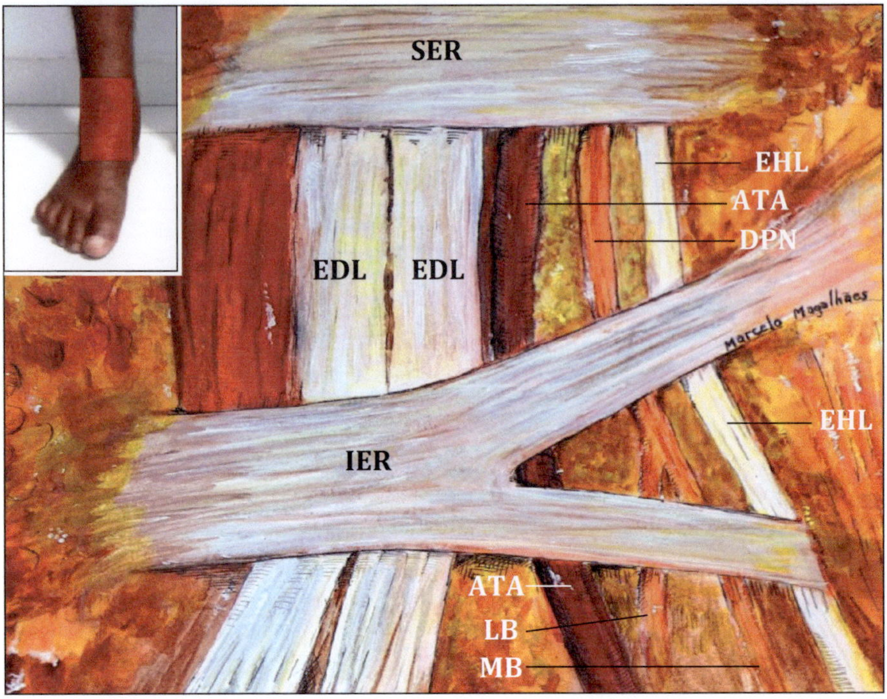

Fig. 8.3 Anterior tarsal tunnel in the right lower limb. *ATA* = anterior tibial artery, *DPN* = deep peroneal nerve, *EDL* = extensor digitorum longus, *EHL* = extensor hallucis longus, *IER* = inferior extensor retinaculum, *LB* = lateral branch, *MB* = medial branch, *SER* = superior extensor retinaculum. Note that the deep peroneal nerve passes under the superior and inferior extensor retinaculum. The tendon of the tibialis anterior muscle lies medial to the tendon of the extensor hallucis longus, deep to the overlying adipose tissue depicted in this region

retinaculum can only result in sensory impairment of the first interdigital space and paresis of extensor hallucis brevis and extensor digitorum brevis muscles.

As the DPN presents a trajectory of almost 90° at the ankle level, to avoid the effect of bowstring on the nerve, the superior and inferior extensor retinaculum act by fixing the nerve [5, 6].

8.2.2 Anatomy of the Anterior Tarsal Tunnel

The anterior tarsal tunnel can be conceptualized as a space of flattened dimensions positioned between the fascia of the navicular and talus bones (ventral) and the inferior extensor retinaculum of the foot [10].

In an anatomical study conducted with 18 formalized cadavers, it was shown that the lateral length of the tarsal tunnel is around 21.7 ± 4.2 mm and the medial length 55.0 ± 9 mm. The width of the anterior tarsal tunnel at the level of the lower edge

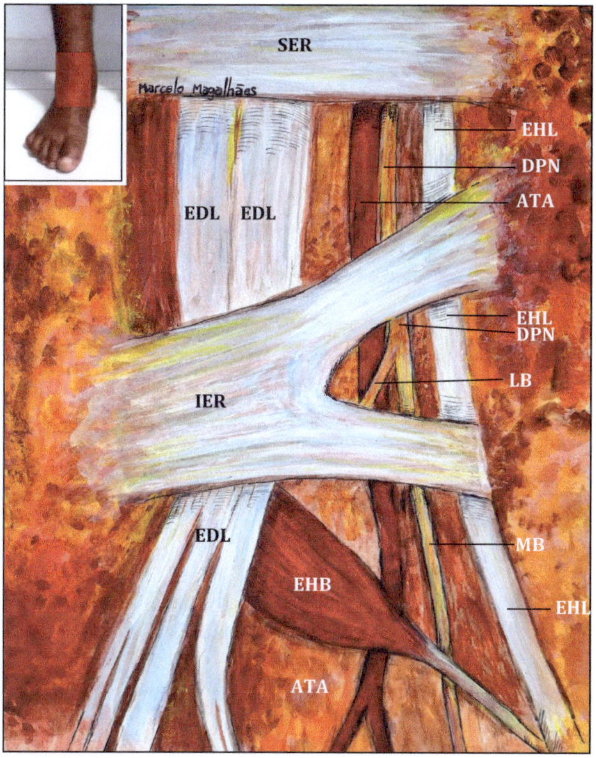

Fig. 8.4 Anterior tarsal tunnel in the right lower limb. *ATA* = anterior tibial artery, *DPN* = deep peroneal nerve, *EDL* = extensor digitorum longus, *EHB* = extensor hallucis brevis, *EHL* = extensor hallucis longus, *IER* = inferior extensor retinaculum, *LB* = lateral branch, *MB* = medial branch, *SER* = superior extensor retinaculum. Note that distally, the deep peroneal nerve passes under the tendon of the extensor hallucis brevis muscle. The tendon of the tibialis anterior muscle lies medial to the tendon of the extensor hallucis longus, deep to the overlying adipose tissue depicted in this region

between the tendons of the extensor hallucis longus and extensor digitorum longus muscles presents 12.6 ± 2.1 mm [7]. The presence of fibrotic bands over the DPN and dorsal artery of the foot, at the level of the anterior tarsal tunnel, is described in about 61.1% of studied specimens [7].

8.3 Etiology of the Anterior Tarsal Tunnel Syndrome

Despite being a rare disease, the anterior tarsal tunnel syndrome presents a wide variety of etiologies described in the medical literature. The most commonly cited cause is local trauma, at the level of the ATT, which includes fractures, dislocations, and sprains. The trauma at this anatomical point would cause local fibrosis or modify the configuration of this tunnel [2]. Other etiologies are described, such as talonavicular osteophytosis, fibrotic bands, use of high-heeled shoes, use of tight shoes, local edema, abnormal posture, pes cavus and ganglia [11–13], use of nitrofurantoin [14], hypertrophy of the extensor digitorum brevis muscle in athletes [4], irritation of the tendon of extensor hallucis brevis muscle [4], and Hansen's disease [14] (Fig. 8.5).

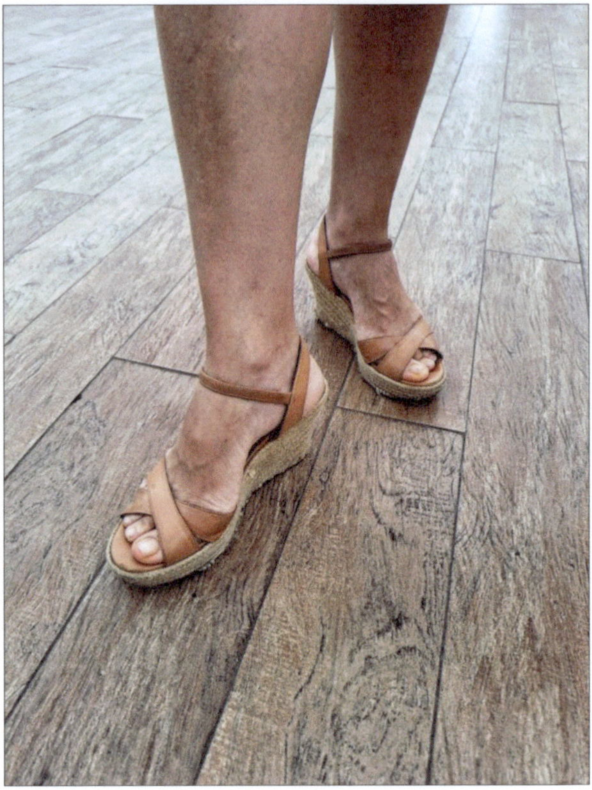

Fig. 8.5 Sandals with tape over the anterior tarsal tunnel. The use of these shoes acts as a risk factor for ATT syndrome. In this case, the deep peroneal nerve suffers compression at the level of the ATT

8.4 Symptoms and Clinical Signs of the Anterior Tarsal Tunnel Syndrome

Patients with this compressive syndrome usually present with sensitivity changes such as pain, hypoesthesia, hyperesthesia, paresthesia of first interdigital space [1, 2]. It is observed that the pain tends to be accentuated with certain positions, like those that require plantar extension of the foot. In more severe clinical cases, the patient may experience atrophy of the extensor hallucis brevis and toes muscles.

Motor symptoms, such as paresis for extension of the hallux and toes, are usually not as evident, since the function of the extensor hallucis brevis muscle can be partly compensated by the preserved motor activity of the extensor hallucis longus and extensor digitorum longus muscles [2].

In the physical examination, digital percussion on the extensor hallucis brevis muscle can reproduce a positive Tinel's sign and the passive movement of plantar extension of the foot and inversion can trigger the symptoms [5, 15].

8.5 Differential Diagnoses of Anterior Tarsal Tunnel Syndrome

Anterior tarsal tunnel syndrome is a relatively rare disease, and therefore, the health professional should exclude other diseases as cause of the symptoms. Among the main differential diagnoses are lumbar disc hernias, Morton's neuroma, CPN compressive syndrome, SPN compressive syndrome, gout, fractures, sprains, vascular disease, anterior compartment syndrome of exercise, primary nerve tumors [4, 13, 16], and inflammatory diseases [4].

Radiculopathy of L5 and S1 spinal nerves resulting from a lumbosacral disc hernia causes pain that radiates from the lumbar spine to the lower limb and usually presents a positive Lasègue's sign. The radiculopathy of the S1 spinal nerve can result in Achilles tendon areflexia, weakness to perform plantar extension of the foot, and changes in sensitivity that involves the plantar region. On the other hand, the radiculopathy of the L5 spinal nerve can result in preserved lower limb reflexes, paresis for dorsiflexion of the foot, and changes in sensitivity in the lateral region of the leg and dorsum of the foot [13, 15–18].

In the CPN tunnel syndrome, the patient may present impairment of the muscles innervated by the superficial and deep peroneal branches. In this case, the patient may present with paresis for eversion of the foot, dorsiflexion of the foot, and extension of the toes. It can also evolve with changes in sensitivity in the lateral region of the leg and dorsum of the foot, including the first interdigital space [19].

The SPN compressive syndrome causes changes in sensitivity on the dorsum of the foot and does not cause muscle atrophy. The percussion of the SPN can promote paresthesia and pain [1].

Patients with clinical symptoms of Morton's neuroma usually present, especially, with pain for walking, particularly when wearing pointed shoes. The pain tends to be unilateral and occurs especially in the third interdigital space and more rarely in the second interdigital space. The Mulder's sign, which consists of painful manual palpation of the interdigital space, may be present [20].

In the sensorimotor polyneuropathy of the lower limbs, resulting from Diabetes Mellitus, patients usually present with symmetric symptoms, in which distal neuropathic pain predominates. Some patients may present with trophic changes of the nails, skin, appendages, as well as motor symptoms, such as paresis, muscle atrophy, and areflexia [21].

8.6 Diagnosis and Additional Tests

Anterior tarsal tunnel syndrome is diagnosed by performing the patient's anamnesis, in which it is possible to identify the risk factors for this disease through the performance of the neurological physical examination. The diagnosis becomes more likely when the patient presents changes in sensitivity or pain in the skin located in the first interdigital space of the foot and when maneuvers that promote the extension of the foot accentuate the symptoms.

The diagnosis of this syndrome in the electroneuromyography examination of the lower limbs is performed through the following findings [22]:

Motor distal latency of the peroneal nerve greater than three standard deviations above the average (normality value 3.87 ± 0.44 ms) and, if unilateral, greater than 130% of the contralateral value.

Or

M response of the extensor digitorum brevis muscle absent.

Or

Electromyographic abnormalities (abnormal spontaneous activity and/or abnormal morphology of the motor unit action potential and firing pattern and reduction of volitional activity) confined to the extensor digitorum brevis muscle.

A simple radiograph of the foot and ankle can assist in identifying osteophytes and pes cavus [4].

Magnetic resonance imaging (MRI) is a test that allows the evaluation of the presence of masses and inflammatory processes of soft tissues.

Ultrasound is a less expensive option compared to MRI that can also evaluate the DPN and other structures in the ATT.

MRI neurography is a test that has been useful for evaluating the compressive mononeuropathies of the lower limb [23, 24].

To exclude inflammatory causes, it is important to request the tests for antinuclear antibody (ANA) and rheumatoid factor. In male patients, the HLA-B7 test should be requested, as this test is positive in patients with clinical symptoms of ankylosing spondylitis [4].

8.7 Conservative Treatment of Patients with Anterior Tarsal Tunnel Syndrome

Conservative treatment should always be the first measure to be faced with a patient with this compressive syndrome. Thus, it is advised that the patient avoid sports activities that lead to trauma to the ATA region, such as soccer and other activities that require plantar extension of the foot [25]. Another relevant guidance is the use of appropriate footwear. Among this last measure, it is advised that women avoid wearing high heels and sandals that require the lace to create compression points on the anterior tarsal tunnel region.

It is cited in the literature the performance of physiotherapy, especially for patients with frequent sprains and reduced proprioception sensitivity [1].

Among the medications described in the literature, tricyclic antidepressants, anticonvulsants, non-steroidal anti-inflammatory drugs [1] are identified. It is also mentioned in the literature, the use of corticosteroid injections that given the risk of peripheral nerve injury during infiltration, this conservative treatment modality should be evaluated very carefully [26].

8.8 Open Surgical Treatment of Patients with Anterior Tarsal Tunnel Syndrome

Surgery is indicated only when symptoms persist after conservative treatment. The patient is positioned in dorsal decubitus and subjected to general anesthesia or spinal anesthesia. The lower extremity should undergo trichotomy, followed by rigorous asepsis. The use of a tourniquet may provide better hemostasis, but it is not mandatory. Among the incision options available, there is the longitudinal and the "Lazy S-shaped" incision that starts proximally to the ankle and distally follows the space located between the first and second tarsometatarsal joints.

After the skin incision and opening of the subcutaneous plane, the tendons of the extensor hallucis longus and extensor digitorum longus muscles are identified. Once the nerve is identified, decompression is performed along its length, by opening the superior and inferior extensor retinaculum, allowing the nerve to be without compression points.

In the distal incision, it is important that the tendon of the extensor hallucis brevis muscle is sectioned for decompression of the medial branch of the DPN that passes under it.

The closure of the subcutaneous plane should be performed, followed by the skin. The patient should rest and not support the foot on the ground for a period of 2 weeks. Keeping the limb elevated will assist in reducing edema in the postoperative period [1] (Figs. 8.6, 8.7, 8.8, and 8.9; Video 8.1)

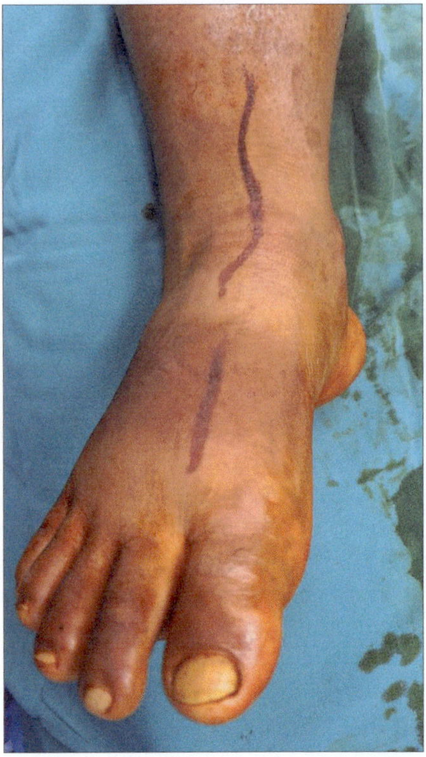

Fig. 8.6 Incisions for decompression of the DPN. The distal incision allows the location of the tendon of the flexor hallucis brevis muscle to be cut, with the aim of decompressing the medial branch of the DPN. The proximal incision allows the release of the nerve at the level of the anterior tarsal tunnel

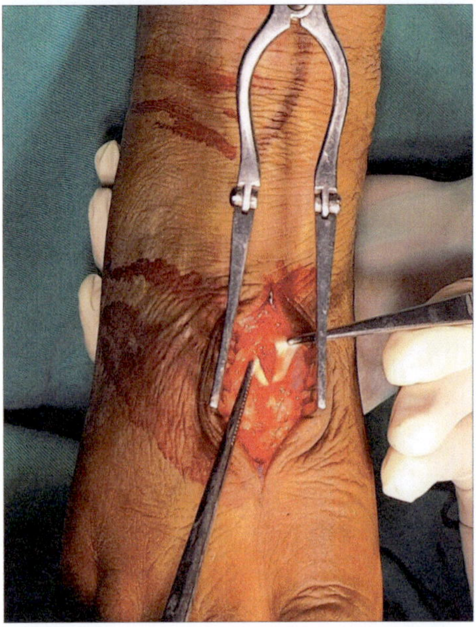

Fig. 8.7 Identification of the tendons of the extensor hallucis brevis muscle (on the left) and the tendon of the extensor hallucis longus (on the right). The tendon of the extensor hallucis brevis has a smaller diameter

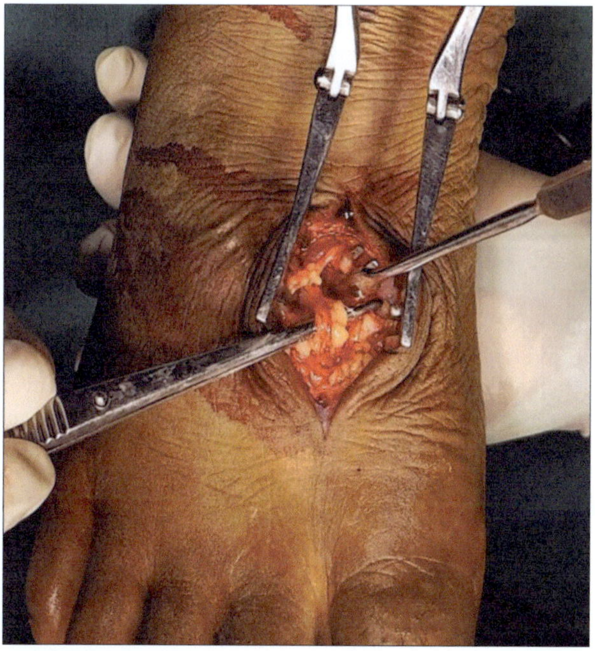

Fig. 8.8 Exposure of the medial branch of the deep peroneal nerve at the level of the distal incision after the section of the flexor hallucis brevis tendon

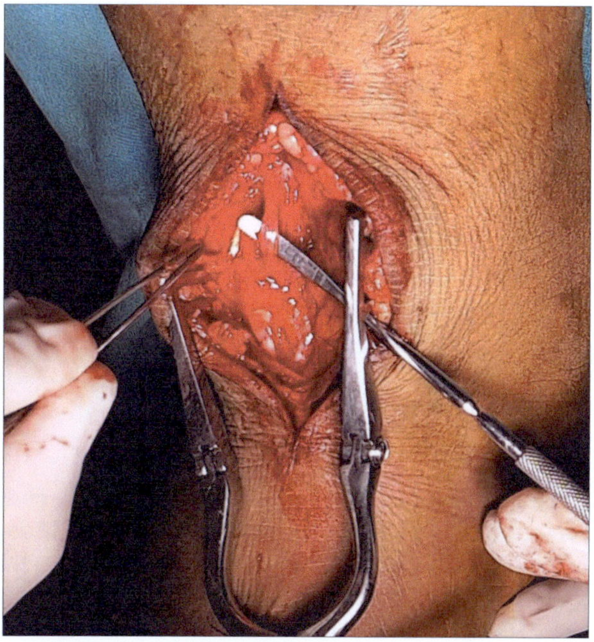

Fig. 8.9 Exposure of the deep peroneal nerve at the level of the proximal incision, after the opening of the inferior and superior extensor retinaculum

8.9 Endoscopic Surgical Treatment of Patients with Anterior Tarsal Tunnel Syndrome

The endoscopic technique for the treatment of patients with this rare mononeuropathy still needs better definition of its role. However, below is the technique based on a case report, in which the patient was successful in her endoscopic treatment.

The endoscopic technique for the treatment of this neuropathy is contraindicated in patients with local fibrosis and expansive lesions inside the anterior tarsal tunnel. However, this surgical modality has a relative contraindication for patients with the presence of osteophytes from the talonavicular joint [27–30].

With the patient in supine position, the ankle is placed in subtalar pronation. A small longitudinal incision should be made, at the level of the tarsometatarsal joint, on the dorsum of the foot of 1 cm, lateral to the tendon of the extensor hallucis longus muscle. The use of a tourniquet on the lower limb is recommended, with the aim of improving hemostasis. The anterior tarsal tunnel is identified by the introduction of a delicate blunt tip dissector, in the disto-proximal direction. Through the system called Agee Single Portal Carpal Tunnel Release System-3M Healthcare, St. Paul MN® bands present in the deep retinaculum are released [27].

8.10 Surgical Complications in the Treatment of Patients with Anterior Tarsal Tunnel Syndrome

Described as complications of the surgical treatment of patients with anterior tarsal tunnel syndrome are nerve structure injury, extensor digitorum brevis injury, surgical wound infection, surgical wound dehiscence, persistence of pain or pre-surgical symptoms, need for a new surgical procedure, revision of surgery, and formation of hypertrophic scar [31].

In the endoscopic technique, worsening of paresthesia in the immediate postoperative period is described, but with subsequent improvement. In a case report, good pain control was noted at 19 months postoperatively [27].

8.11 Prognosis

In the literature, in three published series, it was observed that pain control after surgery was satisfactory, despite the studies being constituted by small samples. It is important to mention that in these 3 series, the technique performed was open surgery [31].

8.12 Conclusion

The anterior tarsal tunnel syndrome is a rare compressive neuropathy of the lower limb whose diagnosis is clinical and corroborated by complementary exams, such as the electroneuromyography. It is a syndrome that can initially be treated conservatively and surgically after the failure of conservative management.

References

1. DiDomenico LA, Masternick EB. Anterior tarsal tunnel syndrome. Clin Podiatr Med Surg. 2006;23(3):611–20. https://doi.org/10.1016/j.cpm.2006.04.007. PMID: 16958392.
2. Logullo F, Ganino C, Lupidi F, Perozzi C, Di Bella P, Provinciali L. Anterior tarsal tunnel syndrome: a misunderstood and a misleading entrapment neuropathy. Neurol Sci. 2014;35(5):773–5. https://doi.org/10.1007/s10072-013-1601-8. Epub 2013 Dec 12. PMID: 24337947.
3. Yassin M, Garti A, Weissbrot M, Heller E, Robinson D. Treatment of anterior tarsal tunnel syndrome through an endoscopic or open technique. Foot (Edinb). 2015;25(3):148–51.
4. Dreyer MA, Gibboney MD. Anterior tarsal tunnel syndrome. [Updated 2023 May 23]. In: StatPearls [Internet]. Treasure Island: StatPearls Publishing; 2023. Available from: https://www.ncbi.nlm.nih.gov/books/NBK538488/.
5. Adelman KA, Wilson G, Wolf JA. Anterior tarsal tunnel syndrome. J Foot Surg. 1988;27(4):299–302. PMID: 3225388.
6. Sarrafian S. The anatomy of the foot and ankle. Philadelphia: J.B. Lippincott; 1983.
7. Aktan Ikiz ZA, Ucerler H, Uygur M. Dimensions of the anterior tarsal tunnel and features of the deep peroneal nerve in relation to clinical application. Surg Radiol Anat. 2007;29(7):527–30. https://doi.org/10.1007/s00276-007-0229-x. Epub 2007 Jul 3. PMID: 17607504.
8. Dellon AL. Deep peroneal nerve entrapment on the dorsum of the foot. Foot Ankle. 1990;11(2):73–80. https://doi.org/10.1177/107110079001100203. PMID: 2265812.
9. Standring S, editor. Gray's anatomy. 39th ed. Spain: Churchill Livingstone; 2005. p. 1505.
10. Liu Z, Zhou J, Zhao L. Anterior tarsal tunnel syndrome. J Bone Joint Surg Br. 1991;73(3):470–3. https://doi.org/10.1302/0301-620X.73B3.1670452. PMID: 1670452.
11. Gessini L, Jandolo B, Pietrangeli A. The anterior tarsal syndrome. Report of four cases. J Bone Joint Surg Am. 1984;66(5):786–7. PMID: 6725331.
12. Krause KH, Witt T, Ross A. The anterior tarsal tunnel syndrome. J Neurol. 1977;217(1):67–74. https://doi.org/10.1007/BF00316318. PMID: 75254.
13. Kennedy JG, Baxter DE. Nerve disorders in dancers. Clin Sports Med. 2008;27(2):329–34. https://doi.org/10.1016/j.csm.2008.01.001. PMID: 18346547.
14. Santos DFD, Pereira RC, Goulart IMB. Anterior tarsal tunnel syndrome: an atypical involvement in primary neural leprosy. Arq Neuropsiquiatr. 2019;77(10):754–5. https://doi.org/10.1590/0004-282X20190114. PMID: 31664354.
15. Kanbe K, Kubota H, Shirakura K, Hasegawa A, Udagawa E. Entrapment neuropathy of the deep peroneal nerve associated with the extensor hallucis brevis. J Foot Ankle Surg. 1995;34(6):560–2. https://doi.org/10.1016/S1067-2516(09)80078-1. PMID: 8646207.
16. Hirose CB, McGarvey WC. Anterior tarsal tunnel syndrome. Foot Ankle Clin N Am. 2004;9:255–69.
17. Kravette MA. Peripheral nerve entrapment syndromes in the foot. J Am Podiatry Assoc. 1971;61(12):457–72. https://doi.org/10.7547/87507315-61-12-457. PMID: 4330101.
18. Delgado-López PD, Rodríguez-Salazar A, Martín-Alonso J, Martín-Velasco V. Natural history, role of physical examination, timing of surgery, treatment options and conflicts of

interests. Neurocirugia (Astur). 2017;28(3):124–34. Spanish. https://doi.org/10.1016/j.neucir.2016.11.004. Epub 2017 Jan 25. PMID: 28130015.
19. Craig A. Entrapment neuropathies of the lower extremity. PM R. 2013;5(5 Suppl):S31–40. https://doi.org/10.1016/j.pmrj.2013.03.029. Epub 2013 Mar 28. PMID: 23542774.
20. Mak MS, Chowdhury R, Johnson R. Morton's neuroma: review of anatomy, pathomechanism, and imaging. Clin Radiol. 2021;76(3):235.e15–23. https://doi.org/10.1016/j.crad.2020.10.006. Epub 2020 Nov 7. PMID: 33168237.
21. Chang MC, Yang S. Diabetic peripheral neuropathy essentials: a narrative review. Ann Palliat Med. 2023;12(2):390–8. https://doi.org/10.21037/apm-22-693. Epub 2023 Feb 8. PMID: 36786097.
22. Logullo F, Di Bella P, Danni MC, Pagelli P, Angeleri F. Intraobserver intertrial reliability in motor nerve conduction studies. Riv It EEG Neurofisiol Clin. 1991;14:175–82.
23. Garwood ER, Duarte A, Bencardino JT. MR imaging of entrapment neuropathies of the lower extremity. Radiol Clin North Am. 2018;56(6):997–1012.
24. Chari B, McNally E. Nerve entrapment in ankle and foot: ultrasound imaging. Semin Musculoskelet Radiol. 2018;22(3):354–63.
25. Swathi, Nellithala GG, Athavale SA. Mid-foot retinaculum: an unrecognized entity. Anat Cell Biol. 2017;50(3):171–4.
26. Crowe CS, Shin AY, Pulos N. Iatrogenic nerve injuries of the upper extremity: a critical analysis review. JBJS Rev. 2023;11(1):e22. https://doi.org/10.2106/JBJS.RVW.22.00161. PMID: 36722824.
27. Lui TH. Endoscopic anterior tarsal tunnel release: a case report. J Foot Ankle Surg. 2014;53(2):186–8. https://doi.org/10.1053/j.jfas.2013.12.005. PMID: 24556485.
28. Lui TH. Arthroscopic triple arthrodesis in patients with Müller Weiss disease. Foot Ankle Surg. 2009;15(3):119–22. https://doi.org/10.1016/j.fas.2008.08.010. Epub 2008 Nov 14. PMID: 19635417.
29. Lui TH, Chan LK. Safety and efficacy of talonavicular arthroscopy in arthroscopic triple arthrodesis. A cadaveric study. Knee Surg Sports Traumatol Arthrosc. 2010;18(5):607–11. https://doi.org/10.1007/s00167-010-1098-0. Epub 2010 Mar 9. PMID: 20217388.
30. Oloff L, Schulhofer SD, Fanton G, Dillingham M. Arthroscopy of the calcaneocuboid and talonavicular joints. J Foot Ankle Surg. 1996;35(2):101–8; discussion 186–7. https://doi.org/10.1016/s1067-2516(96)80025-1. PMID: 8722876.
31. Ferkel E, Davis WH, Ellington JK. Entrapment neuropathies of the foot and ankle. Clin Sports Med. 2015;34(4):791–801.

Chapter 9
Posterior Tarsal Syndrome

9.1 Introduction

The posterior tarsal tunnel syndrome (PTTS) is conceptualized as a compressive neuropathy of the tibial nerve or its plantar branches within the tarsal tunnel that can be idiopathic or present diverse etiology, often associated with lesions that occupy the space of this osteofibrous tunnel [1–4].

The first historical description of this neuropathy was made by Pollock and Davis in 1933, in which a patient presented the symptomatology of the syndrome after a traumatic compression of the tibial nerve [5]. In 1960, Koppel and Thompson described the clinical characteristics resulting from PTTS, and in 1962, Keck coined the term tarsal tunnel syndrome when publishing a case report [6, 7].

As occur in other lower limb neuropathies, the etiologies associated with PTTS are varied. Among the most cited causes in the literature are those of traumatic, infectious, inflammatory, tumoral, vascular, and idiopathic [8]. In a systematic review conducted in 1990, Cimino W.R. observed that 20% of PTTS cases have an idiopathic etiology, in the remaining cases it was possible to identify an underlying etiology [9].

The aim of this chapter is to describe the concept of posterior tarsal tunnel syndrome, its historical aspects, anatomy, pathophysiology, symptoms and clinical signs, diagnostic methods, conservative and surgical treatment, endoscopic treatment, surgical complications, and prognosis.

M. J. S. Magalhães, *Lower Extremity Nerve Entrapments*,
https://doi.org/10.1007/978-3-031-90058-7_9

9.2 Anatomy of the Tibial Nerve

The sciatic nerve is composed of nerve fibers originating from the spinal nerves L4-S3. It is the peripheral nerve of the human body with the largest diameter. The sciatic nerve is responsible for the origin of the common peroneal and tibial nerves, at the level of the distal third of the thigh [10] (Figs. 9.1 and 9.2). The tibial nerve is a mixed type nerve that has fibers with autonomic, motor, and sensory functions. Its constitution includes nerve fibers originating from the spinal nerves L4-S3 [10]. The tibial nerve is responsible for the motility of the following lower limb muscles:

- Soleus muscle
- Tibialis posterior muscle
- Gastrocnemius muscle
- Flexor hallucis longus muscle
- Flexor digitorum longus muscle
- Popliteus muscle
- Quadratus plantae muscle
- Adductor hallucis muscle
- Flexor hallucis brevis muscle
- Flexor digitorum brevis muscle
- Lumbricales I–IV muscles
- Abductor digiti minimi muscle

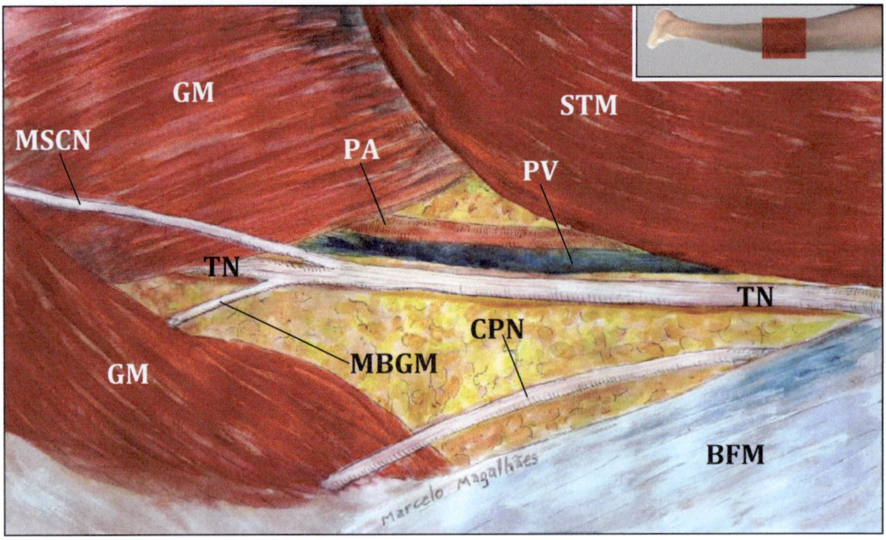

Fig. 9.1 Right lower limb popliteal fossa. *BFM* = biceps femoris muscle, *CPN* = common peroneal nerve, *GM* = gastrocnemius muscle, *MBGM* = muscle branch for gastrocnemius muscle, *MSCN* = medial sural cutaneous nerve, PA = popliteal artery, *PV* = popliteal vein, *STM* = semitendinosus muscle, *TN* = tibial nerve

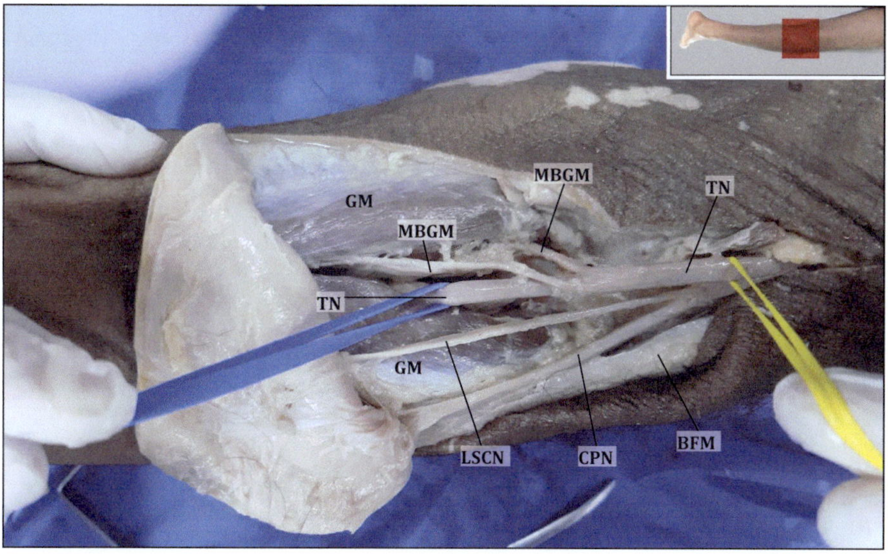

Fig. 9.2 Anatomy of the popliteal fossa in the right lower limb of a formalin-fixed specimen. Blue and yellow tapes highlight the tibial nerve in the popliteal fossa. *CPN* = common peroneal nerve, *BFM* = biceps femoris muscle, *GM* = gastrocnemius muscle, *LSCN* = lateral sural cutaneous nerve, *MBGM* = muscle branch for gastrocnemius muscle, *TN* = tibial nerve

- Flexor digiti minimi brevis muscle
- Interossei muscles

The sensory fibers of the tibial nerve run through the sural, medial plantar, lateral plantar, and calcaneal nerves. It is noted that the sensory territory of the tibial nerve corresponds to the lateral portion of the foot, sole, and a small portion of skin located distally on the dorsum of the toes, excluding the skin located in the first interdigital space, which is made by the deep peroneal nerve.

After the tibial nerve passes through the popliteal fossa, it follows a trajectory over the popliteus muscle. It then reaches a deep trajectory in relation to the soleus muscle and superficial in relation to the tibialis posterior muscle. At the level of the medial malleolus, it penetrates the tarsal tunnel. The tibial nerve at the level of this osteofibrous tunnel emits the following branches: calcaneal, medial plantar, and lateral plantar [10] (Figs. 9.3, 9.4, and 9.5).

Complete proximal injury of the tibial nerve causes the following changes: anesthesia of the plantar region, lateral portion of the foot, and a small portion of skin located distally on the dorsum of the toes, excluding the skin located in the first interdigital space, plegia for foot extension, toe flexion, and foot inversion [9].

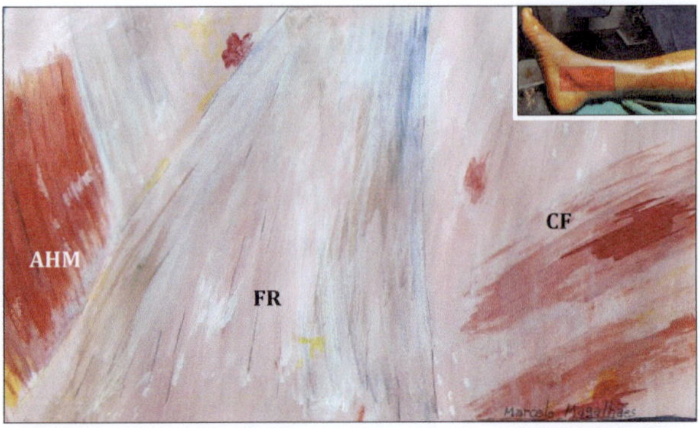

Fig. 9.3 Right ankle with preserved crural fascia and flexor retinaculum. *AHM* = abductor hallucis muscle, *CF* = crural fascia, *FR* = flexor retinaculum

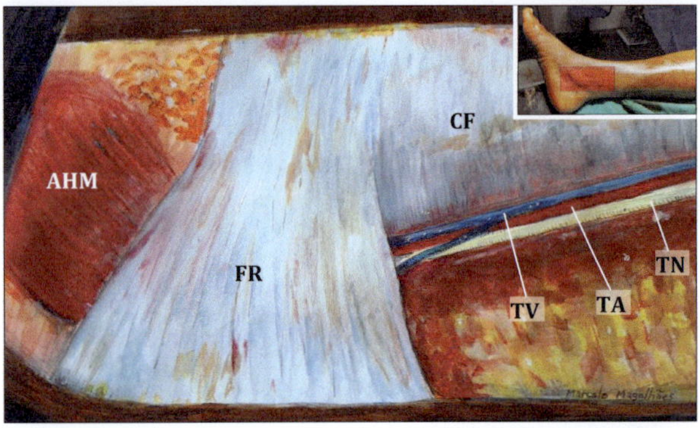

Fig. 9.4 Right ankle after opening the crural fascia. *AHM* = abductor hallucis muscle, *CF* = crural fascia, *FR* = flexor retinaculum, *TA* = tibial artery, *TN* = tibial nerve, *TV* = tibial veins

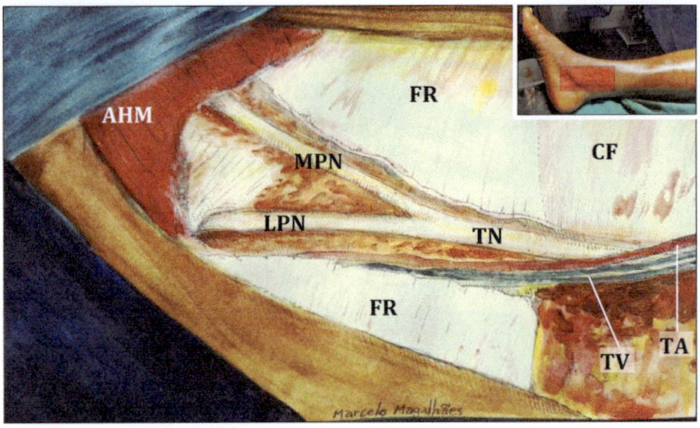

Fig. 9.5 Right ankle after opening the crural fascia and flexor retinaculum. *AHM* = Abductor hallucis muscle, *CF* = crural fascia, *FR* = flexor retinaculum, *LPN* = lateral plantar nerve, *MPN* = medial plantar nerve, *TA* = tibial artery, *TN* = tibial nerve, *TV* = tibial veins

9.2.1 Anatomy of the Posterior Tarsal Tunnel

The posterior tarsal tunnel (PTT) has as its roof, the flexor retinaculum that attaches to the medial malleolus and calcaneus. Inside the tunnel are the tendons of the tibialis posterior muscle, flexor digitorum longus, flexor hallucis longus, tibial nerve, tibial artery, and tibial veins [9]. The posterior limit of the PTT is the posterior process of the talus, the superior limit is the medial malleolus, the lateral limit is constituted by the calcaneus, and the inferior limit is the abductor hallucis muscle. The flexor retinaculum is also called the lancinate ligament or internal annular ligament [11].

9.3 Etiology of Posterior Tarsal Tunnel Syndrome

As with other neuropathies of the lower limb, the etiologies associated with PTTS are varied. Among the most cited causes in the literature are those of traumatic, infectious, inflammatory, tumoral, vascular, and idiopathic origin. It is emphasized that in some cases, no specific alteration is identified in the imaging exams.

The os sustentaculi is an accessory bone located in the foot that connects through a fibrotic band or fibrocartilage to the talus. This accessory bone is positioned between the talus and the calcaneus, which can cause compression of the tibial nerve and/or its branches positioned inside the tarsal tunnel [12–14].

Tarsal coalition is a cause of PTTS described in the literature. It is a bridge of bone, fibrous, or cartilaginous origin that unites two or more tarsal bones. It is estimated that the incidence in the general population is around 1%. It is known that calcaneonavicular and talocalcaneal coalitions are the most frequently identified. The diagnosis can be made by radiography [15, 16].

A Baker's cyst develops from the growth of the bursa gastrocnemius-semimembranosus. This is a usually asymptomatic injury that presents in the popliteal fossa region and can be the cause of thrombophlebitis, compartment syndrome, and compressive neuropathy. The literature describes the rupture of a Baker's cyst with leakage of cystic content to the calf region with compression of the tibial nerve [17]. The initial symptom is described as abrupt intense pain located in the popliteal fossa region [17].

The presence of accessory muscles in the ankle region as a risk factor for PTTS is described in the literature. It is believed that these muscles act as an expansive lesion, which would trigger the neuropathy [18]. The accessory muscle most associated with this compressive neuropathy is the flexor digitorum accessorius longus; however, the muscle tibiocalcaneus internus and accessory soleus are also described [18].

Between 17% and 43% of patients, it is possible to identify in their histories some type of local trauma to the ankle/foot such as fractures, ankle sprains, and ligament injuries [19]. Chronic instability of the medial ankle is described as a risk factor for PTTS and may be associated with frequent sprains that can lead to ligament laxity [20].

In 10% of cases, it is possible to identify a history of inflammatory processes such as osteoarthritis, rheumatoid arthritis, and tenosynovitis [19, 21, 22].

The medical literature describes the onset of PTTS after surgical procedures to correct foot deformities, such as cavovarus feet. It is believed that the reduction of the posterior tarsal tunnel after the procedure would lead to compression of the tibial nerve by the flexor retinaculum [23–25].

Tumors like schwannoma can be a cause of posterior tarsal tunnel syndrome. This tumor is most commonly identified in the skull, spinal nerves, and brachial plexus, rarely affecting nerves in the lower limb. The most commonly affected nerve in the lower limb by schwannoma is the tibial nerve. Usually, tumors of this nature grow slowly and produce non-painful asymptomatic masses. When symptomatic, they produce symptoms of numbness and pain [26–28].

The medical literature describes distinct tumors from the nerve lineage as a cause of tibial neuropathy, such as B cell lymphoma [29].

Intraneural ganglion cyst can lead to PTTS, especially when it affects the tibial nerve at the level of the tarsal tunnel. Intraneural ganglion cysts originate within the nerve, from the epineurium. There is a fibrous capsule filled with a thick mucinous fluid. They occur most commonly between the third and fourth decade of life. It is believed to originate from the degeneration of perineural connective tissue, more rarely, its genesis occurs by filling with synovial joint fluid via the articular branch [30–32].

Among the bone tumors that can cause posterior tarsal tunnel syndrome, osteochondroma stands out. This lesion is the most common benign bone tumor, accounting for about 30% of all tumors of this nature. It commonly presents as a bulge on the surface of the bone that has a cavity inside, with continuity with the bone marrow structure. Despite being the most common benign bone tumor, its location in the foot is rare. It does not have a gender preference and occurs most commonly in children and adolescents [33, 34].

Other causes of this neuropathy are endocrine diseases such as hypothyroidism, mucopolysaccharidoses, gout, and dyslipidemias. It is also described PTTS after intense physical activities like those present in the sports activities of marathon runners [35].

9.4 Symptoms and Clinical Signs of Posterior Tarsal Tunnel Syndrome

The patient's symptomatology will depend on the point of nerve compression. If the tibial nerve is compressed at the level of the tarsal tunnel, before the bifurcation into its medial and lateral plantar branches, the symptoms will compromise the entire distal sensory territory. On the other hand, if the compression occurs more distally, compromising a specific plantar branch, the symptomatology will be restricted only to the territory innervated by that branch. When the compression occurs only in one of the plantar branches, it is called distal tarsal syndrome [35]. It should be noted that when only the calcaneal branch is compromised, only a sensory area of the heel will be compromised [35].

The patient with PTTS usually presents with symptoms of paresthesia, pain, dysesthesia, and allodynia in the territories innervated by the plantar branches of the tibial nerve.

Performing compression on the nerve path at the level of the tarsal tunnel accentuates the paresthesia and causes pain in 60–100% of patients [35]. The Tinel's sign can cause pain that radiates to the patient's plantar region. The maneuver of forced inversion and/or eversion of the foot can intensify the patient's symptoms. Palpation of the tarsal tunnel region is important to detect the presence of bulges that can give clues about the etiology of this neuropathy, such as tumors located in the bones or even inside the osteofibrous tunnel [35].

In a later stage of the disease's evolution, where there is a more pronounced compromise of the neuropathy, the patient may develop some degree of paresis. Usually in these cases, it manifests initially by a paresis of the abductors and later of the short flexors of the fingers. Muscle atrophy and changes in sweating in the plantar skin are late phenomena in the natural evolution of the posterior tarsal tunnel syndrome [35].

It is important to remember that the patient will not develop paresis for the inversion of the foot, nor paresis for plantar flexion of the foot, since the branches responsible for the innervation of these muscles originate at a point proximal to the tarsal tunnel.

9.5 Differential Diagnosis of Posterior Tarsal Tunnel Syndrome

There are several diseases compromising the peripheral nerves that mimic the symptoms of PTTS, especially neuropathies and inflammatory processes that cause pain, numbness in the plantar region of the patient. The distinction between posterior tarsal tunnel syndrome and these diseases is of fundamental importance to avoid failure in the management of the patient's disease. The differential diagnosis for this neuropathy may include diabetic polyneuropathy, lumbar radiculopathy, deep flexor compartment syndrome, Morton's neuroma, calcaneal spur, inflammatory changes in the plantar fascia, and foot ligaments (Fig. 9.6).

In sensory motor polyneuropathy of the lower limbs resulting from Diabetes Mellitus, patients usually present with symmetrical symptoms, in which distal neuropathic pain predominates. The symptomatology tends to intensify during the night. Some patients may have trophic changes in the nails, skin, and appendages, as well as motor symptoms, such as paresis, muscle hypotrophy, and areflexia [35, 36]. Electroneuromyography of the lower limbs can easily confirm the diagnosis of polyneuropathy resulting from diabetes mellitus [36].

Radiculopathy of spinal nerves L5 and S1 resulting from a lumbar disc herniation causes pain that radiates from the lumbar spine to the lower limb and often presents a positive Lasègue sign in its physical examination. S1 spinal nerve

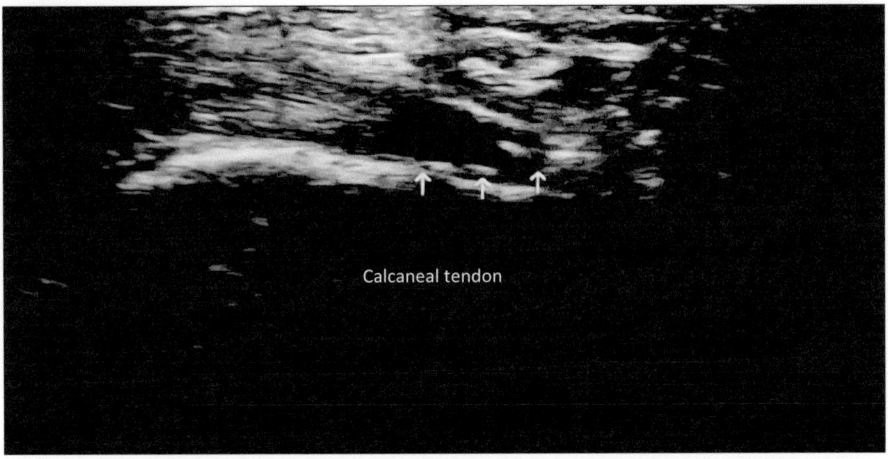

Fig. 9.6 Ultrasound performed with a high-frequency linear transducer (8–12 MHz) of the ankle. Examination reveals calcaneal tendinopathy in a 69-year-old female patient with heel pain. The examination (white arrows) shows the presence of insertional fibers with anechoic intrasubstantial areas suggestive of tendon microtear and echogenic foci of fibrosis

radiculopathy may present with Achilles tendon areflexia, weakness to perform plantar extension of the foot, and changes in sensitivity that involve the plantar region. On the other hand, radiculopathy of the L5 spinal nerve presents with preserved lower limb reflexes and may present with paresis for dorsiflexion of the foot and changes in sensitivity in the lateral region of the leg and dorsum of the foot [35, 37–39].

Patients with clinical symptoms of Morton's neuroma especially have pain when walking, especially when wearing pointed shoes. The pain tends to be unilateral and occurs especially in the third interdigital space and more rarely in the second interdigital space. The Mulder sign may be present, which consists of manual palpation of the interdigital space causing intense pain and radiation [40].

9.6 Clinical Diagnosis of Posterior Tarsal Tunnel Syndrome

The patient's diagnosis is based on the clinical history collected during the anamnesis and neurological physical examination. The symptom that usually predominates is the pain located in the region posterior to the medial malleolus that can radiate to the region of the plantar arch, including also the heel region. The patient may also complain of paresthesia, a feeling of tightness or hypoesthesia in the territory innervated by the tibial nerve. It is important to note that sensory complaints can affect any of the branches of the tibial nerve (medial plantar, lateral plantar, or calcaneal). A point that reinforces the diagnosis is the report that the pain worsened during the night, after daytime work where it was necessary to remain standing carrying heavy objects. Generally, the elevation of the foot can reduce the patient's symptoms [41].

On physical examination, the Tinel sign may be positive along the course of the nerve.

Provocative maneuvers such as the dorsiflexion-eversion test can be useful, by inducing or accentuating the pain [42]. To perform this maneuver, the doctor performs for a period of 5–10 seconds the dorsiflexion of the foot and metatarsophalangeal joints simultaneously to eversion of the foot [43]. Kinoshita et al. (2001) showed that the dorsiflexion-eversion test aggravated the pain in 36 of the 44 feet (82%) with PTTS. On the other hand, in the control group of healthy individuals, the same maneuver did not cause pain [42, 44].

Another semiological maneuver that can be used is the Trepman test, in which the examining doctor performs the passive movement of plantar flexion associated with inversion of the foot, which can cause an increase in pain [45].

The maneuver triple compression stress test consists of the association of the Tinel sign associated with the Trepman maneuver, in which the examiner applies digital pressure on the tibial nerve during plantar flexion and inversion of the foot. Aboueleta et al. (2012) reveal a positivity of this test in 93.8% of symptomatic patients [46].

Inspection is essential for visualization of bulging in the region of the posterior tarsal tunnel, where expansive diseases can develop, such as tumors and cysts. It is possible in chronic cases to identify the hypotrophy of the short flexor muscle of the hallux [41].

9.7 Additional Tests in Posterior Tarsal Tunnel Syndrome

Among the most requested complementary exams are radiography, computed tomography, ultrasonography with and without Doppler, magnetic resonance imaging, and electroneuromyography.

Radiography in profile and antero-posterior incidences are useful for assessing the presence of bone tumors such as chondroma, tarsal coalition, fractures, and bone deformities [41].

Ultrasonography is an exam that has increasingly proven useful due to its versatility and low cost. It is possible through this diagnostic method to identify varicose veins, ganglia, tumors, tenosynovitis, as well as talocalcaneal coalition [41]. Linear transducers of >15 MHz are suitable for nerve visualization. Through Doppler, venous and arterial vascular structures of the tunnel are correctly visualized. The dynamic images of ultrasonography also allow the identification of the presence of ligament laxity, as well as tendon subluxation [47]. It is known that the process of compression of peripheral nerves results in typical echographic changes, in which there is an increase in the transverse area of the nerve proximal to the point of compression, as well as changes in its echogenicity [43]. Therimadasamy et al. (2011) revealed that the transverse area of the posterior tibial nerve in healthy limbs was

10 mm^2, and in limbs affected by PTTS, it was 17 mm^2 [48]; on the other hand, Lee et al. (2005), in a study involving patients with tibial neuropathy due to diabetes mellitus, revealed a transverse area of 24 mm^2 and in patients with healthy limbs, a tibial nerve area of 12 mm^2 [49].

The finding of electroneuromyography most associated with PTTS is the prolongation of distal motor latencies of the abductor digiti minimi muscle which corresponds to the compressive process of the lateral plantar nerve [50] (Fig. 9.7). The most accepted electroneuromyographic findings for diagnosis are:

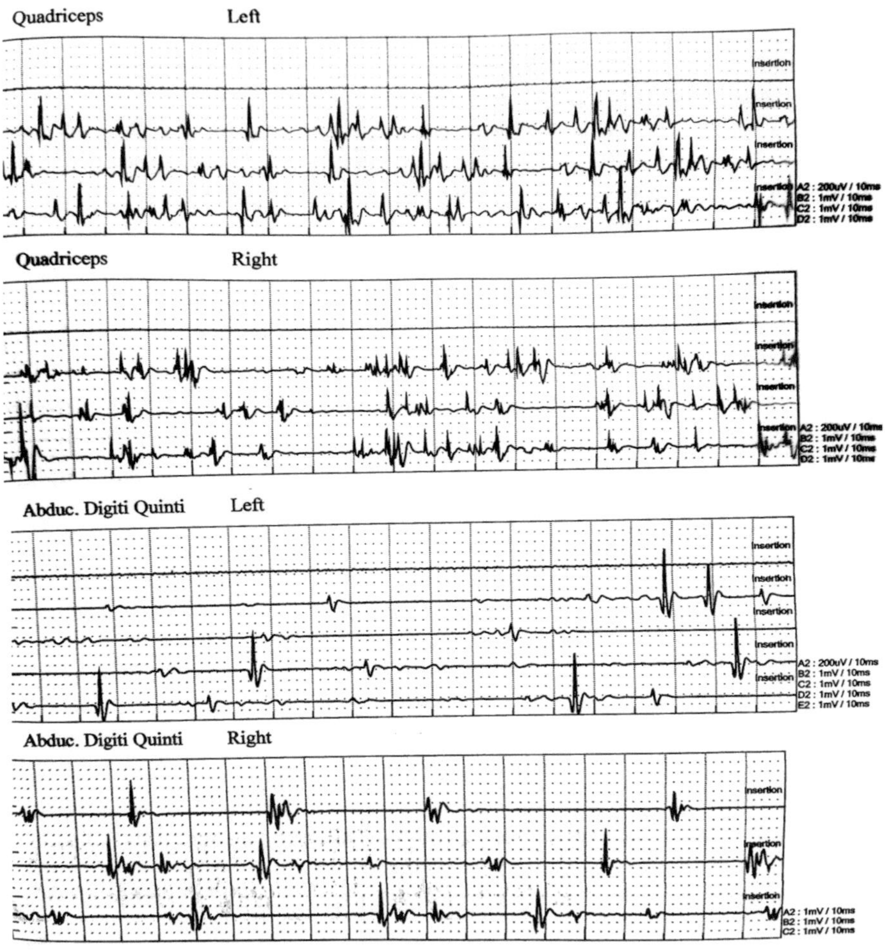

Fig. 9.7 Electromyography of the lower limbs of a patient with a clinical picture of tibial nerve neuropathy at the level of the posterior tarsal tunnel. EMG (with muscle contraction): Voluntary activation showed motor unit potentials (MUP) with normal recruitment and morphological characteristics in the quadriceps muscle, except in the abductor digiti minimi muscles, whose MUPs are neuropathic and have reduced recruitment

1. Prolonged distal motor latency
   - Terminal latency of the abductor hallucis muscle greater than 5.8 milliseconds (ms)
   - Terminal latency of the abductor digiti minimi muscle greater than 6.3 ms
   - Differences between limbs of the same studied branch greater than 1 ms
2. Record of conduction speed less than 41 ms
3. Record of the amplitude of the compound muscle action potential (CMAP) less than 4 millivolts (mv) for the abductor hallucis muscle or less than 3 mv for the abductor digiti minimi muscle
4. Variation of the record between sides, with a decrease in amplitude greater than 50% for the same studied nerve branch [51]

Magnetic resonance imaging is the gold standard exam for identifying masses located inside the PTTS [43].

Finally, computed tomography is an exam that assists in identifying bone deformities [49].

9.8 Conservative Treatment of Posterior Tarsal Tunnel Syndrome

It is important to define that conservative treatment should be the first choice as a management modality for PTTS, unless the patient already presents signs of muscle atrophy or motor involvement of the tibial nerve [11].

The literature cites various medications as an option for the conservative management of this syndrome: tricyclic antidepressants, B vitamin complexes, GABA analog drugs, opioids, and non-steroidal anti-inflammatory drugs [52].

Conservative treatment consists of correcting the underlying conditions that in some way contribute to the clinical picture, such as inflammatory processes. The treatment of rheumatoid arthritis (RA) in a patient with concomitant PTTS may alleviate their pain symptoms. The same applies to endocrinological syndromes such as diabetes mellitus and hypothyroidism [35]. Resting the affected limb may help relieve symptoms.

The use of corticosteroid infiltration inside the tarsal tunnel is also described as a form of treatment. It is important to emphasize that infiltration should be performed with the aid of ultrasonography, with the aim of reducing the risk of inadvertent puncture of the tibial nerve, which will result in worsening pain for the patient [35, 53]. Magalhães et al. (2022) in a systematic review identified that physiotherapy can be an option as a form of conservative treatment [54]. In this same systematic review, it was demonstrated that ultrasound-guided pulsed radiofrequency was an option for cases where open surgery did not control pain symptoms [54].

Cimino WR (1990) in a systematic review observed that only 16% patients who were treated conservatively achieved symptom control. This same author recommended the use of orthopedic insoles as the treatment for PTTS only for patients who had foot deformities, achieving a result of symptom control in 34% of cases [9].

The literature still does not present data with satisfactory scientific evidence for the conservative management of PTTS regarding the time and modality of these therapies [35].

9.9 Surgical Treatment

9.9.1 Open Surgical Treatment of Posterior Tarsal Tunnel Syndrome

Surgical treatment is indicated when conservative treatment fails or when at the time of diagnosis, the presence of expansive lesions inside the PTT is identified (Figs. 9.8, 9.9, 9.10, 9.11, 9.12, and 9.13).

The patient should undergo anesthesia, preferably without the use of a muscle blocker, as in this way, if a neurophysiological study is used, the tibial nerve can be evaluated. The use of a tourniquet on the lower limb is at the surgeon's discretion. The most ergonomic surgical position for the surgeon is when the patient is in the supine position, with a small cushion under the knee of the limb to be operated on, in addition to a slight flexion of the knee, associated with a slight external rotation of the foot.

The most recommended incision is one that is approximately 5–7 cm in length, with an arciform aspect, retro-posterior to the medial malleolus. In general, the incision follows the path of the tibial nerve. After opening the skin, it is common to identify several veins located in the subcutaneous plane, on the surface of the PTT that usually bleed a lot when injured. It is necessary to open the crural fascia and the

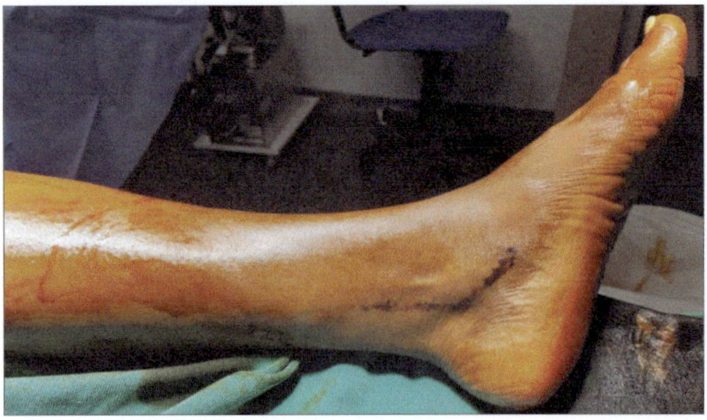

Fig. 9.8 Marking of the arcuate incision for access to the posterior tarsal tunnel in the left lower limb. The incision line should start straight about 3 cm proximal to the medial malleolus, on the axis between the medial malleolus and the Achilles tendon. It presents a slight curve passing below the medial malleolus for approximately 2 cm

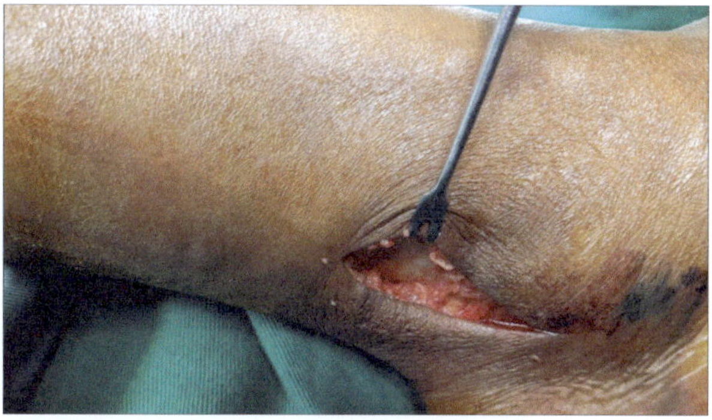

Fig. 9.9 Incision for access to the posterior tarsal tunnel in the left lower limb. Note the exposure of the crural fascia

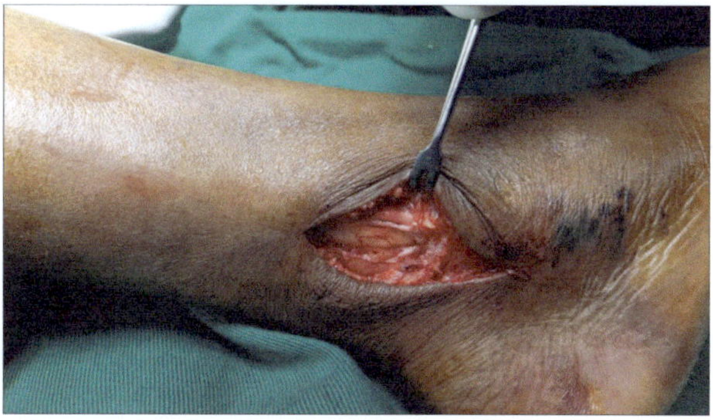

Fig. 9.10 Incision for access to the posterior tarsal tunnel of the left lower limb after opening the crural fascia. At this moment, it is important to identify the vascular bundle, tendon of the tibialis posterior muscle, and tibial nerve. Sometimes it will be possible to identify the sensory branch for the calcaneus

PTT so that the tibial nerve can be identified, as well as its distal branches and medial and lateral plantar branch [11]. In the postoperative period, the patient should be instructed to elevate the foot that underwent surgical treatment when at rest and to use a crutch to walk, thus avoiding foot support on the ground.

When the patient presents an intraneural ganglion cyst as the cause of PTTS, it is important to try to identify the existence of an articular branch as the exit point of synovial fluid from the joint to the cyst. If identified, the removal of the articular branch may reduce the chance of recurrence of the cystic lesion [31, 55, 56].

In those cases where the patient presents schwannoma as the etiology of PTTS, surgery should be performed to remove the tumor by dissecting the fascicles, sacrificing only that fascicle that originated the tumor. The performance of a prior biopsy for the confirmation of schwannoma should not be performed due to the risk of causing worsening pain or even motor deficit. The use of neurophysiological monitoring during the surgery to remove the tibial nerve tumor is mandatory, to thus reduce the chances of motor deficit. Through monitoring, it is possible for the surgeon to open the epineurium in a region without motor fascicles [57].

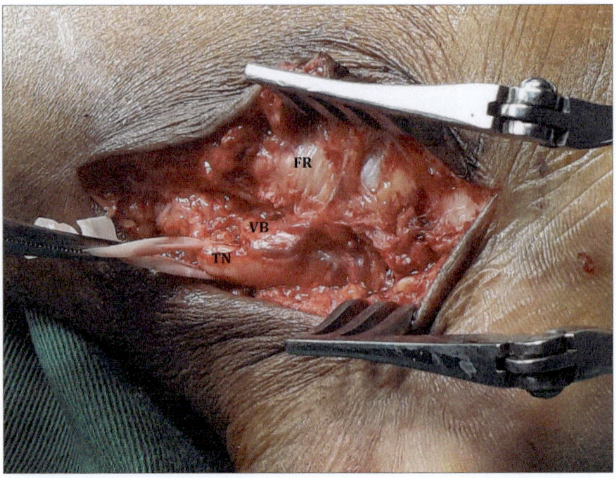

Fig. 9.11 Incision for access to the posterior tarsal tunnel in the left lower limb after opening the crural fascia and the flexor retinaculum (FR). Note that the tibial nerve (TN) was isolated by a surgical tape. Also note the presence of the vascular bundle represented by the acronym VB. At this moment, it is important to identify the vascular bundle, tendon of the tibialis posterior muscle, and tibial nerve. Sometimes it will be possible to identify the sensory branch for the calcaneus

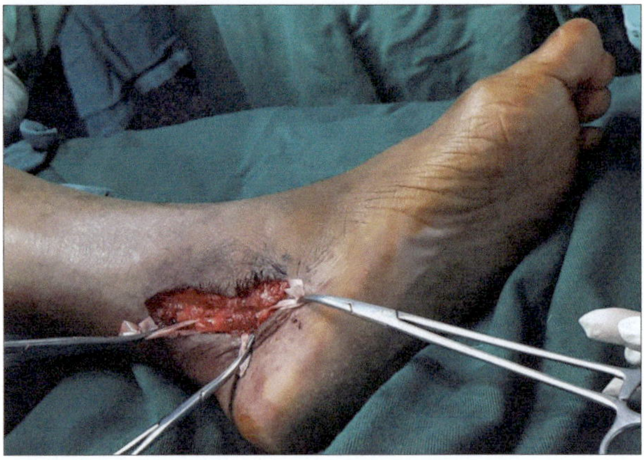

Fig. 9.12 Incision for access to the posterior tarsal tunnel in the left lower limb after opening the crural fascia, flexor retinaculum, and decompression of the tibial nerve and its medial and lateral plantar branches. The three nerves were isolated by surgical tapes. The vascular bundle was preserved

9.9.2 *Endoscopic Surgical Treatment of Posterior Tarsal Tunnel Syndrome*

Endoscopic surgery is an option for the treatment of PTTS, but the medical literature does not have scientific studies with large series of cases.

According to Yoshida A. et al. (2015), the patient is subjected to local anesthesia with lidocaine, without the use of a tourniquet and through a small 1 cm incision made proximally in the medial region of the foot, the endoscope is introduced. The

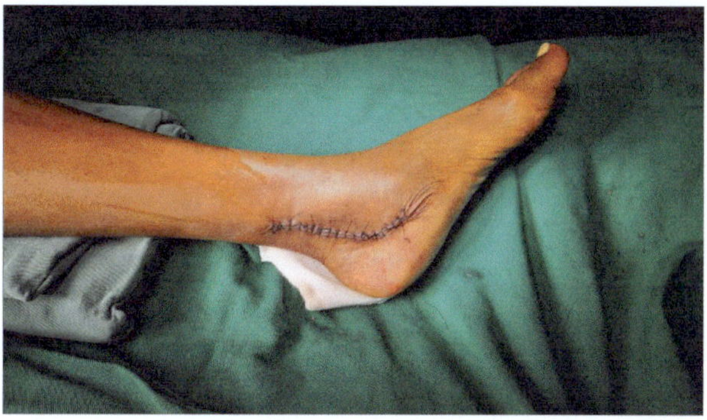

Fig. 9.13 Surgical access to the posterior tarsal tunnel in the left lower limb. Skin suture by simple stitches of mononylon 3-0

next step is to visualize the vessels, the tibial nerve, and its branches. After identifying the vasculonervous elements, a specific cutting instrument is introduced into the work field to section the flexor retinaculum. Once released from compression, the vasculonervous elements are evaluated again. In case of bleeding, at least three options can be used: bipolar in the work field to perform hemostasis and ligate the bleeding vessel through the skin or mechanical compression. These authors recommend not suturing the skin so that the endoscope entry point serves for drainage of bleeding. The authors recommend as postoperative care not to support the foot on the ground for a period of 1 week [58].

9.9.3 Surgical Treatment of Posterior Tarsal Tunnel Syndrome by the Lipografting Technique

Morandi E.M. et al. (2016) describe the case report of a patient who had already undergone simple decompression of the PTT with persistence of symptoms. Imaging exams revealed the emergence of fibrosis with thickening of the tibial nerve at the old surgical site. The patient underwent a surgical revision in which adipose tissue from the abdominal region was placed over the nerve, promoting good postoperative pain control [54].

9.9.4 Ultrasound-Guided Decompression of the Posterior Tarsal Tunnel

Gibello A.F. et al. (2018) published a study conducted on a cadaver in which the PTT is evaluated by 13 MHz ultrasound, and through a small incision, the surgical instrument is introduced to perform the opening of the flexor retinaculum [59].

9.9.5 Surgical Complications in the Treatment of Patients with Posterior Tarsal Tunnel Syndrome

Numerous post-surgical complications such as hypertrophic scarring, surgical wound dehiscence, persistent pain, and increased pain are described in the literature [6, 54]. Performing multiple surgeries can lead to a worsening of the clinical picture [58].

9.10 Prognosis

A systematic review comparing conservative and surgical treatment of PTTS revealed symptom control in 68% (n = 204) of cases undergoing open surgery, 100% (n = 8) of cases undergoing endoscopic treatment, and 7% (n = 2) of cases undergoing conservative treatment [3, 54, 60–66]. It is important to note that the groups undergoing conservative treatment and endoscopic surgery consisted of a small number of patients [19]. Antoniadis G. et al. (2008), in a review on the subject, revealed that success rates in the surgical treatment of PTTS varied between 75% and 91% [1, 9, 66–68].

In a systematic review conducted by Magalhães et al. (2022), it was revealed that the highest success rates in surgeries occurred in cases where there were structures causing nerve compression located inside the tunnel, such as bone prominence, varicose veins, ganglia, talocalcaneal coalition, and trauma [54]. Lau J. et al. (1998) showed in their study that some factors negatively influenced success rates, such as advanced age, the presence of a deficit at the time of surgery, the presence of fibrotic epineural scar on the tibial nerve, and chronic symptoms [69]. Sammarco G.J. et al. (2003) found in their study that patients with symptoms with less than 12 months of evolution had higher success rates in symptom control [63].

9.11 Conclusion

PTTS is a rare compressive neuropathy of the lower limb that can cause pain in the plantar region. It is a syndrome that has numerous underlying causes and therefore requires imaging tests during the diagnostic process. The initial management of these patients should be conservative, with surgery indicated only in refractory cases. The literature describes various therapeutic approaches and indicates that patients with identifiable etiology inside the posterior tarsal tunnel have a better prognosis when treated surgically, compared to those whose etiology is idiopathic.

References

1. Bailie DS, Kelikian AS. Tarsal tunnel syndrome: diagnosis, surgical technique, and functional outcome. Foot Ankle Int. 1998;19:65–72.
2. Shirokane K, Kim K, Akimoto M, Isu T, Kokubo R, Koketsu K, Ideguchi M, Murai Y. Zig-zag skin incision for treatment of tarsal tunnel syndrome. J Nippon Med Sch. 2024;91(4):357–61. https://doi.org/10.1272/jnms.JNMS.2024_91-404. PMID: 39231638.
3. Takakura Y, Kitada C, Sugimoto K, et al. Tarsal tunnel syndrome. Causes and results of operative treatment. J Bone Joint Surg. 1991;73:125–8.
4. Garchar DJ, Lewis JE, DiDomenico LA. Hypertrophic sustentaculum tali causing a tarsal tunnel syndrome: a case report. J Foot Ankle Surg. 2001;40:110–2.
5. Pollock L, Davis L. Peripheral nerve injuries. Am J Surg. 1932;18:361.
6. Koppel HP, Thompson WA. Peripheral entrapment neuropathies of the lower extremity. N Engl J Med. 1960;262:56–60.
7. Keck C. The tarsal-tunnel syndrome. J Bone Joint Surg. 1962;44A:180–2.
8. Dellon AL. The four medial ankle tunnels: a critical review of perceptions of tarsal tunnel syndrome and neuropathy. Neurosurg Clin N Am. 2008;19(4):629–48, vii. https://doi.org/10.1016/j.nec.2008.07.003. PMID: 19010287.
9. Cimino WR. Tarsal tunnel syndrome: a review of the literature. Foot Ankle Int. 1990;11:47–52.
10. Siqueira MG, Martins RS. Anatomia cirúrgica das vias de acesso aos nervos periféricos (Portuguese version). Brasil: Ed. Dilivros; 2005.
11. Fortier LM, Leethy KN, Smith M, McCarron MM, Lee C, Sherman WF, Varrassi G, Kaye AD. An update on posterior tarsal tunnel syndrome. Orthop Rev (Pavia). 2022;14(4):35444. https://doi.org/10.52965/001c.35444. PMID: 35769658; PMCID: PMC9235437.
12. Bencardino J, Rosenberg Z, Beltran J, et al. Os sustentaculi: depiction on MR images. Skeletal Radiol. 1997;26:505–6.
13. Kose O. The accessory ossicles of the foot and ankle; a diagnostic pitfall in emergency department in context of foot and ankle trauma/Ayak ve ayak bilegi cevresinde gorulen aksesuar kemikcikler; acil serviste ayak ve ayak bilegi travma hastalarinda tanisal tuzak. J Acad Emerg Med. 2012;11:106–15.
14. Kraft H. Assimilated accessory skeletal element of the foot (os sustentaculi) as cause for frequently recurring disorders. Arch Orthop Unfallchir. 1958;49:652.
15. Stormont DM, Peterson HA. The relative incidence of tarsal coalition. Clin Orthop Relat Res. 1983;181:28–36.
16. Taniguchi A, Tanaka Y, Kadono K, et al. C sign for diagnosis of talocalcaneal coalition. Radiology. 2003;228:501–5.
17. Lee JH, Jun JB, Lee HS, Yun HR, Choi CH, Park SB, Hong EK, Yoo DH, Kim SY. Posterior tibial neuropathy by a Baker's cyst: case report. Korean J Intern Med. 2000;15(1):96–8.
18. Cheung Y. Normal variants: accessory muscles about the ankle. Magn Reson Imaging Clin N Am. 2017;25(1):11–26. https://doi.org/10.1016/j.mric.2016.08.002.
19. Oh S, Meyer R. Entrapment neuropathies of the tibial nerve. Neurol Clin. 1999;17:593–615.
20. Alshalawi S, Galhoum AE, Alrashidi Y, et al. Medial ankle instability: the deltoid dilemma. Foot Ankle Clin. 2018;23(4):639–57. https://doi.org/10.1016/j.fcl.2018.07.008.
21. Mummenthaler M, Stöhr M, Müller-Vahl, editors. Läsion peripherer Nerven und radikuläre Syndrome. Stuttgart: Thieme Verlag; 2003.
22. Tackmann W, Richter HP, Stöhr M, editors. Kompressionssyndrome peripherer Nerven. Heidelberg: Springer; 1989.
23. Stødle AH, Molund M, Nilsen F, Hellund JC, Hvaal K. Tibial nerve palsy after lateralizing calcaneal osteotomy. Foot Ankle Spec. 2019;12(5):426–31. https://doi.org/10.1177/1938640018816363.
24. Willis AR, Samad AA, Prado GT, Gabisan GG. Heterotopic ossification and entrapment of the tibial nerve within the tarsal tunnel: a case report. J Foot Ankle Surg. 2016;55(5):1106–9. https://doi.org/10.1053/j.jfas.2016.01.032.

25. Cody EA, Greditzer HG, Macmahon A, Burket JC, Sofka CM, Ellis SJ. Effects on the tarsal tunnel following Malerba Z-type osteotomy compared to standard lateralizing calcaneal osteotomy. Foot Ankle Int. 2016;37(9):1017–22. https://doi.org/10.1177/1071100716651966.
26. Albert P, Patel J, Badawy K, Weissinger W, Brenner M, Bourhill I, Parnell J. Peripheral nerve schwannoma: a review of varying clinical presentations and imaging findings. J Foot Ankle Surg. 2017;56:632–7. https://doi.org/10.1053/j.jfas.2016.12.003.
27. Nawabi DH, Sinisi M. Schwannoma of the posterior tibial nerve: the problem of delay in diagnosis. J Bone Joint Surg Br. 2007;89-6:814–6. https://doi.org/10.1302/0301-620X.89B6.19077.
28. Hallahan K, Vinokur J, Demski S, Faulkner-Jones B, Giurini J. Tarsal tunnel syndrome secondary to schwannoma of the posterior tibial nerve. J Foot Ankle Surg. 2014;53-1:79–82. https://doi.org/10.1053/j.jfas.2012.12.020.
29. Moussa A, Chakhachiro Z, Sawaya RA. Posterior tibial nerve lymphoma presenting as tarsal tunnel syndrome: a case report. J Foot Ankle Surg. 2018;57(1):167–9. https://doi.org/10.1053/j.jfas.2017.07.004.
30. Spinner RJ, Hébert-Blouin M-N, Maniker AH, Amrami KK. Clock face model applied to tibial intraneural ganglia in the popliteal fossa. Skeletal Radiol. 2009;38(7):691–6.
31. Spinner RJ, Atkinson JL, Tiel RL. Peroneal intraneural ganglia: the importance of the articular branch. A unifying theory. J Neurosurg. 2003;99(2):330–43.
32. Spinner RJ, Amrami KK, Wolanskyj AP, et al. Dynamic phases of peroneal and tibial intraneural ganglia formation: a new dimension added to the unifying articular theory. J Neurosurg. 2007;107:296–307.
33. Kitsoulis P, Galani V, Stefanaki K, Paraskevas G, Karatzias G, Agnantis NJ, Bai M. Osteochondromas: review of the clinical, radiological and pathological features. In Vivo. 2008;22(5):633–46.
34. Herrera-Perez M, Aciego De Mendoza M, De Bergua-Domingo JM, Pais-Brito JL. Osteochondromas around the ankle: report of a case and literature review. Int J Surg Case Rep. 2013;4(11):1025–7.
35. Hirose CB, McGarvey WC. Anterior tarsal tunnel syndrome. Foot Ankle Clin N Am. 2004;9:255–69.
36. Chang MC, Yang S. Diabetic peripheral neuropathy essentials: a narrative review. Ann Palliat Med. 2023;12(2):390–8. https://doi.org/10.21037/apm-22-693. Epub 2023 Feb 8. PMID: 36786097.
37. Kanbe K, Kubota H, Shirakura K, Hasegawa A, Udagawa E. Entrapment neuropathy of the deep peroneal nerve associated with the extensor hallucis brevis. J Foot Ankle Surg. 1995;34(6):560–2. https://doi.org/10.1016/S1067-2516(09)80078-1. PMID: 8646207.
38. Kravette MA. Peripheral nerve entrapment syndromes in the foot. J Am Podiatry Assoc. 1971;61(12):457–72. https://doi.org/10.7547/87507315-61-12-457. PMID: 4330101.
39. Delgado-López PD, Rodríguez-Salazar A, Martín-Alonso J, Martín-Velasco V. Natural history, role of physical examination, timing of surgery, treatment options and conflicts of interests. Neurocirugia (Astur). 2017;28(3):124–34. Spanish. https://doi.org/10.1016/j.neucir.2016.11.004. Epub 2017 Jan 25. PMID: 28130015.
40. Mak MS, Chowdhury R, Johnson R. Morton's neuroma: review of anatomy, pathomechanism, and imaging. Clin Radiol. 2021;76(3):235.e15–23. https://doi.org/10.1016/j.crad.2020.10.006. Epub 2020 Nov 7. PMID: 33168237.
41. Ahmad M, Tsang K, Mackenney PJ, Adedapo AO. Tarsal tunnel syndrome: a literature review. Foot Ankle Surg. 2012;18(3):149–52. https://doi.org/10.1016/j.fas.2011.10.007. Epub 2011 Dec 21. PMID: 22857954.
42. Kinoshita M, Okuda R, Morikawa J. The dorsiflexion eversion test for diagnosis of tarsal tunnel syndrome. J Bone Joint Surg. 2001;83-A(12):1835–9.
43. McSweeney SC, Cichero M. Tarsal tunnel syndrome-a narrative literature review. Foot (Edinb). 2015;25(4):244–50. https://doi.org/10.1016/j.foot.2015.08.008. Epub 2015 Sep 12. PMID: 26546070.

44. Doneddu PE, Coraci D, Loreti C, Piccinini G, Padua L. Tarsal tunnel syndrome: still more opinions than evidence. Status of the art. Neurol Sci. 2017;38(10):1735–9. https://doi.org/10.1007/s10072-017-3039-x.
45. Trepman E, et al. Effect of foot and ankle position on tarsal tunnel compartment pressure. Foot Ankle Int. 1999;20(11):721–6.
46. Abouelela AA, Zohiery AK. The triple compression stress test for diagnosis of tarsal tunnel syndrome. Foot (Edinb). 2012;22(3):146–9. https://doi.org/10.1016/j.foot.2012.02.002. Epub 2012 Mar 8. PMID: 22405941.
47. Kerasnoudis A, Tsivgoulis G. Nerve ultrasound in peripheral neuropathies: a review. J Neuroimaging. 2015;25(4):528–38. https://doi.org/10.1111/jon.12261. Epub 2015 May 21. PMID: 25996962.
48. Therimadasamy A, et al. Combination of ultrasound and nerve conduction studies in the diagnosis of tarsal tunnel syndrome. Neurol India. 2011;59(2):296.
49. Lee M, et al. Tarsal tunnel syndrome caused by talocalcaneal coalition. Clin Imaging. 2002;26(2):140–3.
50. Alan USPD, Sendromu HTT. Tarsal tunnel syndrome in a patient on longterm peritoneal dialysis: case report. Turk Neurosurg. 2007;17(4):283–5.
51. Preston D, Shapiro B. Nerve conduction studies normal adults' values. In: 674 Electromyography and neuromuscular disorders. Clinical-electrophysiologic 675 correlations. 2nd ed. Philadelphia: Elsevier Butterworth Heineman; 2005.
52. McSweeney SC, Cichero M. Tarsal tunnel syndrome-a narrative literature review. Foot. 2015;25(4):244–50. https://doi.org/10.1016/j.foot.2015.08.00.
53. Crowe CS, Shin AY, Pulos N. Iatrogenic nerve injuries of the upper extremity: a critical analysis review. JBJS Rev. 2023;11(1):e22. https://doi.org/10.2106/JBJS.RVW.22.00161. PMID: 36722824.
54. Magalhães MJS, Ribeiro ICV, Cardoso MM, Gepp RA. Surgical treatment compared to conservative treatment in remission of pain and hyposthesia in tarsal tunnel syndrome – systematic review. Arq Bras Neurocir. 2022;41(2):e145–e152. https://doi.org/10.1055/s-0042-1742425.
55. Silveira CRS, Vieira CGM, Pereira BM, Pinto Neto LH, Chhabra A. Cystic degeneration of the tibial nerve: magnetic resonance neurography and sonography appearances of an intraneural ganglion cyst. Skeletal Radiol. 2017;46(12):1763–7.
56. Spinner RJ, Dellon AL, Rosson GD, Anderson SR, Amrami KK. Tibial intraneural ganglia in the tarsal tunnel: is there a joint connection? J Foot Ankle Surg. 2007;46(1):27–31.
57. Magalhães MJS, Pereira DVM, Oliva HNP, Durães DTS, Caiado FL, Araújo GM, Freitas Junior ETF. Peripheral nerve schwannomas: a literature review. Arq Bras Neurocir. 2019;38:308–14.
58. Yoshida A, Okutsu I, Hamanaka I. Endoscopic tarsal tunnel syndrome surgery using the universal subcutaneous endoscope system. Asia-Pac J Sport Med Arthrosc Rehabil Technol. 2016;3:1–5. https://doi.org/10.1016/j.asmart.2015.09.001.
59. Fernández-Gibello A, Moroni S, Camuñas G, et al. Ultrasound-guided decompression surgery of the tarsal tunnel: a novel technique for the proximal tarsal tunnel syndrome—part II. Surg Radiol Anat. 2019;41:43–51. https://doi.org/10.1007/s00276-018-2127-9.
60. Flores LP. Resultados do tratamento cirúrgico da síndrome do túnel do tarso posterior idiopática. Arq Bras Neurocir. 2005;24:144–50.
61. Krishnan GK, Pinzer T, Schackert G. A novel endoscopic technique in treating single nerve entrapment syndromes with special attention to ulnar nerve transposition and tarsal tunnel release: clinical application. Oper Neurosurgery. 2006;59:89–100.
62. Settanni FA, Leandro LM, Zuleta JA, Neri EA. Management of tarsaltunnel syndrome. Report of seven cases. Arq Neuropsiquiatr. 1994;52(04):530–4.
63. Sammarco GJ, Chang L. Outcome of surgical treatment of tarsal tunnel syndrome. Foot Ankle Int. 2003;24(02):125–31.
64. Kavlak Y, Uygur F. Effects of nerve mobilization exercise as an adjunct to the conservative treatment for patients with tarsal tunnel syndrome. J Manip Physiol Ther. 2011;34(07):441–8.

65. Baba H, Wada M, Annen S, Azuchi M, Imura S, Tomita K. The tarsaltunnel syndrome: evaluation of surgical results using multivariate analysis. Int Orthop. 1997;21(02):68–71 (SICOT).
66. Pfeiffer WH, Cracchiolo A III. Clinical results after tarsal tunnel decompression. J Bone Joint Surg Am. 1994;76(08):1222–30.
67. Skalley TC, Schon LC, Hinton RY, Myerson MS. Clinical results following revision tibial nerve release. Foot Ankle Int. 1994;15:360–7.
68. Antoniadis G, Scheglmann K. Posterior tarsal tunnel syndrome: diagnosis and treatment. Dtsch Arztebl Int. 2008;105(45):776–81. https://doi.org/10.3238/arztebl.2008.0776.
69. Lau J, Daniels T. The effects of tarsal tunnel release and stabilization procedures on tibial nerve tension in a surgically created pes planus foot. Foot Ankle Int. 1998;19:770–7.

Chapter 10
General Aspects of Meralgia Paresthetica

10.1 Introduction

Meralgia paresthetica (MP) is the neuropathy resulting from the impairment of the lateral femoral cutaneous nerve (LFCN) that presents symptoms such as neuropathic pain, paresthesia, and dysesthesia in the lateral region of the thigh.

This syndrome was initially described in the 1880s independently by two authors, Bernhardt and Roth. The term meralgia was first coined by Roth, whose words *meros* and *algos* mean in Greek thigh and pain, respectively [1].

Regarding its epidemiological characteristics, MP can occur at any time in life; however, this syndrome is most commonly manifested in the fifth decade of life. It is a neuropathy that tends to occur more in males and be unilateral [1, 2].

The diagnosis of this disease is typically made from the neurological clinical examination and the patient's clinical history, associated with electroneuromyography (ENM) and imaging exams. The treatment is usually carried out conservatively, and surgical treatment is reserved for cases where symptoms persisted, despite the implementation of conservative treatment [1].

The aim of this chapter is to discuss the epidemiology, pathophysiology, signs, symptoms, and exams of MP.

10.2 Anatomy of the Lateral Femoral Cutaneous Nerve

This is a purely sensory nerve originating from fibers coming from the posterior division of the spinal nerves L2 and L3 of the lumbar plexus. It provides sensory innervation to the anterior and lateral portion of the thigh (Fig. 10.1).

It follows a path that begins inside the pelvis, in the retroperitoneum, and ends its course after reaching the lateral region of the thigh [3].

M. J. S. Magalhães, *Lower Extremity Nerve Entrapments*,
https://doi.org/10.1007/978-3-031-90058-7_10

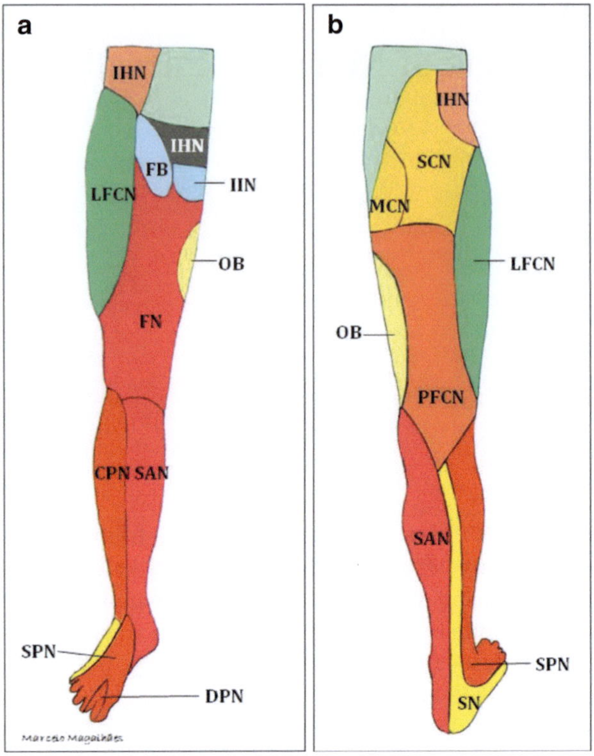

Fig. 10.1 Anterior and posterior view of the sensory territories of the main nerves of the lower limb. Note in dark green the skin area innervated by the LFCN. *CPN* = common peroneal nerve, *DPN* = deep peroneal nerve, *FB* = femoral branch- genitofemoral nerve, *FN* = femoral nerve, *IHN* = iliohypogastric nerve, *IIL* = ilioinguinal nerve, *LFCN* = lateral femoral cutaneous nerve, *MCN* = medial cluneal nerve, *OB* = obturator nerve, *SAN* = saphenous nerve, *SCN* = superior cluneal nerve, *SPN* = superficial peroneal nerve, *SN* = sural nerve. * The area of the ilioinguinal nerve also has sensory branches from the genital branch of the genitofemoral nerve

Inside the pelvis, the LFCN emerges on the lateral edge of the psoas major muscle, shortly after its formation, and follows an infero-lateral path over this same muscle. On this path over the psoas major muscle, the nerve is located between the two layers of the superficial iliac fascia [4]. At a more distal point in the pelvis, the LFCN is crossed by the deep circumflex iliac vessels, and after crossing the aponeuroticofascial tunnel, also known as the iliopubic tract, it reaches the inguinal ligament (IL) [5]. After passing the IL, this nerve leaves the pelvis and reaches the lateral portion of the thigh.

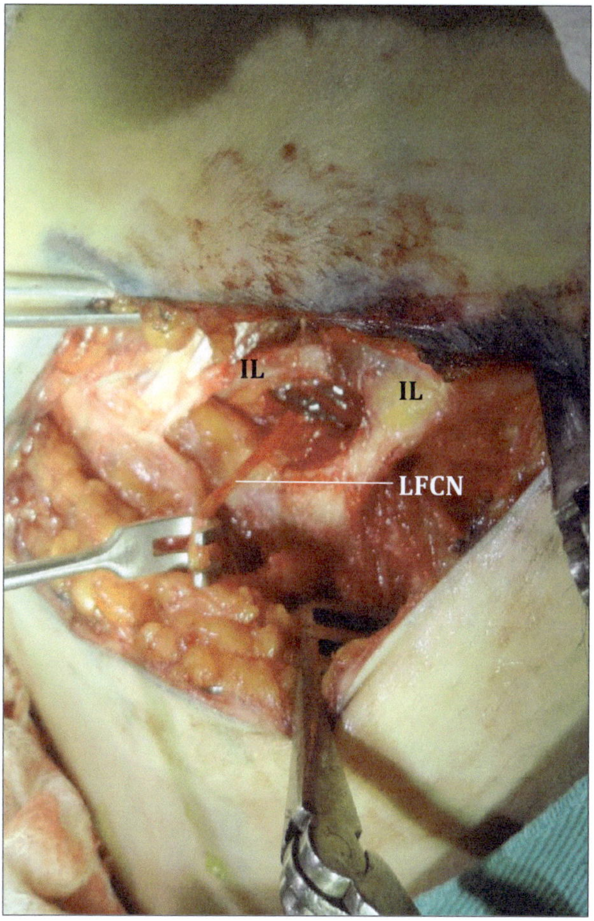

Fig. 10.2 Lateral femoral cutaneous nerve in the right lower limb. *IL* = inguinal ligament. *LFCN* = lateral cutaneous femoral nerve

According to Siqueira MG et al., the LFCN is easily identifiable between 5 and 25 mm medial to the anterior superior iliac spine (ASIS) [6]. The authors Tomaszewski et al. (2016) in their review of the literature mention that the nerve is identified 19 mm medial to the ASIS [3], and Grothaus et al. (2005) describe that this distance varies between 6 and 73 mm [5].

After leaving the inguinal ligament, the LFCN follows a path under the fascia lata that crosses over or through the fibers of the sartorius muscle. After passing the sartorius muscle, the nerve divides into anterior and posterior branches. Both branches pierce the fascia lata to reach the subcutaneous plane (Figs. 10.2, 10.3, and 10.4).

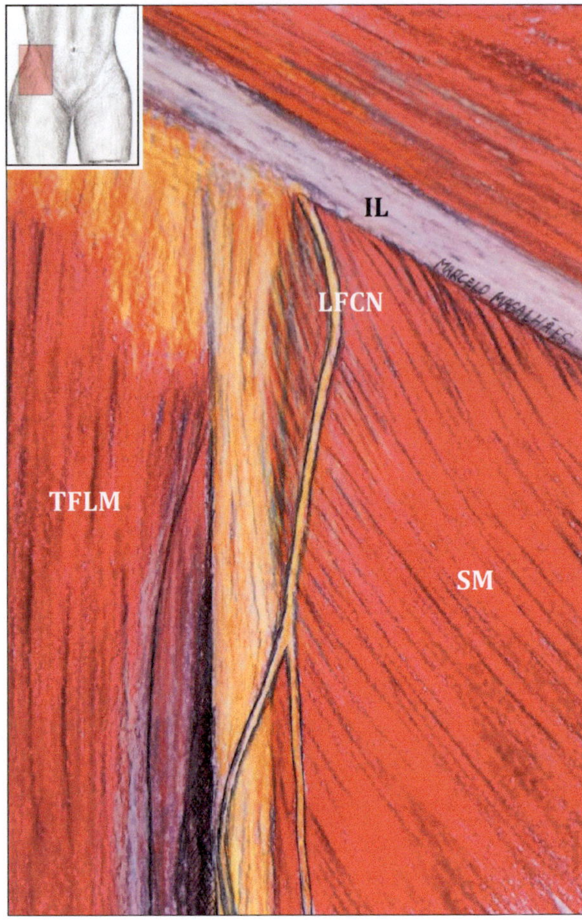

Fig. 10.3 Lateral femoral cutaneous nerve in the right lower limb. *IL* = inguinal ligament, *LFCN* = lateral cutaneous femoral nerve, *SM* = sartorius muscle, *TFLM* = tensor fascia lata muscle

10.2.1 Anatomical Variations of the LFCN

The authors Aszmann et al. (1997) described at least five anatomical variations of the course of the LFCN in the vicinity of the ASIS. Three of these anatomical variations are more susceptible to compressive processes for the development of MP [7, 8].

Type A: In 4% of cases, the LFCN follows a path posterior to the ASIS.
Type B: In 27% of cases, the LFCN follows a path anterior to the ASIS, superficial to the sartorius muscle (SM), however, within the fibers of the IL.
Type C: Makes up 23% of all cases. The LFCN follows a path anterior to the ASIS and is enveloped by the tendinous origin of the SM.

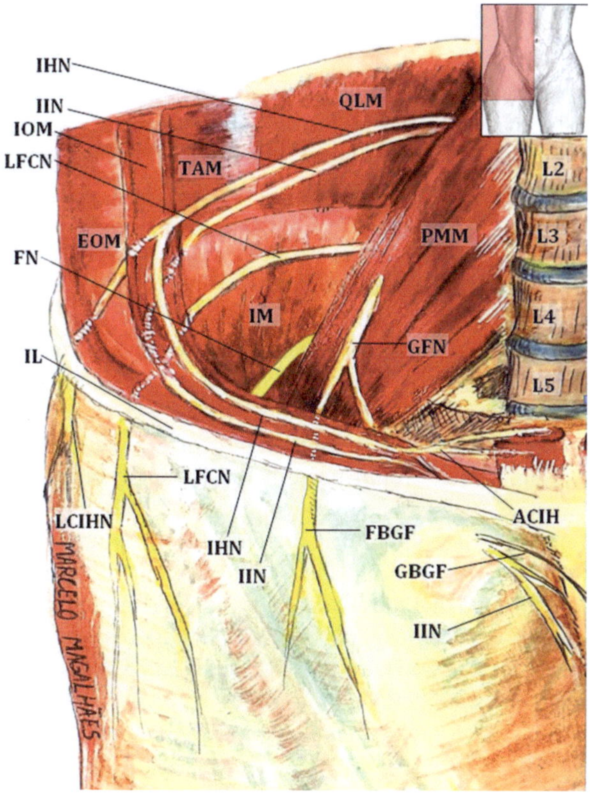

Fig. 10.4 Anatomy of the main nerves of the inguinal region and anterior region of the thigh. *ACIH* = anterior cutaneous branch of iliohypogastric nerve, *AEOM* = abdominal external oblique muscle, *AIOM* = abdominal internal oblique muscle, *FBGN* = femoral branch of genitofemoral nerve, *FN* = femoral nerve, *GBGF* = genital branch of genitofemoral nerve, *GFN* = genitofemoral nerve, *IHN* = iliohypogastric nerve, *IIN* = ilioinguinal nerve, *IL* = inguinal ligament, *IM* = iliacus muscle, *LCIH* = lateral cutaneous branch of iliohypogastric nerve, *LFCN* = lateral femoral cutaneous nerve, *PMM* = psoas major muscle, *QLM* = quadratus lumborum muscle, *TAM* = transverse abdominal muscle

Type D: Responsible for 26% of cases. In this subtype, the LFCN is positioned medial to the origin of the SM, in the interval between the tendon of the SM and the thick fascia of the iliopsoas muscle, deep to the IL.

Type E: 20% of cases correspond to this anatomical variation. The LFCN is positioned more medially, in a loose tissue, deep to the IL, over the fascia of the iliopsoas muscle with branches that contribute to the formation of the femoral nerve and genitofemoral nerve.

10.3 Symptoms of MP

Patients with MP may develop symptoms manifested in the region of the skin innervated by the LFCN, which corresponds to the anterolateral and lateral portion of the thigh. In 73% of cases, the symptoms of MP occur on the lateral part of the thigh and in 26% in the anterior region [9].

A study involving a large number of patients showed no tendency for this neuropathy to occur on a specific side [9].

The most commonly identified complaints include pain, burning, vibration sensation (like the vibration of a cell phone), cold sensation, and paresthesias. The pain, when present, can be mild, with spontaneous resolution, or it can be of great intensity, persisting over time [10]. The symptoms of MP tend to intensify when the patient walks or remains in orthostatism and relieve when the patient sits. Hypothetically, the tension of the inguinal ligament is reduced when the patient is in a seated position, which would explain the relief of symptoms in this position [11].

The symptoms can vary greatly in their duration. Symptoms that persist for 15 days are described; on the other hand, periods as long as 20 years are described in the literature. It is noted that the average duration of symptoms is 34 months [11].

Regarding the persistence of symptoms, 36% of patients with MP report that the symptoms persisted for a period between 12 months and 5 years [11]. Between 10% and 18% of patients have bilateral symptoms [9, 12, 13].

In cases where MP occurred as a result of surgical iatrogenesis, the symptoms set in within the first 12 hours of surgery in 92% of cases [12, 14].

10.4 Differential Diagnosis of MP

Various diseases can progress with pain, paresthesia, and hypoesthesia in the anterolateral region of the thigh, such as radiculopathy resulting from lumbar disc herniation and lumbar stenosis. Trummer et al. (2000) described the case report of a 67-year-old female patient, with a case of disc herniation at the L2/L3 level that caused L3 radiculopathy mimicking the symptoms of MP. The patient's treatment was performed through microsurgery via lateral transmuscular approach, which showed good control of the symptoms [14].

10.5 Pathophysiology of MP

In most cases of MP, the compression point of the LFCN occurs at the level of the IL; however, compressions of this nerve at a point proximal to this ligament are described in the medical literature.

Tumors located in the abdominal region, pelvis, lower limb, and spine have been described as the cause of MP in numerous case reports [15–25].

The histopathological study of the nerve in patients with this disease shows internodal changes in the LFCN, such as edema, as well as vascular thickening and perineural thickening [25]. These changes suggest a mechanism of focal demyelination and Wallerian degeneration [26].

Ruiter et al. (2018) performed the histopathological study of 39 patients undergoing surgery for the treatment of MP, with 10 patients reporting failure of pain control after initial neurolysis and 29 patients in which the initial surgery was neurectomy of the LFCN [27]. These authors showed that the histopathological findings did not reveal changes in the thickness of the perineurium, collagen percentage, and mucoid material percentage between patients with >1 year and those with <1 year of MP symptoms [27]. Another point of interest in this study was the absence of a typical intraneural finding in the histopathological examination at the compression point [27]. This suggests that MP is a dynamic disease from the point of view of the compressive process [27].

10.6 Risk Factors for Meralgia Paresthetica

Numerous risk factors have been described in the literature: pregnancy, diabetes mellitus (DM), obesity with a body mass index (BMI) $\geq$ 30, Hansen's disease, acquired immunodeficiency syndrome, iatrogenesis, long periods in the prone position, direct local trauma, toxins (alcohol, lead), intra-abdominal and lower limb tumors, tight clothing such as police uniforms, and belt use [26, 28–41].

Ramírez Huaranga et al. (2013) described a renal tumor as the cause of MP [15]. Magalhães et al. (2019) identified a bone tumor in the pelvis, adjacent to the CIAS as the cause of MP [16].

Arabi et al. (2015) published a case report in which a 50-year-old male patient presented with MP resulting from intradural schwannoma at the level of L2 that evolved with symptom control after its resection [17].

Rau et al. (2010) described a case report in which a 50-year-old woman presented with pain in the right lower limb whose etiology was associated with the presence of a lipoma located on the sartorius muscle. The patient underwent resection of the lesion, evolving with complete symptom control [18]. Makris et al. (2002) published a case report of a 67-year-old man, with LFCN schwannoma. The symptoms were controlled after tumor resection; however, this control occurred progressively over a period of three months [19].

Non-tumoral diseases located in the abdominal region have also been described as the etiology of MP. Noh et al. (2015) described a case report in which the pancreatic pseudocyst was involved as the cause of MP [20]. Kodama et al. (2015) described a case report of a 7-year-old girl, with a clinical picture of acute appendicitis associated with leukemia, who during the chemotherapy period developed symptoms of MP. There was symptom control only with antibiotic therapy [21].

Among the vascular diseases associated with MP is angiomyomatosis. Yamamoto et al. (2001) published a case report of a 15-year-old male patient, with a clinical picture of pelvic hemangiomatosis as the cause of MP. The patient underwent LFCN neurolysis and partial excision of pelvic hemangiomatosis, obtaining control of the painful symptoms [22].

MP has also been associated with pregnancy or the childbirth process. Chung et al. (2010) described a case report in which a patient 29 years old, two days after a cesarean delivery, evolved with MP [23]. Sax et al. (2006) also mention the association between the pregnancy and MP, commenting that in general, there is spontaneous regression of the disease [24].

Patients who remain in the prone position for lumbar or thoracic laminectomy are at greater risk of developing postoperative MP, especially if they have a high BMI and if the surgery lasts longer than 3.5 hours [42–44]. Gupta et al. showed that the incidence of MP in 110 patients who underwent lumbar surgery with posterior approach was 12% [13, 45]. In addition to spine surgery, MP is described as a complication resulting from gynecological obstetric surgery, endoscopic laparoscopy, cesarean delivery, and bone grafting from the ASIS [46–49].

MP is also described after hip arthroplasty surgeries. Goulding et al. mention that out of 132 patients who underwent two different hip arthroplasty techniques ($N = 55$), anterior total hip arthroplasty, and ($N = 77$) hip resurfacing, 107 (81%) developed MP [50].

10.7 Physical Examination and Semiological Maneuvers

10.7.1 Pelvic Compression Test

Pelvic compression test is a maneuver described by Nouraei et al. (2007), which consists of applying compression to the patient's pelvis when they are in a lateral decubitus position with the affected side positioned upwards. The examiner should maintain the compression for 45 seconds. If there is relief from pain located in the anterolateral region, the test is considered positive [51]. According to these same authors, the sensitivity of the test is 95% and the specificity 93.3%.

Another semiological sign performed for the investigation of MP is the Tinel sign over the LFCN. Parmar et al. (2003) reported their clinical experience in investigating the symptoms of MP through percussion of the LFCN, when the nerve leaves the IL [52]. However, there are no clinical studies that have made a comparison between a positive Tinel sign and ENM exams of the affected limb.

10.7.2 Nerve Block Test with Anesthetic

Another possibility for diagnosing MP is performing an anesthetic block, with 1% lidocaine in the subcutaneous plane, in the vicinity of the LFCN, when this nerve leaves the IL. The infiltration point is located approximately 1 cm medial and inferior to the ASIS. The test is considered positive if the patient has symptom control for about 30 minutes [10, 36].

10.8 Additional Tests

10.8.1 Ultrasound in MP

Ultrasound (US) can be a tool that assists in the diagnosis of MP. One measure used is the cross-sectional area of the LFCN near the ASIS. Powell et al. (2020) published that the expected area of the LFCN for healthy patients is 3 mm^2 and patients with MP 9 mm^2 (standard deviation of ± 2.3 mm^2) [53, 54]. On the other hand, Suh et al. (2013) state that the cross-sectional area of the LFCN is 11 mm^2 [55]. Despite these cited values, Powell et al. (2020) mention that 30% of patients with suspected MP do not show changes in the US of the LFCN.

The US can also reveal signs associated with a compressive process, such as the presence of fibrotic tissue surrounding the nerve, in addition to the change in its caliber [53]. The authors Mallouhi et al. (2006) state that with the advent of 18 MHz US, it was possible to identify other changes suggestive of a compressive process, such as indistinguishable perineurium, which results in a hypoechoic appearance and increased intraneural vascularization [56].

Finally, the US also assists in identifying regional diseases that may be the etiology of MP, such as lipomas and schwannomas [18].

10.8.2 Magnetic Resonance Neurography of the LFCN

Chhbra et al. (2013) conducted a controlled study that evaluated the diagnostic accuracy of MR neurography (MRN) for the investigation of MP. This study utilized a 3-tesla magnetic resonance imaging (MRI) scanner. A total of 28 patients were included as the control group, while 11 patients with MP constituted the intervention group. The MRN demonstrated a diagnostic accuracy of 90% or higher, enabling the detection of neuromas and signal alterations in the LFCN structure [57].

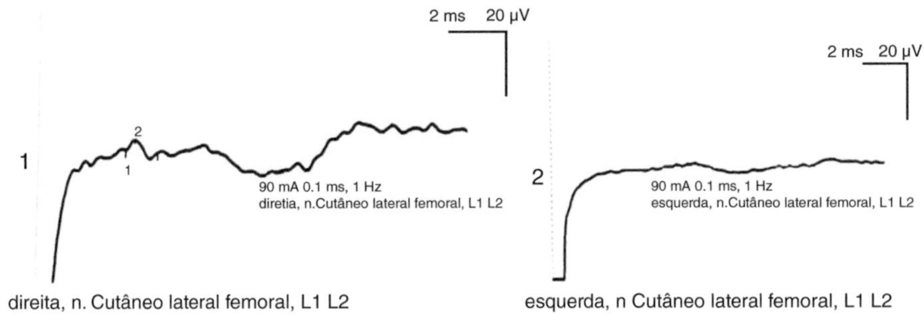

Fig. 10.5 Electroneuromyography of the lower limbs revealing involvement of the left LFCN in a patient with MP, where the diagnosis was previously confirmed by anesthetic block. Note the absence of sensory nerve action potential in the graph on the right

10.8.3 Electroneuromyography of the Lower Limbs

The ENM exam in general is difficult to perform due to the small nerve caliber. This study may reveal that the orthodromic conduction of the LFCN presents a unilaterally abnormal sensory nerve action potential (SNAP). The ss amplitude ratio with a value greater than 2.3 has a specificity of 98.3% for the diagnosis of MP and the amplitude of the SNAP less than 3 μVolts specificity of 73.5% [9] (Fig. 10.5).

10.9 Conclusion

MP is a neuropathy resulting from the impairment of the LFCN, characterized by neuropathic pain, paresthesia, and dysesthesia in the lateral thigh region. Its diagnosis is essentially clinical, but it can be confirmed through tests such as ENM and US. Conservative treatment is the initial approach, with surgery reserved for refractory cases.

The anatomy of the LFCN reveals a complex course with anatomical variations that may predispose to nerve compression and the subsequent development of MP. Symptoms vary in intensity and duration, sometimes persisting for years in some patients.

Different conditions, such as lumbar radiculopathies, tumors, and iatrogenic compressions, must be considered in the differential diagnosis. The pathophysiology of MP involves compression and histopathological changes in the LFCN, potentially leading to focal demyelination and Wallerian degeneration.

Various risk factors, including DM, obesity, pregnancy, and tight clothing, are associated with MP development. Physical examination, including specific tests such as the pelvic compression test and anesthetic nerve block, assists in diagnosis.

Complementary exams, such as US and ENM, can confirm the diagnosis and guide therapeutic management.

Despite its benign nature, MP can significantly impact patients' quality of life, making accurate diagnosis and appropriate therapeutic approaches essential.

References

1. Gomez YC, Remotti E, Momah DU, Zhang E, Swanson DD, Kim R, Urits I, Kaye AD, Robinson CL. Meralgia Paresthetica review: update on presentation, pathophysiology, and treatment. Health Psychol Res. 2023;11:71454.
2. Madiraca Glasović D, Šlaus N, Šitum M, Poćina M. Meralgia Paresthetica – lateral femoral cutaneous nerve entrapment. Rad Hrvatske akademije znanosti i umjetnosti Medicinske znanosti. 2021;54–55:56–63.
3. Tomaszewski KA, Popieluszko P, Henry BM, et al. The surgical anatomy of the lateral femoral cutaneous nerve in the inguinal region: a meta-analysis. Hernia. 2016;20:649–57. https://doi.org/10.1007/s10029-016-1493-7.
4. Dias Filho LC, Valença MM, Guimarães Filho FAV, et al. Lateral femoral cutaneous neuralgia: an anatomical insight. Clin Anat. 2003;16:309–16. https://doi.org/10.1002/ca.10106.
5. Grothaus MC, Holt M, Mekhail AO, Ebraheim NA, Yeasting RA. Lateral femoral cutaneous nerve: an anatomic study. Clin Orthop Relat Res. 2005;437:164–8. https://doi.org/10.1097/01.blo.0000164526.08610.97.
6. Siqueira MG, Martins RS. Anatomia cirúrgica das vias de acesso aos nervos periféricos. (Portuguese version) Ed. Dilivros, Brasil 2005.
7. Aszmann OC, Dellon ES, Dellon AL. Anatomical course of the lateral femoral cutaneous nerve and its susceptibility to compression and injury. Plast Reconstr Surg. 1997;100(3):600–4.
8. Swezey E, Bordoni B. Anatomy, bony pelvis and lower limb: lateral femoral cutaneous nerve. 2023. In: StatPearls [Internet]. Treasure Island: StatPearls Publishing; 2024.
9. Seror P, Seror R. Meralgia paresthetica: clinical and electrophysiological diagnosis in 120 cases. Muscle Nerve. 2006;33(5):650–4.
10. Grossman MG, Ducey SA, Nadler SS, et al. Meralgia paresthetica: diagnosis and treatment. J Am Acad Orthop Surg. 2001;9(5):336–44.
11. Cheatham SW, Kolber MJ, Salamh PA. Meralgia paresthetica: a review of the literature. Int J Sports Phys Ther. 2013;8(6):883–93.
12. Zhou L, Siao P. Lateral femoral cutaneous neuropathy caused by prone positioning to treat COVID-19-associated acute respiratory distress syndrome. Muscle Nerve. 2021;63(6):E50–2.
13. Ecker AD. Diagnosis of Meralgia Paresthetica. JAMA. 1985;253(7):976.
14. Trummer M, Flaschka G, Unger F, Eustacchio S. Lumbar disc herniation mimicking meralgia paresthetica: case report. Surg Neurol. 2000 Jul;54(1):80–1.
15. Ramírez Huaranga MA, Ariza Hernández A, Ramos Rodríguez CC, González García J. What meralgia paresthetica can hide: renal tumor as an infrequent cause. Reumatol Clin. 2013;9(5):319–21.
16. Magalhães LVB, Massardi FR, Pereira SAC. Pelvic osteochondroma causing meralgia paresthetica. Neurol India. 2019;67(3):928–9.
17. Arabi H, Khalfaoui S, El Bouchti I, Rokhsi R, Benhima MA, Saidi H, Elktaibi A. Meralgia paresthetica with lumbar neurinoma: case report. Ann Phys Rehabil Med. 2015;58(6):359–61.
18. Rau CS, Hsieh CH, Liu YW, Wang LY, Cheng MH. Meralgia paresthetica secondary to lipoma. J Neurosurg Spine. 2010;12(1):103–5.
19. Makris AP, Makris D. Schwannoma of the lateral femoral cutaneous nerve, an unusual cause of Meralgia Paresthetica: a case report. J Orthop Case Rep. 2020;10(8):80–3.

20. Noh KH, Kim DS, Shin JH. Meralgia paresthetica caused by a pancreatic pseudocyst. Muscle Nerve. 2015;52(4):684–5.
21. Nishimura M, Kodama Y, Fukano R, Okamura J, Ogaki K, Sakaguchi Y, Migita M, Inagaki J. Meralgia Paresthetica as a presentation of acute appendicitis in a girl with acute lymphoblastic leukemia. J Pediatr Hematol Oncol. 2015;37(3):e182–3.
22. Yamamoto T, Kurosaka M, Marui T, Mizuno K. Hemangiomatosis presenting as meralgia paresthetica. J Pediatr Surg. 2001;36(3):518–20.
23. Chung KH, Lee JY, Ko TK, Park CH, Chun DH, Yang HJ, Gill HJ, Kim MK. Meralgia paresthetica affecting parturient women who underwent cesarean section – a case report. Korean J Anesthesiol. 2010;59 Suppl(Suppl):S86–9.
24. Sax TW, Rosenbaum RB. Neuromuscular disorders in pregnancy. Muscle Nerve. 2006;34(5):559–71.
25. Payne RA, Harbaugh K, Specht CS, Rizk E. Correlation of histopathology and clinical symptoms in Meralgia Paresthetica. Cureus. 2017;9(10):e1789.
26. Harney D, Patijn J. Meralgia paresthetica: Diagnosis and management strategies. Pain Med. 2007;8(8):669–77.
27. Ruiter GCW, Lim J, Thomassen BJW, van Duinen SG. Histopathologic changes inside the lateral femoral cutaneous nerve obtained from patients with persistent symptoms of meralgia paresthetica. Acta Neurochir. 2019;161(2):263–9.
28. Khalil N, Nicotra A, Rakowicz W. Treatment for meralgia paraesthetica. Cochrane Database Syst Rev. 2012;12:CD004159.
29. Glasović DM, Šlaus N, Šitum M, Pećina M. Review article RAD 547. Med Sci. 2021;547:54–5.
30. Yoshida S, Oya S, Matsui T. Risk factors of meralgia paresthetica after prone position surgery: possible influence of operating position, laminectomy level, and preoperative thoracic kyphosis. J Clin Neurosci. 2021;89:163–7.
31. Parisi TJ, Mandrekar J, Dyck PJ, et al. Meralgia paresthetica: relation to obesity, advanced age, and diabetes mellitus. Neurology. 2011;77(16):1538–42.
32. Beresford HR. Meralgia paresthetica after seat-belt trauma. J Trauma. 1971;11(7):629–30.
33. Blake SM, Treble NJ. Meralgia paraesthetica–an addition to 'seatbelt syndrome'. Ann R Coll Surg Engl. 2004;86(6):W6–7.
34. Fargo MV, Konitzer LN. Meralgia paresthetica due to body armor wear in U.S. soldiers serving in Iraq: a case report and review of the literature. Mil Med. 2007;172(6):663–5.
35. Goel A. Meralgia paresthetica secondary to limb length discrepancy: case report. Arch Phys Med Rehabil. 1999;80(3):348–9.
36. Haim A, Pritsch T, Ben-Galim P, et al. Meralgia paresthetica: a retrospective analysis of 79 patients evaluated and treated according to a standard algorithm. Acta Orthop. 2006;77(3):482–6.
37. Jiang GX, Xu WD, Wang AH. Spinal stenosis with meralgia paraesthetica. J Bone Joint Surg Br. 1988;70(2):272–3.
38. Korkmaz N, Ozcakar L. Meralgia paresthetica in a policeman: the belt or the gun. Plast Reconstr Surg. 2004;114(4):1012–3.
39. Mondelli M, Rossi S, Romano C. Body mass index in meralgia paresthetica: a case-control study. Acta Neurol Scand. 2007;116(2):118–23.
40. Moscona AR, Sekel R. Post-traumatic meralgia paresthetica–an unusual presentation. J Trauma. 1978;18(4):288.
41. Park JW, Kim DH, Hwang M, et al. Meralgia paresthetica caused by hip-huggers in a patient with aberrant course of the lateral femoral cutaneous nerve. Muscle Nerve. 2007;35(5):678–80.
42. Yang SH, Wu CC, Chen PQ. Postoperative Meralgia Paresthetica after posterior spine surgery: incidence, risk factors, and clinical outcomes. Spine (Phila Pa 1976). 2005;30(4).
43. Ercan S, Ataizi ZS, Ertilav K. The correlation of Meralgia Paresthetica and spinal surgery in prone position. Turk Neurosurg. 2020;30:89–93.

44. Yoshida S, Oya S, Matsui T. Risk factors of meralgia paresthetica after prone position surgery: possible influence of operating position, laminectomy level, and preoperative thoracic kyphosis. J Clin Neurosci. 2021;89:292–6.
45. Gupta A, Muzumdar D, Ramani PS. Meralgia paraesthetica following lumbar spine surgery: a study in 110 consecutive surgically treated cases. Neurol India. 2004;52:66.
46. Yamamoto T, Nagira K, Kurosaka M. Meralgia paresthetica occurring 40 years after iliac bone graft harvesting: case report. Neurosurgery. 2001;49(6):1455–7.
47. Kavanagh D, Connolly S, Fleming F, et al. Meralgia paraesthetica following open appendicectomy. Ir Med J. 2005;98(6):183–5.
48. Polidori L, Magarelli M, Tramutoli R. Meralgia paresthetica as a complication of laparoscopic appendectomy. Surg Endosc. 2003;17(5):832.
49. Paul F, Zipp F. Bilateral meralgia paresthetica after cesarian section with epidural analgesia. J Peripher Nerv Syst. 2006;11(1):98–9.
50. Goulding K, Beaule PE, Kim PR, et al. Incidence of lateral femoral cutaneous nerve neuropraxia after anterior approach hip arthroplasty. Clin Orthop Relat Res. 2010;468(9):2397–404.
51. Nouraei SA, Anand B, Spink G, et al. A novel approach to the diagnosis and management of meralgia paresthetica. Neurosurgery. 2007;60(4):696–700.
52. Parmar MS. Hiphuggers' tingly thighs. CMAJ. 2003;168(1):16.
53. Shi X, Liu F, Liu F, Chen Z, Zhu J. Sonographic features of the lateral femoral cutaneous nerve in meralgia paresthetica. Quant Imaging Med Surg. 2021;11(10):4269–74.
54. Powell GM, Baffour FI, Erie AJ, Puffer RC, Spinner RJ, Glazebrook KN. Sonographic evaluation of the lateral femoral cutaneous nerve in meralgia paresthetica. Skeletal Radiol. 2020;49:1135–40.
55. Suh DH, Kim DH, Park JW, Park BK. Sonographic and electrophysiologic findings in patients with meralgia paresthetica. Clin Neurophysiol. 2013;124:1460–4.
56. Mallouhi A, Pülzl P, Trieb T, Piza H, Bodner G. Predictors of carpal tunnel syndrome: accuracy of gray-scale and color Doppler sonography. AJR Am J Roentgenol. 2006;186:1240–5.
57. Chhabra A, Del Grande F, Soldatos T, et al. Meralgia paresthetica: 3-Tesla magnetic resonance neurography. Skeletal Radiol. 2013;42:803–8.

Chapter 11
Management of Meralgia Paresthetica

11.1 Introduction

Meralgia paresthetica (MP) is the disease resulting from the impairment of the lateral femoral cutaneous nerve (LFCN) in which the most commonly identified symptoms are neuropathic pain, paresthesia, dysesthesia in the lateral region of the thigh.

This syndrome was initially described in the 1880s independently, by two authors, Bernhardt and Roth. The term meralgia was coined initially by Roth, whose words *meros* and *algos* mean in Greek thigh and pain, respectively [1, 2].

Regarding its epidemiological characteristics, MP can occur at any time of life; however, this syndrome manifests more commonly in the 5th decade of life. It is a neuropathy that tends to occur more in males and be unilateral [1, 2].

The diagnosis is typically made from the neurological clinical examination and the clinical history of the patient associated with electroneuromyography (ENM) and imaging exams. The treatment is usually performed conservatively and surgical treatment is reserved only for cases where symptoms persisted, despite the conservative treatment [1].

The objective of this chapter is to discuss the conservative and surgical management of patients diagnosed with MP.

Supplementary Information The online version contains supplementary material available at https://doi.org/10.1007/978-3-031-90058-7_11.

M. J. S. Magalhães, *Lower Extremity Nerve Entrapments*,
https://doi.org/10.1007/978-3-031-90058-7_11

11.2 Treatment of the Patient with MP

11.2.1 Natural Course of the Disease

Little is known about the natural evolution of patients with MP. What is known is based on a few available studies. There is an observational study conducted in 1938 by Ecker et al. (1938) involving 29 patients, in which 18 of them (62%) evolved with spontaneous improvement [3]. Another study addressing the same theme, conducted by researchers Chhuttani et al. (1966), involved 115 patients with MP and revealed that 16 patients (27%) evolved with symptom control and 18 (30%) with persistent symptoms. In this study, there was a loss of follow-up of 55 patients (48%), which compromised its result [4].

11.2.2 Conservative Treatment of the Patient with MP

Several studies cite the use of various medications for the conservative treatment of the sensation of paresthesia, pain, and burning in patients with MP. Medication treatment should be the first option for the management of these patients [4–8].

Evaluating the systematic review of Kalil et al. (2012), it is possible to identify different medication options for the treatment of these patients. These include nonsteroidal anti-inflammatory drugs (NSAIDs), amitriptyline, carbamazepine, phenytoin, as well as the use of local ice for symptom control [4–8]. The implementation of physiotherapy as a form of MP treatment has also been described in medical literature [9].

The rates of refractoriness of pain control with the use of medications revolve around 10 to 15% of patients [9, 10].

11.3 Minimally Invasive Treatment of the Patient with MP

11.3.1 Pulsed Radiofrequency

Pulsed radiofrequency (PRF) is a minimally invasive option for the treatment of patients with MP. The electrocardiogram monitor and blood pressure monitor should be available during the procedure. The technique consists of positioning the patient in supine position, with the affected limb slightly externally rotated. The area that should be subjected to asepsis includes the skin between the umbilical scar and the proximal third of the thigh. It consists of locating the LFCN near the anterior superior iliac spine (ASIS) through stimulation 50 Hz, with voltage between 0.3 and 0.5 V. If the electrode is positioned correctly, the patient will present pain in the territory innervated by the NCFL. The voltage should reach the value of 2 V with the aim of excluding motor activity. Remember that not far from the LFCN is the femoral nerve. Once the LFCN is identified, the lesion by radiofrequency is performed with a voltage of 45 V, reaching the temperature of 42 °C for a period of 2 minutes [9, 10].

11.3.2 Extended Pulsed Radiofrequency

Another technique cited in the literature for the treatment of patients with MP is extended pulsed radiofrequency (EPRF) [11]. However, it is little used and described in the literature. Mishra et al. (2020) described a case report of a 38-year-old male patient, who was initially subjected to conservative treatment with medication and later, with pulsed radiofrequency. As symptoms returned after two months, extended pulsed radiofrequency was chosen, which showed pain control, even after six months of treatment [10]. Ghai et al. (2018) described a series of cases where EPRF was used for the treatment of MP [12]. It is important to note that this technique is already used for the treatment of other neuropathies and the targets are the trigeminal ganglion, trigeminal nerve, and the geniculate nerve [13, 14].

The electrocardiogram monitor and blood pressure monitor should be available during the procedure. The technique consists of positioning the patient in supine position, with the affected limb slightly externally rotated. The area that should be subjected to asepsis includes the skin between the umbilical scar and the proximal third of the thigh. The technique initially consists of locating the LFCN near the ASIS, through 50 Hz stimulation with voltage between 0.3 and 0.5 V. If the electrode is correctly positioned through physical contact with the LFCN, the patient will present pain in the anterolateral portion of the thigh. The voltage should reach the value of 2 V with the aim of excluding motor activity. Remember that not far from the LFCN is the femoral nerve. Once the nerve is identified, the radiofrequency lesion is performed at a maximum temperature of 42 °C with an approximate duration of 8 minutes [10].

11.3.3 LFCN Neurolysis by Alcoholization

Among other possible minimally invasive techniques for the treatment of MP is neurolysis by alcoholization [15]. The technique consists of positioning the patient in supine position, with the affected limb slightly externally rotated. The electrocardiogram monitor and blood pressure monitor should be available during the procedure. The area that should be subjected to asepsis includes the skin between the umbilical scar and the proximal third of the thigh. The identification of the LFCN should be performed with the help of ultrasound. It is important to stress that the nerve generally presents its anatomical position up to about 1 cm medial to the ASIS. The LFCN is located between the plane of the iliac fascia/fascia lata and the sartorius muscle. After identifying the nerve, an anesthetic block with 1% lidocaine should be performed medial to the ultrasound transducer. With the introduction of a stimulator, a stimulus with 0.42 mA and 2 Hz should be performed for pain assessment. Once the patient confirms the pain on the lateral face of the thigh through the stimulus, 1 ml of 0.9% SF should be injected between the space of the two fascias to perform hydrodissection after a negative aspiration with the syringe. Then, 2.5 ml of anesthetic and 0.5% bupivacaine should be injected with 2.5 ml of 90% alcohol [12].

Before the use of radiofrequency neurolysis for nerve ablation, the technique of neurolysis with the use of alcohol was well disseminated for the treatment of spasticity, oncological pain, and chronic pain [16, 17]. Ethanol at low concentrations such as 5%–10% can be used as a local anesthetic by reducing the conductance of sodium and potassium ions. However, at high concentrations, ethanol causes protein denaturation and cell injury through the precipitation and dehydration of the cytoplasm [18].

11.4 Surgical Treatment

11.4.1 Laparoscopic Neurolysis of the LFCN

Laparoscopic neurolysis is a technique that is not widely used and is rarely described in medical literature. Its execution requires the use of a 10 mm infra-umbilical portal and two other 5 mm portals in the same location used for inguinal hernia repair. The LFCN is identified through the transparency of the peritoneum, which is incised near the point where the inguinal ligament (IL) inserts into the ASIS. Once the nerve is identified, the posterior leaflet of the IL is divided, promoting nerve release. Any point of nerve adhesion with tissues along its path should be released using a diathermic hook [19].

11.4.2 LFCN Neurolysis

LFCN neurolysis is among the most commonly used techniques for treating patients with MP. The technique involves positioning the patient in the supine position, with the affected limb slightly externally rotated. A cushion should be placed under the gluteal region ipsilateral to the surgery. The use of an electrocardiogram and blood pressure monitoring during the procedure is recommended. General anesthesia should be performed without the use of muscle relaxants. The area to be sterilized includes the skin between the umbilical scar and the proximal third of the thigh. The incision marking can be facilitated by manually palpating the ASIS and the pubic tubercle. A line can be drawn between these two structures, identifying the path of the IL. The medial incision line should extend from the ASIS, about 5 cm, and should follow the axis of the IL, but slightly inferior to it. The LFCN is located between the plane of the iliac fascia/lata fascia and the sartorius muscle. Once the nerve is identified, it should be released from the adjacent planes in its 360°, using Metzenbaum scissors or Halstead mosquito forceps, including the IL. Some authors suggest opening the ligament to avoid persistent compression points. The closure should include the subcutaneous plane and skin [20].

11.4.3 LFCN Neurectomy

LFCN neurectomy is also among the most commonly used techniques for treating patients with MP in medical literature. This procedure involves positioning the patient in the supine position, with the affected limb slightly externally rotated. A cushion should be placed under the gluteal region, ipsilateral to the surgery. The use of an electrocardiogram and blood pressure monitoring during the procedure is recommended. General anesthesia should be performed without the use of muscle relaxants. The area to be sterilized includes the skin between the umbilical scar and the proximal third of the thigh. The incision marking can be facilitated by manually palpating the ASIS and the pubic tubercle. A line can be drawn between these two structures, identifying the path of the IL. The incision line should extend medially from the ASIS to about 5 cm, following the axis of the IL, but slightly inferior to it.

In some patients, it will be necessary to use adhesive tape to pull the abdominal skin away from the surgical site. For this, micropore tape can be used. The LFCN is located deep, between the plane of the iliac fascia/lata fascia and the sartorius muscle. Once the nerve is identified, it should be released from the adjacent planes in its 360°, using Metzenbaum scissors, or Halstead mosquito forceps.

Then the LFCN should undergo transection, with the proximal stump of the nerve positioned in a space inside the pelvis. This maneuver will reduce the chances of forming a painful neuroma in the late postoperative period. The closure should include the subcutaneous plane and skin [20] (Figs. 11.1, 11.2, 11.3, 11.4, and 11.5, Video 11.1).

11.4.4 LFCN Neurolysis and Medial Transposition

The technique of neurolysis and medial transposition of the LFCN is a less commonly used option compared to LFCN neurolysis and neurectomy.

The technique involves positioning the patient in the supine position, with the affected limb slightly externally rotated. A cushion should be placed under the gluteal region, ipsilateral to the surgery. The electrocardiogram and blood pressure monitoring during the procedure should be used. General anesthesia should be performed, without the use of muscle relaxants. The area to be sterilized includes the

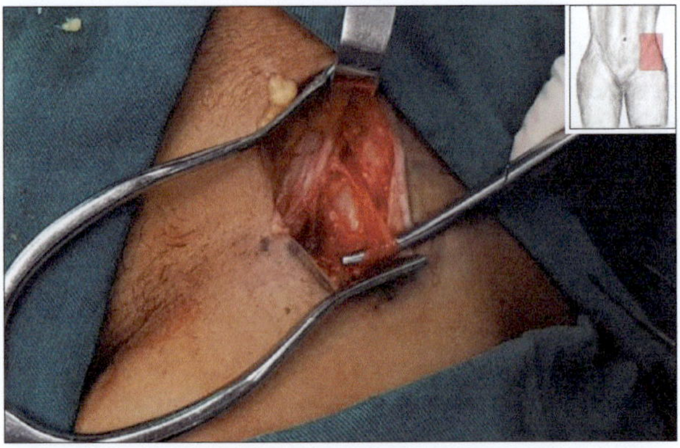

Fig. 11.1 Technique of neurectomy of the LFCN in the left lower limb. Note the nerve already dissected and exposed by the surgical instrument

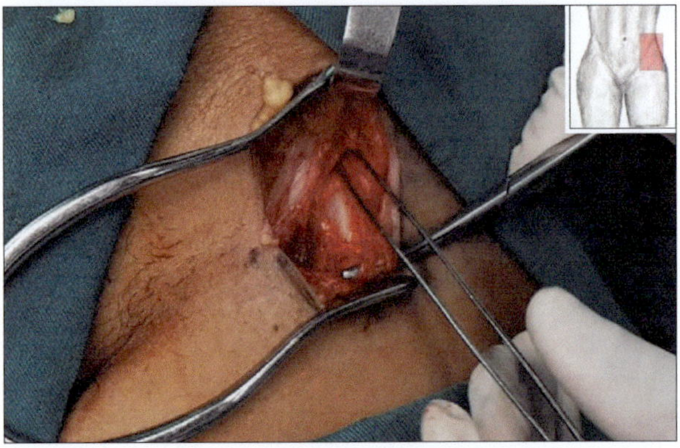

Fig. 11.2 Technique of neurectomy of the LFCN in the left lower limb. After the LFCN is dissected, the canal through which it passes at the level of the IL is enlarged so that after its section, its introduction into the abdominal cavity is facilitated

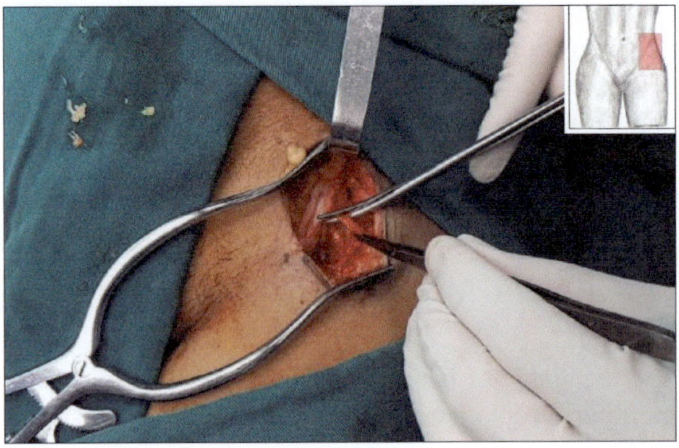

Fig. 11.3 Technique of neurectomy of the LFCN in the left lower limb. Moment when the LFCN was subjected to surgical section

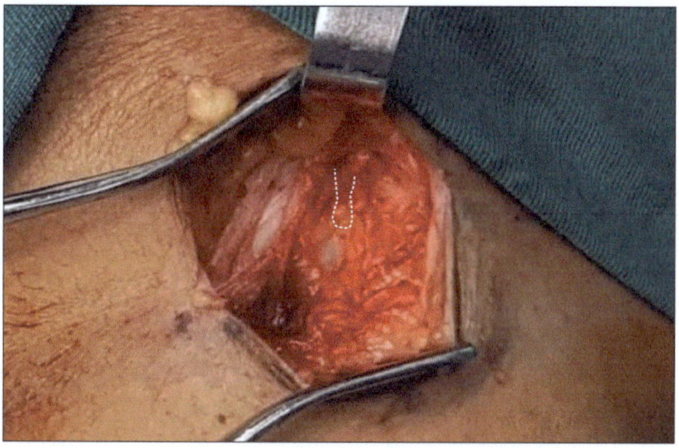

Fig. 11.4 Technique of neurectomy of the LFCN in the left lower limb. Note the nerve already sectioned delimited by the dotted white line

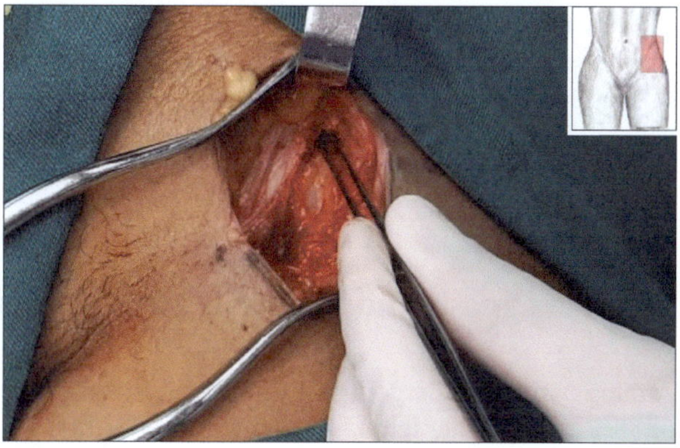

Fig. 11.5 Technique of neurectomy of the LFCN on the left. Note the nerve already sectioned is introduced into the abdominal cavity by the surgical clamp

skin between the umbilical scar and the proximal third of the thigh. The incision marking can be facilitated by manually palpating the ASIS and the pubic tubercle. A line can be drawn between these two structures, identifying the path of the IL. The incision line should extend medially from the ASIS for about 5 cm, following the axis of the IL, but slightly inferior to it. In some patients, it will be necessary to use adhesive tape to pull the abdominal skin away from the surgical site. For this, micropore tape can be used. The LFCN is located deep, between the plane of the iliac fascia/lata fascia and the sartorius muscle. Once the nerve is identified, it should be released from the adjacent planes in its 360° using Metzenbaum scissors or Halstead mosquito forceps. A small cavity should be created medial to the nerve, in the loose tissues present there. Then the LFCN should undergo a medial transposition to its original position. As soon as the nerve is positioned in the desired medial plane, it should be ensured that its structure is completely free and without tension. The distance of medial nerve displacement is approximately 2 cm. A Vycril® 3.0 suture may be used to prevent lateral displacement of the nerve. The closure should include the subcutaneous plane and skin [21].

11.4.5 Comparison Between Neurectomy and Neurolysis as Treatment for MP

Several studies have revealed that neurectomy has more lasting results when compared to neurolysis.

Van Earten et al. (1995) revealed that among 10 patients undergoing neurolysis, only three achieved symptom relief; on the other hand, 9 out of 11 patients undergoing neurectomy achieved pain control [22]. The case series of Williams et al. (1991) demonstrated that 23 out of 24 patients undergoing neurectomy of the LFCN achieved symptom relief [23]. In the case series of Ivins GK (2000), it was revealed that in the group of eight patients undergoing neurolysis as a form of treatment for MP, four experienced symptom relief, of which two had a recurrence of symptoms [24]. Siu and Shandran (2005) in a large case series revealed that in the group of 45 patients undergoing LFCN neurolysis, 43% of cases achieved pain control, 40% partial control, and 17% no pain control [25].

It is important to remember that in neurectomy for the treatment of MP, the patient always presents as a clinical outcome, an area of anesthesia in the anterolateral region of the thigh [20].

11.5 Prognosis and Factors That Influence Surgical Outcome

Among patients undergoing LFCN neurolysis, the success rate reached an average of 88%, on the other hand, in neurectomy 94% [5].

It was possible to identify the influence of symptom duration on surgical outcome [5, 26]. Some studies show that the longer the duration of symptoms, the worse the post-surgical prognosis. Macnicol et al. (1990) revealed in their study involving 25 patients with MP who underwent surgical decompression of the LFCN, a success rate in 15 cases (60%) [26]. In this study, it was identified in the group without symptom control after surgery that the manifestations of neuropathy had already persisted for a period greater than 18 months [26]. Siu et al. (2005) also corroborate that a long duration of symptoms is associated with a worse prognosis [25].

11.5.1 Prognosis of Iatrogenic Meralgia Paresthetica

Iatrogenic MP can result from spinal, abdominal, and pelvic surgeries [5]. Different mechanisms have been raised as etiology of iatrogenic MP. In spinal surgery, the phenomenon would result from the compressive process of the LFCN at the level of the ASIS, due to the prone position of the patient. Kalil et al. (2012) revealed in their extensive systematic review that iatrogenic MP presents complete recovery of symptoms in 97% ($N = 99$) of 102 patients [5]. It should be noted that these results excluded direct injuries that caused axonotmesis or neurotmesis of the LFCN [5].

11.6 Conclusion

MP presents different options for patient management. In general, the patient should initially undergo conservative treatment, through oral medication and physiotherapy. In the failure of pain control by conservative options, the possibility of performing surgical treatment should be evaluated. Among the invasive options, pulsed radiofrequency, neurolysis, and neurectomy stand out.

References

1. Gomez YC, Remotti E, Momah DU, Zhang E, Swanson DD, Kim R, Urits I, et al. Meralgia Paresthetica review: update on presentation, pathophysiology, and treatment. Health Psychol Res. 2023;11:71454.
2. Madiraca Glasović D, Šlaus N, Šitum M, Pećina M. Meralgia Paresthetica – Lateral Femoral Cutaneous Nerve Entrapment. Rad Hrvatske akademije znanosti i umjetnosti Medicinske znanosti. 2021;54–55:56–63.
3. Ecker AD, Woltman HW. Meralgia paraesthetica: a report of one hundred and fifty cases. JAMA. 1938;110:1650–2.
4. Chhuttani PN, Chawla LS, Sharma TD. Meralgia paraesthetica. Acta Neurol Scand. 1966;42(4):483–90.
5. Khalil N, Nicotra A, Rakowicz W. Treatment for meralgia paraesthetica. Cochrane Database Syst Rev. 2012;12:CD004159.
6. Kitchen C, Simpson J, Meralgia paraesthetica. A review of 67 patients. Acta Neurol Scand. 1972;48(5):547–55.
7. Massey EW. Meralgia paresthetica secondary to trauma of bone graft. J Trauma. 1980;20(4):342–3.
8. Stevens H. Meralgia paraesthetica. Arch Neurol Psychiatr. 1957;77:557–74.
9. Byrd D, Mackey S. Pulsed radiofrequency for chronic pain. Curr Pain Headache Rep. 2008;12:37–41.
10. Mishra P, Tandon S, Nath A. Extended pulsed radiofrequency as a part of multimodal pain management in a refractory case of Bernhardt-Roth syndrome. BMJ Case Rep. 2020;13(11):e237864.
11. Philip CN, Candido KD, Joseph NJ, Crystal GJ. Successful treatment of meralgia paresthetica with pulsed radiofrequency of the lateral femoral cutaneous nerve. Pain Physician. 2009;12(5):881–5.
12. Ghai B, Dhiman D, Loganathan S. Extended duration pulsed radiofrequency for the management of refractory meralgia paresthetica: a series of five cases. Korean J Pain. 2018;31:215–20.
13. Thapa D, Ahuja V, Dass C, et al. Management of refractory trigeminal neuralgia using extended duration pulsed radiofrequency application. Pain Physician. 2015;18:433–5.
14. Ahmed A. Prolonged pulsed radiofrequency ablation of Genicular nerves of knee for intractable pain from knee osteoarthritis: a case report. J Pain Relief. 2016;5:275.
15. Chen CK, Phui VE, Saman MA. Alcohol neurolysis of lateral femoral cutaneous nerve for recurrent meralgia paresthetica. Agri. 2012;24(1):42–4.

16. Kong KH, Chua KS. Neurolysis of the musculocutaneous nerve with alcohol to treat post-stroke elbow flexor spasticity. Arch Phys Med Rehabil. 1999;80(10):1234–6.
17. Erdine S. Neurolytic blocks: when, how, why. Agri. 2009;21(4):133–40.
18. Ritchie JM. The aliphatic alcohols. In: Goodman LS, Gilman A, editors. Goodman and Gilman's the pharmacological basis of therapeutics. 6th ed. New York: Macmillan; 1980. p. 376–90.
19. Bhardwaj N, Lloyd DM. Laparoscopic relief of meralgia paraesthetica. Ann R Coll Surg Engl. 2011;93(6):491.
20. Emamhadi M. Surgery for Meralgia Paresthetica: neurolysis versus nerve resection. Turk Neurosurg. 2012;22(6):758–62.
21. Greeneway GP, Page PS, Ammanuel SG, Hanna AS. Lateral femoral cutaneous nerve transposition. Neurosurg Focus Video. 2023;8(1):V8.
22. van Eerten PV, Polder TW, Broere CA. Operative treatment of meralgia paresthetica: resection versus neurolysis. Neurosurgery. 1995;37:63–5.
23. Williams PH, Trzil KP. Management of meralgia paresthetica. J Neurosurg. 1991;74:76–80.
24. Ivins GK. Meralgia paresthetica, the elusive diagnosis: clinical experience with 14 adult patients. Ann Surg. 2000;232:281–6.
25. Siu TL, Chandran KN. Neurolysis for meralgia paresthetica: an operative series of 45 cases. Surg Neurol. 2005;63(1):19–23.
26. Macnicol MF, Thompson WJ. Idiopathic meralgia paresthetica. Clin Orthop Relat Res. 1990;254:270–4.

Chapter 12
Piriformis Syndrome

12.1 Introduction

This is a syndrome described in which the sciatic nerve (SN) in its course under the piriformis muscle/level of the ischial tuberosity undergoes compressive process, triggering pain symptoms in the patient. There is in the literature the citation of several eponyms for this disease, such as deep gluteal syndrome, pelvic outlet syndrome, and infrapiriform foramen syndrome [1, 2].

The first case of sciatica associated with the piriformis muscle was described by Yeoman W. in 1928 when analyzing 100 cases of arthritis of the sacroiliac joint [3]. Only six years later, Mixter and Barr (1934) described the association of sciatica with intervertebral disc herniation [4]. Only later, in 1947, Robson DR coined for the first time the term Piriformis Syndrome (PS) for patients who presented pain in the region of the sacroiliac joint and piriformis muscle [5].

PS is a controversial disease that still leads to heated discussions among scholars of peripheral nerve diseases. Strong skepticism exists about PS among health professionals. A survey conducted in the USA, involving 75 physiatrists, revealed that 72% were confident in the existence of the disease, 55% reported that the diagnosis was overestimated, and 38% believed that the disease was underdiagnosed [6–8]. Several authors believe that PS would result more from a myofascial disorder than a compressive neuropathy [6–8]. It is noted that its clinical manifestations are not very consistent and can present as pain in the gluteal region, as well as symptoms similar to those identified in lumbosciatica, such as pain radiating to the ipsilateral lower limb.

The objective of this chapter is to describe the epidemiology of PS, its pathophysiology, differential diagnoses, etiology, symptoms and clinical signs, complementary exams, and conservative and surgical treatment.

M. J. S. Magalhães, *Lower Extremity Nerve Entrapments*,
https://doi.org/10.1007/978-3-031-90058-7_12

12.2 Anatomy of the Sciatic Nerve and Piriformis Muscle

The sciatic or ischiatic nerve is the peripheral nerve with the largest diameter in the human body, about 2 cm [9]. It is made up of the posterior and anterior divisions of the spinal nerves L4, L5, S1, and S2, in addition to the anterior division of the spinal nerve S3. Anatomically, the posterior divisions are responsible for the formation of the peroneal nerve and the anterior ones of the tibial nerve [10] (Fig. 12.1).

Proximal injuries of this nerve are usually very severe and result in paralysis of all muscles distal to the knee and significant sensory deficits involving the plantar region, lateral face of the leg, and dorsum of the foot.

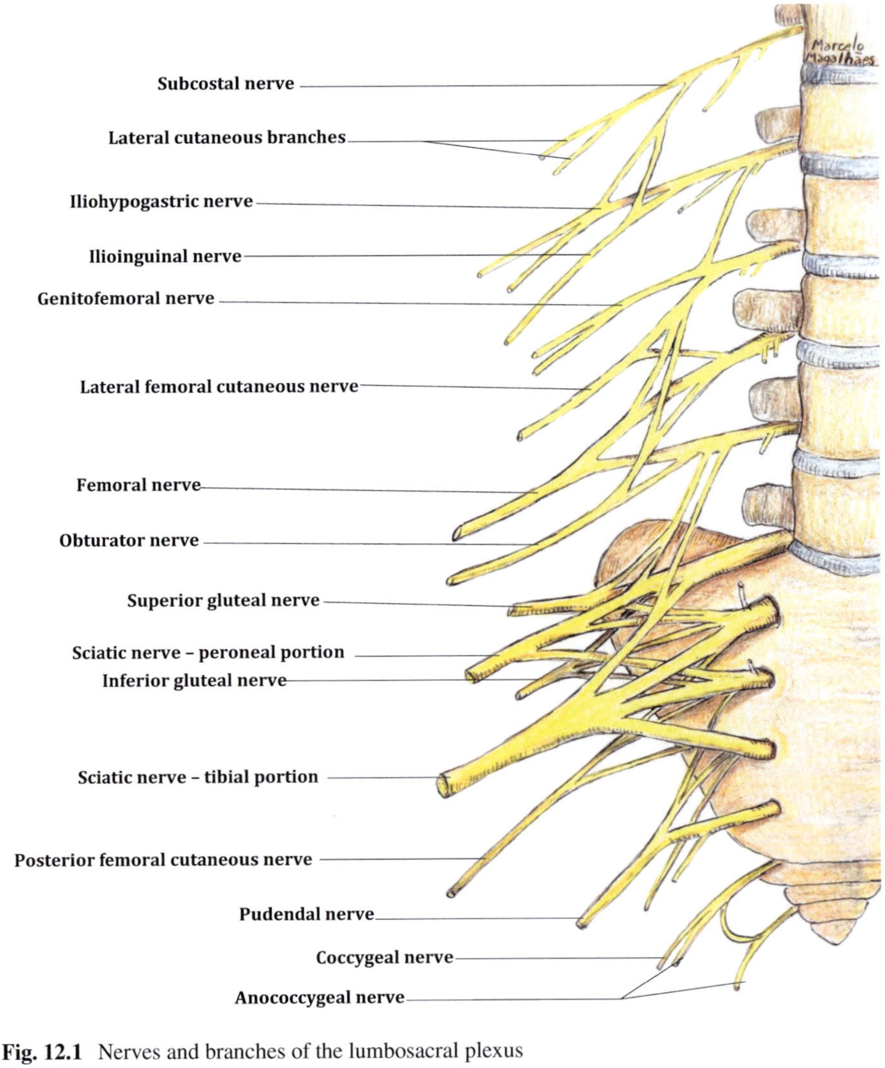

Fig. 12.1 Nerves and branches of the lumbosacral plexus

The SN leaves the pelvis through the greater sciatic foramen presenting a trajectory inferior to the piriformis muscle. Beaton and Anson (1937) described six possible anatomical variations between the SN and the piriformis muscle [11] (Fig. 12.2).

It is important to mention that there is in the medical literature a description of variations of the piriformis muscle in which the classification of Beaton and Anson does not apply [12].

Type I: This is the most commonly identified anatomical variation in which the sciatic nerve. SN presents itself as a single bundle that emerges under the piriformis muscle.

Type II: In this anatomical variation, the SN presents two divisions, one of them has a trajectory through the muscle fibers and another division over the muscle.

Type III: Anatomical variation in which the nerve presents itself as a single bundle that emerges over the piriformis muscle.

Type IV: The SN presents itself divided into two bundles, one transits through the muscle fibers and the other division passes under the muscle.

Type V: Variation in which the nerve is made up of a single bundle that emerges through the muscle fibers.

Type VI: In this anatomical variation, the nerve presents two bundles that pass respectively below and above the muscle [13].

It should be noted that the most commonly identified anatomical variations of the SN in the American population [14] and Eastern European are those of type I-IV [15], types I and II predominate among Indians [16] and Japanese [17, 18], types IV, V, and VI predominate in the Ethiopian population [19] (Fig. 12.2).

Still under the gluteus maximus muscle and after leaving the piriformis muscle, the SN follows a path over the muscles: superior gemellus, obturator internus, inferior gemellus, quadratus femoris, and adductor minimus. After leaving the gluteal

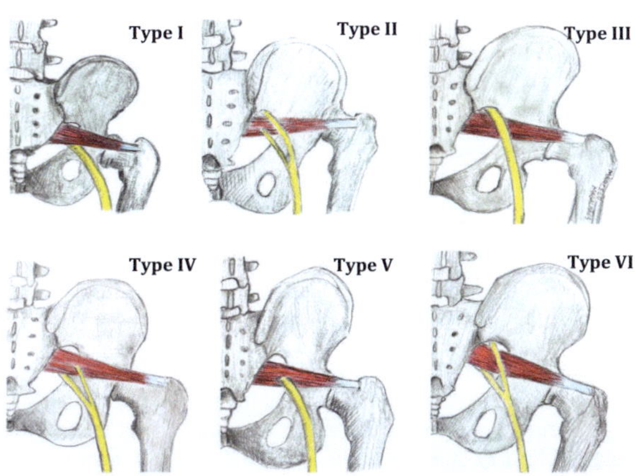

Fig. 12.2 Anatomical variation of the sciatic nerve and its relationship with the piriformis muscle

region, the nerve positions itself posterior to the femur, lateral to the biceps femoris muscle, and medial to the iliotibial tract. Further down the thigh, the biceps femoris muscle crosses over the sciatic nerve to position itself laterally to the nerve and the semitendinosus muscle positions itself medially to the SN [10] (Figs. 12.3, 12.4, and 12.5).

At the thigh level, the tibial division of the SN produces branches for motor innervation of the semitendinosus, semimembranosus, and long head of the biceps femoris muscles and the ischial part of the adductor magnus muscle. The peroneal

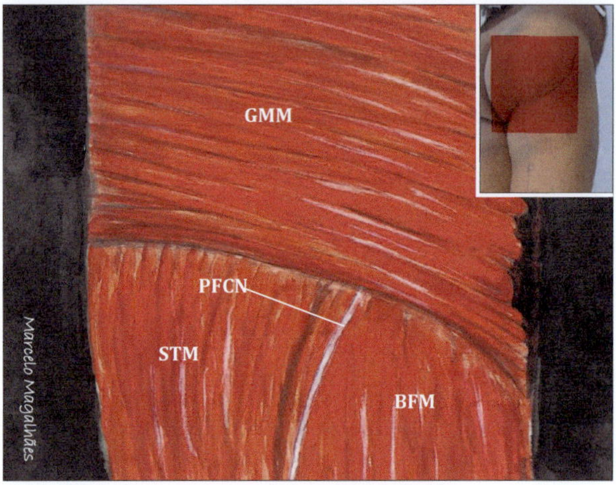

Fig. 12.3 View of the right gluteal region, with exposure of the posterior femoral cutaneous nerve. *BFM* = biceps femoris muscle, *GMM* = gluteus maximus muscle, *PFCN* = posterior femoral cutaneous nerve, *STM* = semitendinosus muscle

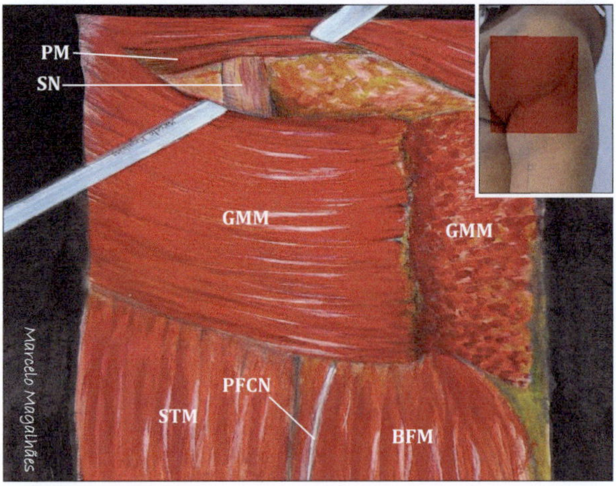

Fig. 12.4 View of the right gluteal region, with exposure of the posterior femoral cutaneous nerve and the sciatic nerve, after opening the fibers of the gluteus maximus muscle. Note the presence of the piriformis muscle over the sciatic nerve. *BFM* = biceps femoris muscle, *GMM* = gluteus maximus muscle, *PFCN* = posterior femoral cutaneous nerve, *PM* = piriformis muscle, *SN* = sciatic nerve, *STM* = semitendinosus muscle

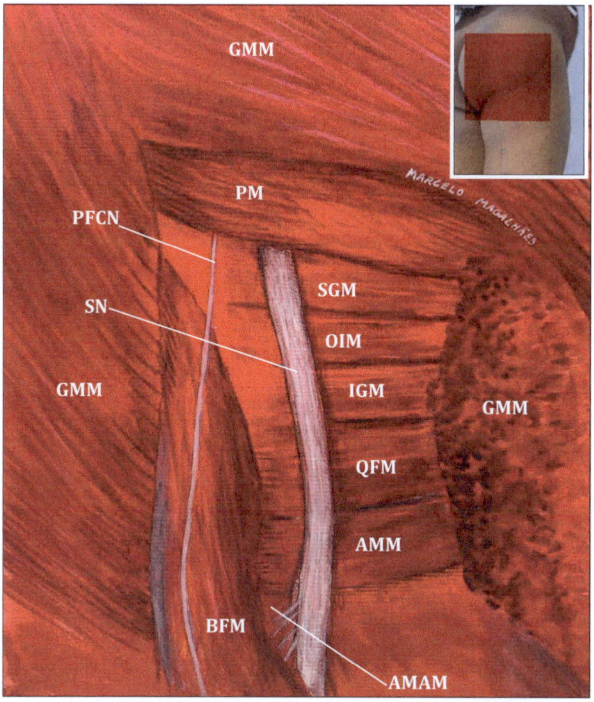

Fig. 12.5 View of the right gluteal region, with exposure of the posterior femoral cutaneous nerve and the sciatic nerve, after sectioning the fibers of the gluteus maximus muscle. Note the presence of the piriformis muscle over the sciatic nerve. *AMAM* = adductor magnus muscle, *AMM* = adductor minimus muscle, *BFM* = biceps femoris muscle, *GMM* = gluteus maximus muscle, *IGM* = inferior gemellus muscle, *OIM* = obturator internus muscle, *PFCN* = posterior femoral cutaneous nerve, *PM* = piriformis muscle, *QFM* = quadratus femoris muscle, *SGM* = superior gemellus muscle, *SN* = sciatic nerve

division, in turn, at the thigh level, innervates only the short head of the biceps femoris muscle. It is important to note that all motor and sensory innervation below the knee is performed by the branches of the SN, with the exception of a medial extension of skin on the leg and foot, whose innervation is performed by the saphenous nerve, a sensory branch of the femoral nerve. In the structure of the sciatic nerve, it is possible to identify the medial (tibial division) and lateral (peroneal division) trunks, which are gathered under the same sheath. Approximately, at the level of the union of the middle third with the distal third of the thigh, the sciatic nerve undergoes the process of division into the common peroneal and tibial nerves [10] (Fig. 12.6a, b).

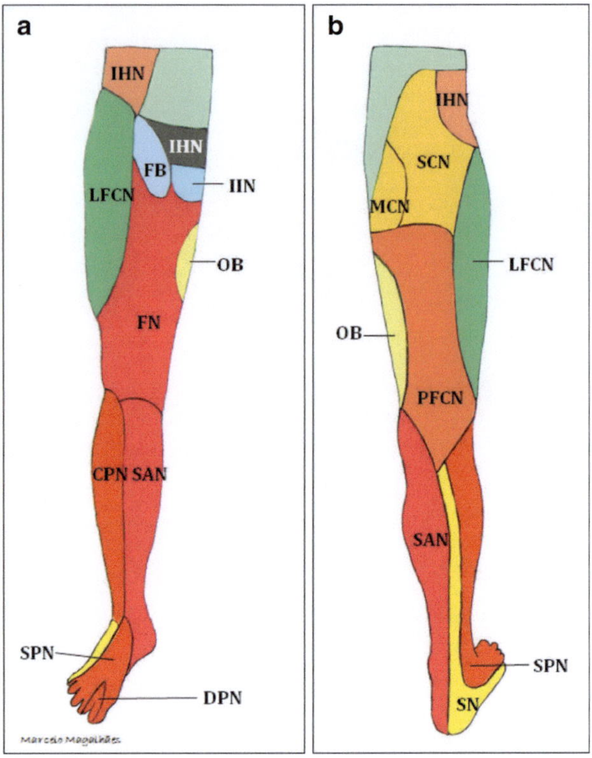

Fig. 12.6 (**a**, **b**) Anterior and posterior view of the sensory territories of the main nerves of the lower limb. *CPN* = common peroneal nerve, *DPN* = deep peroneal nerve, *FB* = femoral branch (genitofemoral nerve), *FN* = femoral nerve, *IHN* = iliohypogastric nerve, *IIN* = ilioinguinal nerve, *LFCN* = lateral femoral cutaneus nerve, *MCN* = medial cluneal nerve, *OB* = obturator nerve, *SAN* = saphenous nerve, *SCN* = superior cluneal nerve, *SPN* = superficial peroneal nerve, *SN* = sural nerve. *The ilioinguinal nerve area also has fibers from the genital branch of the genitofemoral nerve

12.2.1 Vascular Irrigation of the Sciatic Nerve

Georgakis et al. (2008) demonstrated that the arterial nutrition of the SN is performed through the sciatic arteries, which can appear in a number from one to four [20]. It was observed that in 50% of cases, the arteries originated from the medial circumflex femoral artery, 39% from the inferior gluteal artery, 7% from the first perforating artery, and 4% from the internal pudendal artery [20]. The average length of these arteries varied greatly according to their origin.

When the sciatic artery originated from the superior division of the inferior gluteal artery, it had an average length of 15.8 mm, when it originated from direct branches of the inferior gluteal artery 35.9 mm and from the branches of the first perforating artery, 22.7 mm [20]. Stolarczyk et al. (2000) demonstrated the presence of an intrinsic and extrinsic microvascular system in the SN, which are independent and join through anastomoses [21]. Studies carried out on rat sciatic nerves showed that the removal of the epineurium resulted in a 58% reduction in blood flow. This data suggests that most of the blood nutrition of the rat's sciatic nerve originates from the surface of this [21]. Zamir et al. (2012), also in an anatomical study with rat sciatic nerves, carried out by neuroimaging examination and anatomical dissection, corroborated the data from Stolarczyk et al. (2000), in which this intraneural arterial anastomosis system operates bidirectionally providing greater resistance to ischemia in case of interruption of arterial nutrition in one of the systems [21, 22].

12.2.2 Anatomy of the Piriformis Muscle

This is a muscle that originates at the level of S2 and S4, in the ventrolateral portion of the sacrum bone. It inserts into the piriform fossa of the greater trochanter of the femur. This muscle is innervated by the spinal nerves S2 and S3. Anatomical variation is described in the literature between the nerve branches that pass through the PM [23–26]. This muscle has the function of external rotation of the leg and abduction of the thigh when the hip is flexed [27–29] (Figs. 12.4 and 12.5).

12.3 Epidemiology of Piriformis Syndrome

Chang A. et al. (2023) cites that piriformis syndrome (PS) is responsible for 0.3–6% of all cases of low back pain and lumbosciatica [30]. Shane P. and Cass DO (2014) believe that this syndrome occurs in a proportion of 1:6 men/women and that it is more frequent in middle-aged adults [31]. Other authors cite that its prevalence as a cause of sciatica would be around 5–6% [28, 32]. Hopayan et al. (2010) revealed in their systematic review that the average age of patients with PS was 43 years [29].

12.4 Etiology of Piriformis Syndrome

As occurs in other compressive syndromes, PS can be the result of the presence of different underlying diseases, from tumors, local inflammatory processes, traumas, among other causes. Below is a list of risk factors/causes of PS.

- Trauma in the gluteal region [5, 32–39].
- Presence of anatomical variation of the PM [28, 32, 40–42].
- Application of injection in the gluteal region [43, 44].
- Post laminectomy [33, 44–48].

- Bursitis of the PM [49].
- Tumors in the infrapiriform foramen region [50].
- Sciatic nerve schwannoma [2].
- Lipoma [48].
- Abscess [51].
- Hematoma [52, 53].

12.5 Differential Diagnosis of Piriformis Syndrome

Various diseases that can cause pain in the hip and gluteal region potentially can be confused with PS, such as trochanteric bursitis and tendinopathies of the gluteus minimus and medius muscles. Among these diseases stand out injury to the posterior muscles of the thigh, facet syndromes, lumbosacral disc herniation, lumbosacral spondylolisthesis, lumbosacral spondylolysis, sacroiliac joint dysfunction/injury, tumors, and arteriovenous malformation [54]. Kulcu and Naderi (2008) revealed in their work the prevalence of different etiologies of non-discogenic sciatic pain. It is noted that piriformis syndrome accounted for 67.8% of cases, being the most common non-discogenic etiology [55] (Figs. 12.7, 12.8, 12.9, 12.10, and 12.11).

- Piriformis Syndrome 67.8%.
- Compression of distal extraforaminal spinal nerve 6%.
- Compression of the lumbosacral plexus 1.3%.
- Spinal nerve injury post-spinal surgery 1.3%.
- Inadequate decompression of spinal nerve 0.8%.
- Sacral fracture 0.4%.

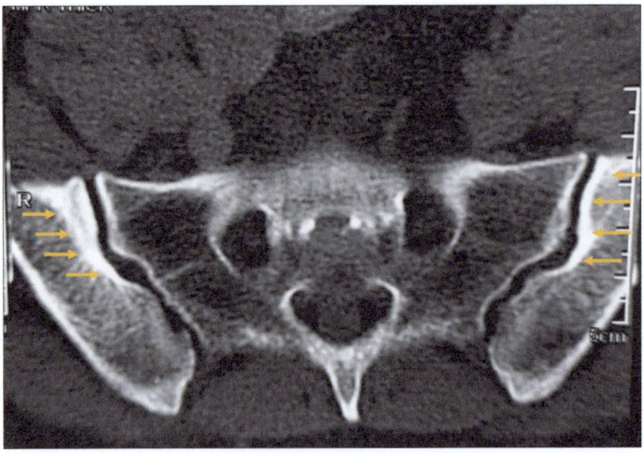

Fig. 12.7 Sacroiliitis. Computed tomography of the sacroiliac joint revealing sacroiliitis (yellow arrows) in a 48-year-old female patient with pain in the buttock region

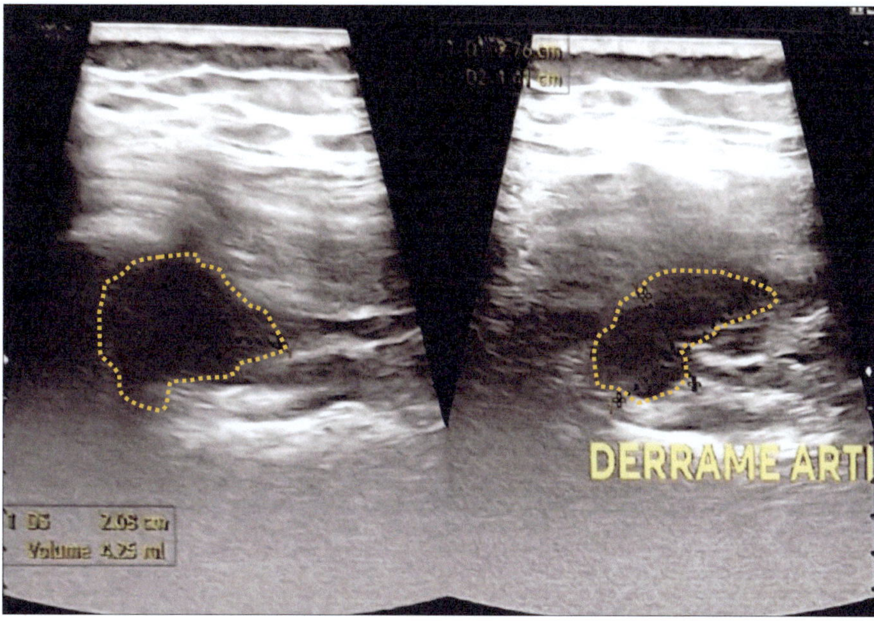

Fig. 12.8 Hip joint effusion secondary to osteoarthritis. Ultrasound of the hip joint of a patient with pain in the buttock region. The patient had previously undergone microdiscectomy for the treatment of lumbosciatica and due to persistent pain in the buttock region, she underwent an ultrasound. The examination revealed joint effusion (dotted yellow line) with a volume of 4.25 cm^3. This finding suggests severe osteoarthritis of the hip joint

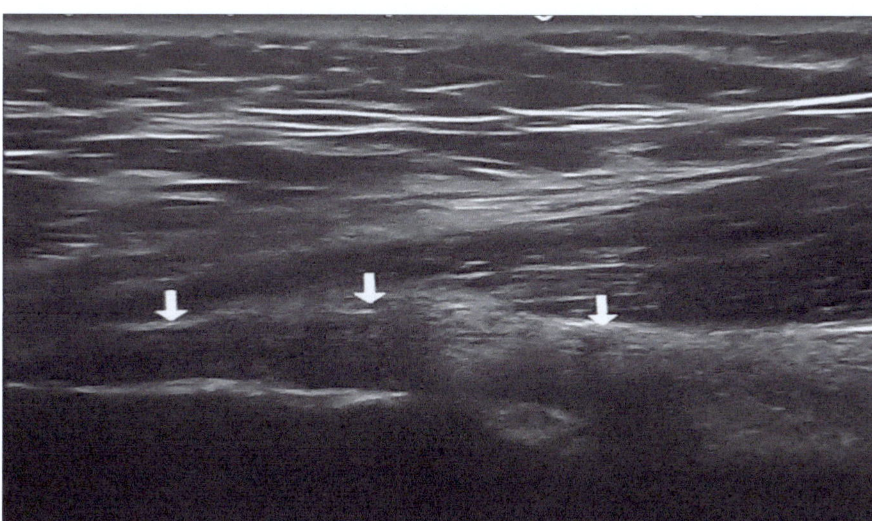

Fig. 12.9 Tendinitis of the gluteus minimus muscle. Ultrasound of the gluteal region reveals a reduction in the fibrillar pattern, a slightly echogenic aspect, and thickening of the tendon of the gluteus minimus muscle (white arrows)

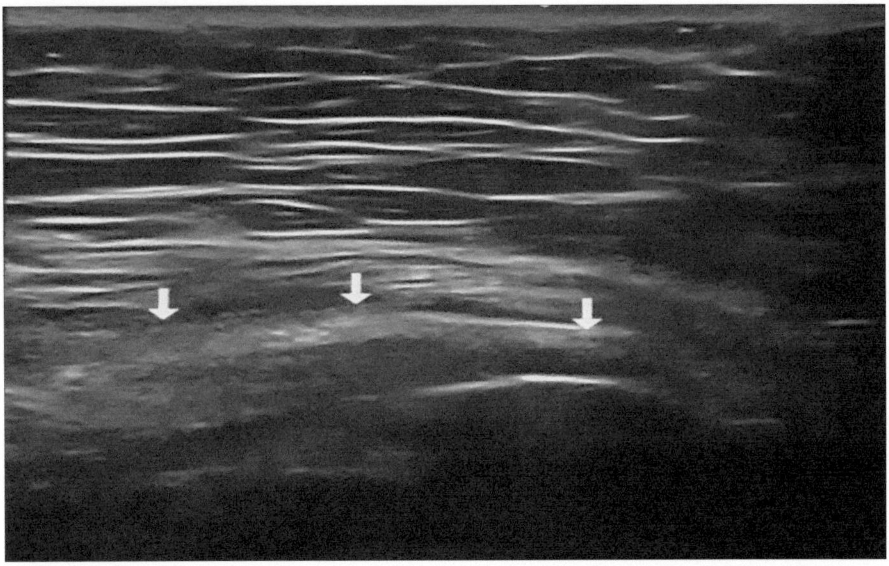

Fig. 12.10 Tendinitis of the gluteus medius muscle. Ultrasound of the gluteal region reveals a reduction in the fibrillar pattern, a slightly echogenic aspect, and thickening of the tendon of the gluteus medius muscle (white arrows)

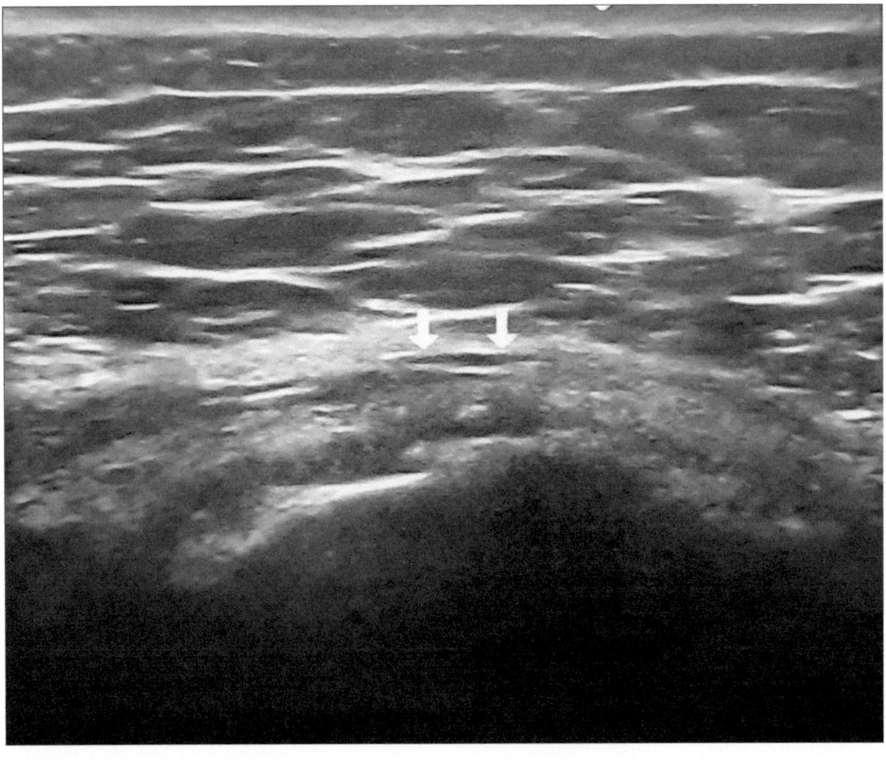

Fig. 12.11 Trochanteric bursitis. Ultrasound of the trochanteric region reveals distension of the trochanteric bursa (white arrows)

12.6 Pathophysiology of Piriformis Syndrome

Various etiologies have been associated with PS, from sports practices to trauma in the gluteal region. The trauma in the region of the PM would lead to the formation of scar tissue that would trigger this syndrome [14, 39, 56]. It is also proposed as pathophysiology that the myofascial syndrome could lead to spasms in the PM triggering the PS [14]. Jankovic et al. (2013) report that PS could be divided into two components, somatic and neuropathic [14]. The somatic component would result from myofascial pain contributed by pain points in the small external rotator muscles and the neuropathic component that would result from direct compression of the sciatic nerve [8, 34, 41, 57, 58]. Another factor that could contribute to PS would be the presence of anatomical variations of the MP and the course of the sciatic nerve. Anatomical variations of other nerves that have a course in the gluteal region were also associated with PS [26, 28, 34, 35, 40, 41, 59–64].

12.7 Symptoms of Piriformis Syndrome

It is important to note that there is no pathognomonic sign for the diagnosis of PS. Patients can present both acute symptoms as insidious. In cases where the manifestations present themselves acutely, they are usually associated with local trauma in the gluteal region. On the other hand, in patients with PS resulting from myofascial pain or overuse of the PM, symptoms tend to present an insidious onset [31].

Among the most commonly identified symptoms is pain in the region of the buttock that may be present in more than 95% of cases [29]. The gluteal pain tends to accentuate with the patient in the sitting or squatting position. The pain in PS can also be present with a pattern of lumbosciatalgia. Low back pain may be present in 18.1% of cases [46, 65]. It is also described in the literature the presence of paresthesia in the region inguinal, lumbar, perineum, buttocks, hip, back of the thigh, calf, feet, and rectum [14]. The literature also comments that among female patients, dyspareunia may be present as a symptom and in men sexual dysfunction [28, 29, 41]. Hopayian et al. (2010) revealed a large variation in the prevalence of dyspareunia that was identified between 13% to 100% [29].

12.8 Physical Examination

Inspection may reveal in more severe cases the presence of hypotrophy of the gluteal region on the affected side [41, 66, 67] (Figs. 12.12 and 12.13).

Palpation of the sacroiliac joint can be painful in 38.5% of patients with PS. Among the semiological maneuvers used for screening, this syndrome is the Freiberg sign, which was present in 32% to 63% of cases, the Pace sign between

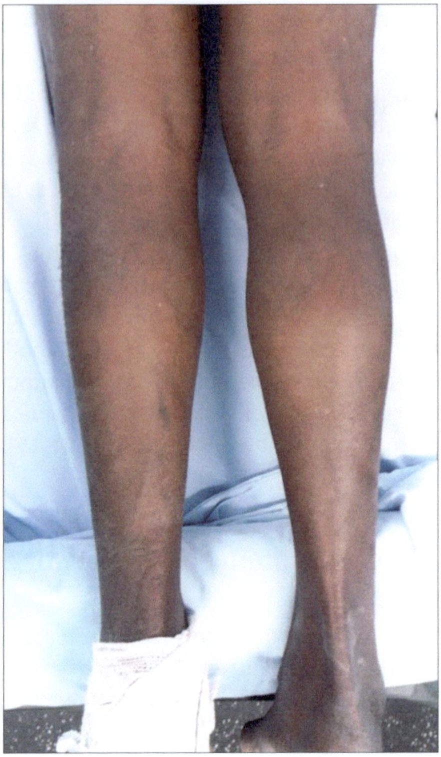

Fig. 12.12 Inspection of the lower limbs. Male patient, 63 years old, with clinical picture of piriformis syndrome in the left lower limb. The patient's main complaint is sciatica. The etiology of the syndrome is associated with trauma in the buttock region. Note the hypotrophy of the left calf

30% and 74%, painful external rotation of the lower limb between 59% and 92%, and internal rotation in 24% of cases [29].

According to Hopayian et al. (2010), three clinical characteristics can be present simultaneously in 22% of cases: buttock pain, pain worsened by sitting, and pain for external rotation of the legs [29].

Various semiological maneuvers have been described with the aim of identifying patients with PS. Such tests usually result in the stretching of the PM with compression of the SN, which reproduces the symptoms of lumbosciatalgia.

- *Freiberg Maneuver*: This consists of forced internal rotation of the patient's affected leg when they are in the supine position [68].
- *FAIR Maneuver*: This maneuver can be performed with the patient in the lateral or dorsal decubitus position. The patient is subjected to hip flexion, adduction, and internal rotation of the limb lower. The maneuver results in paresthesia and pain in the posterior pelvis [69].
- *Active Piriformis Test*: The patient is positioned in lateral decubitus and asked to perform the external rotation and abduction of the hip against the force of the examiner. The test is positive when the patient presents typical pain. This test has a sensitivity of 0.78 and specificity of 0.8 [70].

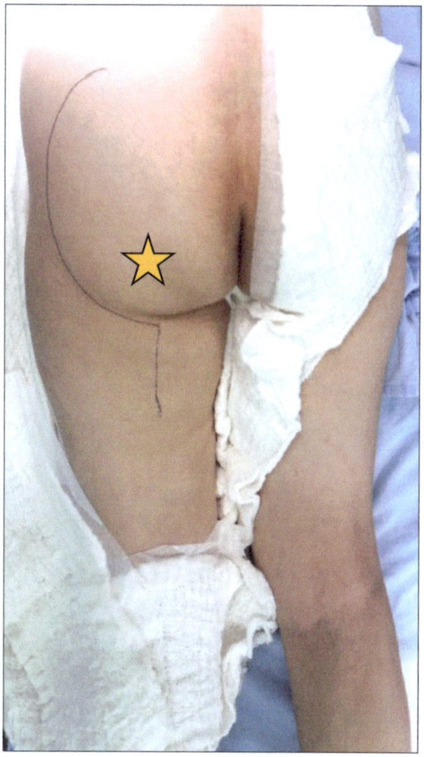

Fig. 12.13 Palpation in the region indicated by the yellow star on the left buttock caused intense pain. Middle-aged female patient with a history of idiopathic piriformis syndrome. She underwent surgical treatment with resolution of symptoms

- *Pace Test*: The patient in a seated position is subjected to leg abduction against the resistance of the examiner. The maneuver when positive causes pain [71].
- *Beatty Test*: The patient is positioned in lateral decubitus with the hip in flexion and then hip abduction is performed against gravity [71].
- *Solheim Sign*: The patient is positioned in dorsal decubitus, with the thigh flexed and adducted. The sign is positive when the patient presents a sensation of pain during the maneuver [72].

12.9 Additional Tests

Pelvic radiography has little value in the investigation of patients with PS as it can identify few findings, the most relevant being the presence of calcification in the muscle or in the piriformis tendon [34, 73] (Fig. 12.14).

Computed tomography (CT) of the pelvis can assist in the evaluation of the anatomical difference of the PM between the affected and non affected side, as well as the aspect of the infrapiriform foramen [59, 74, 75]. The CT of the lumbosacral spine can assist in the detection of herniated disc, spondylolisthesis, and fractures of

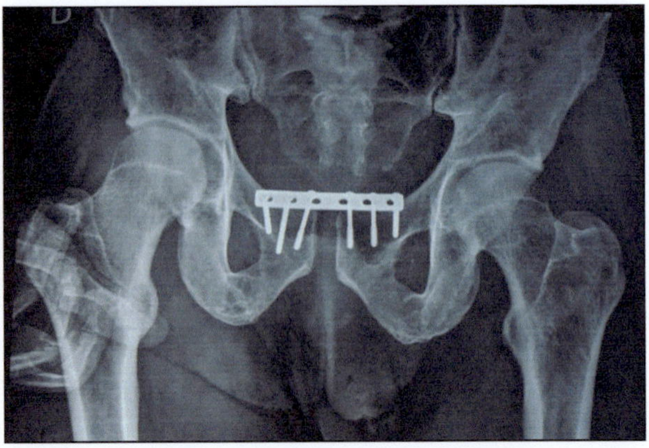

Fig. 12.14 Pelvic radiograph showing pubic symphysis diastasis and fixation. Patient with clinical picture of left piriformis syndrome after a fall from height

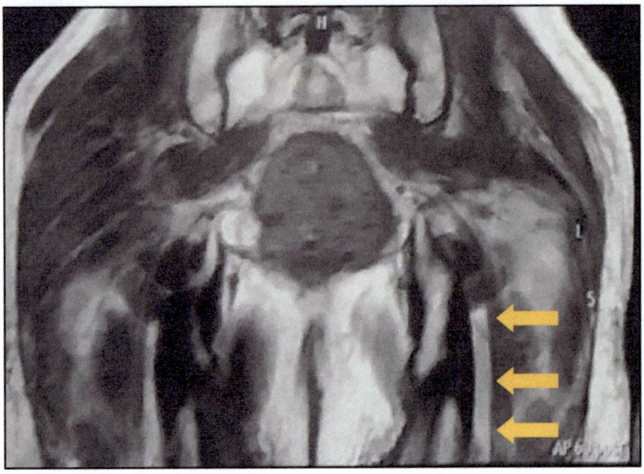

Fig. 12.15 Magnetic resonance imaging of the pelvis in coronal incidence. Note on the left, the thickened sciatic nerve (yellow arrows). Patient victim of trauma in the gluteal region, evolving with left piriformis syndrome

the vertebral column. This exam also assists in the identification of sacroiliitis, which is an important differential diagnosis (Fig. 12.7).

Magnetic resonance imaging (MRI) of the lumbosacral spine is a relevant exam to exclude the presence of herniated disc that promotes symptoms very similar to PS. The MRI of the pelvis can assist in the identification of changes in the sciatic nerve and adjacent tissues [76, 77]. In trauma to the gluteal region, it can also identify signs of denervation of this musculature and thickening of the sciatic nerve (Figs. 12.15 and 12.16). A pathognomonic sign in the MRI of the pelvis for the diagnosis of PS has not yet been described. On the other hand, the MRI of the pelvis can also assist in the identification of anatomical abnormalities that can predispose to PS [78]. This modality of exam assists in the identification of the increase in the volume of the PM, a change that can be present in patients with PS [78, 79]. It is important to mention that this increase in muscle volume is identified in 19% of asymptomatic patients [80].

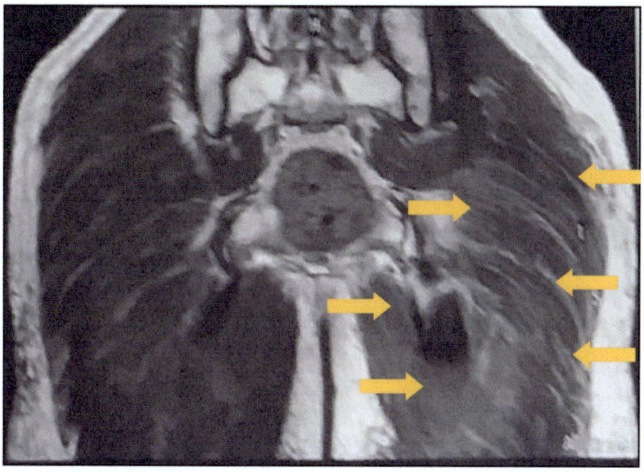

Fig. 12.16 Magnetic resonance imaging of the pelvis in coronal incidence. Note on the left, the presence of hypersignal in the gluteus maximus muscle due to its denervation (yellow arrows) after local trauma occurred many months ago

Neurography by MRI seems to be a promising exam in the diagnosis of PS. Filler et al. (2005) demonstrated that the presence of asymmetry in the MP and hyperintensity in the SN at the level of the MP presented a specificity of 0.93 and sensitivity of 0.64 to predict good-excellent results in the surgery of decompression of the sciatic nerve [47].

Ultrasonography (US) is also a relevant tool in the investigation that can assist in the visualization of trigger points in the PM with increased tone [81–84]. Currently, high-resolution US allows to evaluate the cross-sectional area of nerves in the upper limbs that may be increased in cases of compressive neuropathy; however, for the SN, these parameters are not yet defined [85].

The role of the ENM exam in patients with PS in anatomical position is minimal. In order to improve diagnostic accuracy, the patient during the ENM exam can be positioned on the exam bed with flexion, adduction, and internal rotation of the lower limb [34, 35, 37, 65, 85, 86]. The EMG in these patients can compare the H peroneal and tibial reflex obtained in a position of flexion, adduction, and internal rotation of the lower limb [normal value of prolongation 0.01 (0.61 millisecond)]. Some authors suggest that a prolongation of 1.86 milliseconds in the FAIR test position would be a diagnostic criterion for PS [34, 35, 37, 65, 85, 86]. Fishman and Zybert (1992) describe the delay in the H reflex by internal rotation, adduction, and flexion of the leg affected by pain as a suggestive finding for the diagnosis of PS [87].

12.10 Conservative Treatment

The initial treatment of PS should consist of a conservative approach through noninvasive therapies. The literature cites as an initial medicinal option the use of nonsteroidal anti-inflammatory drug (NSAID), muscle relaxants, and medications for neuropathic pain control, such as pregabalin and gabapentin [88].

Psychotherapy is also mentioned as a treatment option for this group of patients [88].

Physiotherapy can also be used as a treatment modality and focuses on isometric or non-isometric activities that result in the stretching of the PM. Physiotherapists usually use the FAIR position (Flexion, Adduction, and Internal Rotation) for the management of patients with PS. Some articles cite the performance of relaxation techniques after isometric activity as a treatment option [89, 90]. Regarding the control of symptoms in PS with this category of treatment, Shane et al. (2014) state that the success rate of physiotherapy is 51.5% [31].

In addition to oral medications and physiotherapy, therapy performed through local injection has been described and uses different medications such as lidocaine, corticosteroids, and botulinum toxin associated with different imaging methods, as well as, EMG [37, 46, 47, 57, 91–97].

Fishman et al. (2002) described 353 patients with a diagnosis of PS in which the combination of physiotherapy treatment with lidocaine injection with triamcinolone resulted in a reduction of at least 50% of the pain in 79% of the patients after 16 months of treatment [37].

The treatment with the highest success rate described in the studies so far was the infiltration of botulinum toxin into the PM. Lang et al. (2004) in a study involving 20 patients with PS who underwent infiltration of 5000 IU of botulinum toxin B into the PM achieved pain control in 95% of the cases [92]. Botulinum toxin type A is also described in the literature for pain control in these patients, with the recommended dose between 100 and 200 IU associated with 1–1.5 ml of 0.9% NS [34, 57, 98, 99].

Most of the studies whose treatment was performed through infiltration of corticosteroids and/or botulinum toxin involved a small number of patients and therefore the publication of studies with better controls and randomization process would be of great value [31]. Michel et al. (2013) investigated the PS, developing a clinical scoring system for its diagnosis and a treatment strategy. With 250 patients evaluated, a clinical score of 12 points was created, with PS "probable" with a score of 8 or more (sensitivity of 96.4% and specificity of 100%). The combination of medication and rehabilitation resulted in 51.2% cure, while non-responders received botulinum toxin injections, achieving good results in 77% of the cases [100]. Yoon et al. (2007), in a small study, also demonstrated symptom control in patients with PS after the use of botulinum toxin type A compared to conservative treatment with corticosteroids [99].

It is important to mention that the needle puncture technique in the belly of the PM for drug injection does not have reliable anatomical landmarks. In the region where the PM is positioned, very noble structures can be identified, such as the sciatic nerve, posterior femoral cutaneous nerve, inferior gluteal artery, and inferior gluteal nerve. Given this fact, blind injection using only anatomical points is not recommended [14].

Even the use of EMG or neurostimulation with the aim of identifying the PM also has technical limitations. It is proven that the stimulus at the tip of the needle used for this monitoring, even distant from the target, can produce a motor action potential or muscle contraction [101–104].

Even fluoroscopy, when used for the correct positioning of the needle in the belly of the PM, has technical limitations. In a study conducted on a cadaver, in only 30% of the cases, the puncture allowed the needle to be correctly located inside the PM [105].

On the other hand, the use of CT or US for the puncture of the PM showed higher success rates [105]. Studies conducted on cadavers showed a success rate of 95%, when the patient was subjected to puncture of the piriformis muscle through the use of US [105].

12.11 Surgical Treatment of the Piriformis Syndrome

Surgery is indicated as a treatment modality for patients with PS after the failure of conservative treatment has been confirmed. However, there is a lack of studies with an appropriate methodological design to evaluate the role of surgery in these patients [14].

The patient is positioned in the prone position, with the ipsilateral knee slightly flexed. A cushion is positioned under the anterior iliac crest. The incision can be made in the shape of a question mark or an inverted question mark. The incision begins approximately 2–3 cm from the postero-superior iliac crest and follows in the caudal direction, on the lateral edge of the gluteus maximus muscle until it reaches the region of the greater trochanter of the femur, acquiring a crescent shape. From this point, the incision line curves about 2.5 cm medial to the greater trochanter of the femur, on the inferior gluteal line, and follows on the midline posterior of the thigh for about 4–5 cm [10].

The incision should deepen into the skin, reaching the subcutaneous plane and gluteal fascia which should be sectioned. After opening the fascia, the gluteal musculature should be sectioned in a transverse direction of the fibers; usually, the monopolar scalpel can assist in obtaining a more uniform plane and less blood loss. It is important to note that the incision in the gluteal musculature should be in a plane slightly medial to the femoral gluteal tuberosity, so that the surgeon can perform the myorrhaphy after the end of the surgical procedure [10] (Figs. 12.17, 12.18, and 12.19).

After the complete section of the gluteus muscle fibers, it is possible to perform its retraction medially for adequate exposure of the subgluteal space structures.

During the process of medial retraction of the gluteus maximus muscle, avoid excessive traction to prevent injury to the inferior gluteal nerve and inferior gluteal artery [10].

Upon reaching the avascular subgluteal plane, the presence of adipose tissue and the PM over the sciatic nerve is identified. The posterior femoral cutaneous nerve is identified at this time of surgical approach. Then the PM is carefully sectioned, as the SN has a trajectory in its ventral region.

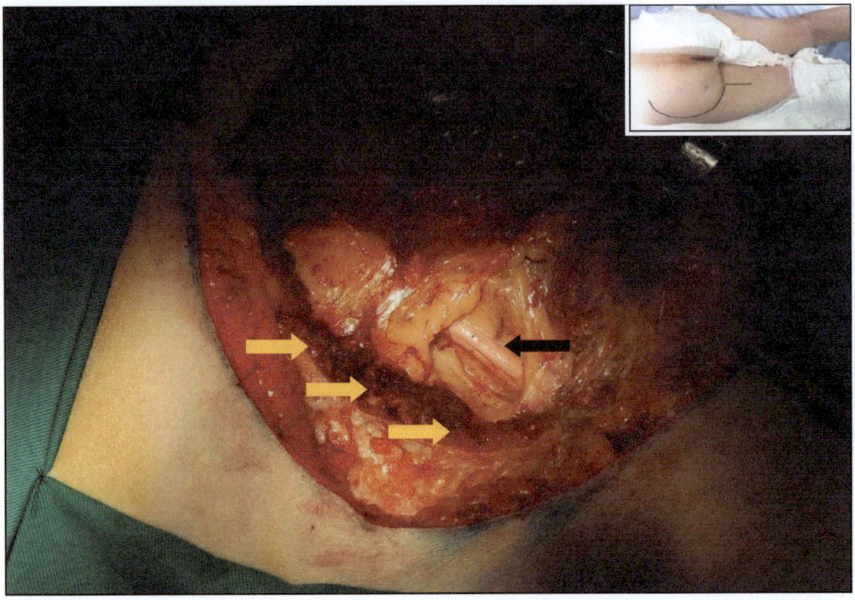

Fig. 12.17 Surgical access to the sciatic nerve at the level of the left gluteal region. Yellow arrows indicate the sectioned fibers of the gluteus maximus muscle (lateral edge). Black arrow indicates sciatic nerve. Note the presence of adipose tissue over the sciatic nerve

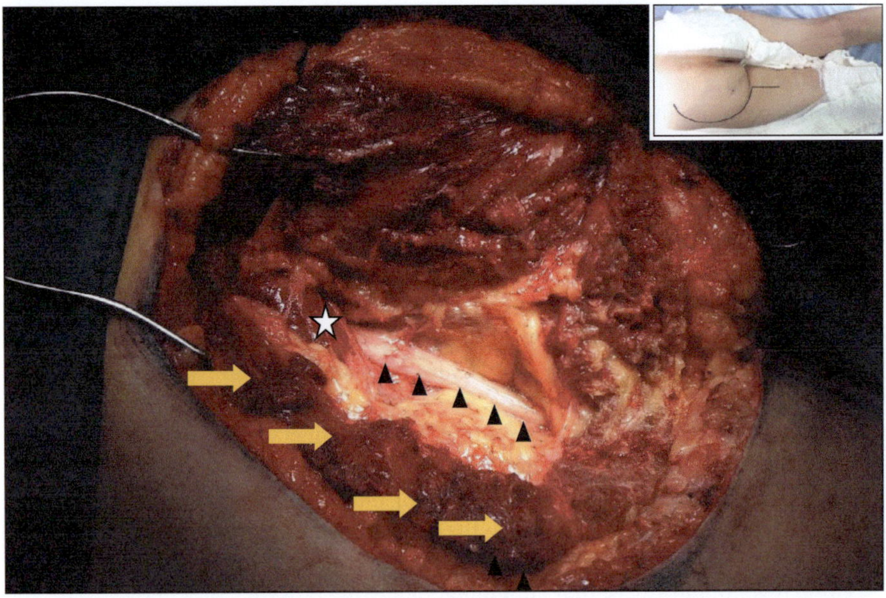

Fig. 12.18 Surgical access to the sciatic nerve at the level of the left gluteal region. Yellow arrows indicate the sectioned fibers of the gluteus maximus muscle (lateral edge). Black arrowheads indicate sciatic nerve. Note that the adipose tissue between the gluteal musculature and the sciatic nerve has been resected. White star indicates the piriformis muscle

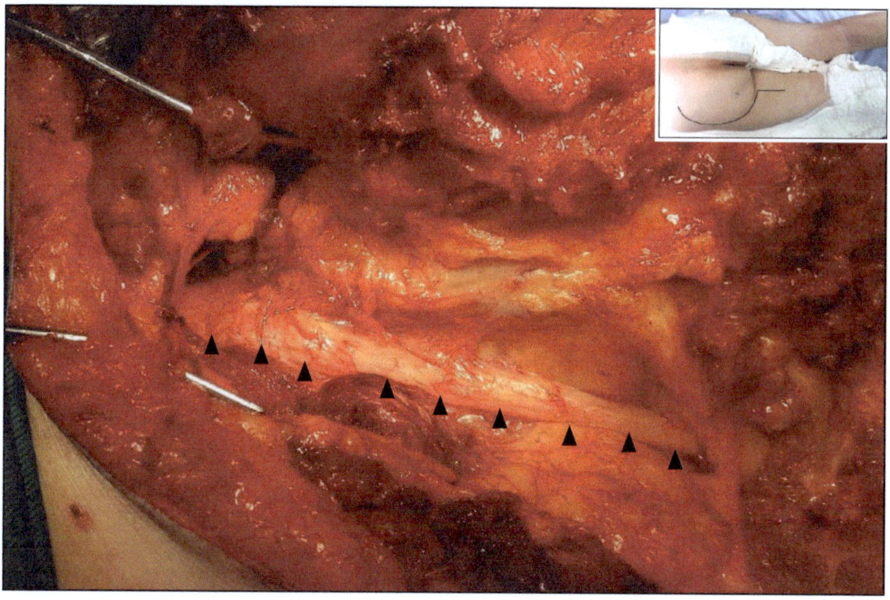

Fig. 12.19 Surgical access to the sciatic nerve at the level of the left gluteal region. The piriformis muscle was sectioned. Black arrowheads indicate the completely decompressed sciatic nerve at the level of the piriformis fossa

12.12 Conclusions

PS is a controversial disease due to the lack of clear and well-established criteria for confirming its diagnosis. The establishment of electroneuromyographic or neuroimaging criteria for disease confirmation will be of great value. Regarding treatment, studies with the best methodological design found that the use of botulinum toxin in the PM, under imaging guidance, provided the best outcomes in pain control. It is important to note that there are still studies needed to evaluate the real role of surgical treatment in patients with PS.

References

1. Hopayian K. Sciatica in the community — not always disc herniation. Int J Clin Pract. 1999;53:197–8.
2. Reichel G, Gaerisch F Jr. Piriformis syndrome. A contribution to the differential diagnosis of lumbago and coccygodynia (German). Zentralbl Neurochir. 1988;49:178–84.
3. Yeoman W. The relation of arthritis of the sacroiliac joint to sciatica, with the analysis of 100 cases. Lancet. 1928;2:111922.
4. Mixter W, Barr J. Rupture of the intervertebral disc with involvement of the spinal canal. N Engl J Med. 1934;211:2105.
5. Robinson DR. Pyriformis syndrome in relation to sciatic pain. Am J Surg. 1947;73:3558.

6. McCrory P. The "piriformis syndrome"–myth or reality? Br J Sports Med. 2001;35(4):209–10.
7. Campbell WW, Landau ME. Controversial entrapment neuropathies. Neurosurg Clin N Am. 2008;19(4):597–vii.
8. Porta M. A comparative trial of botulinum toxin type A and methylprednisolone for the treatment of myofascial pain syndrome and pain from chronic muscle spasm. Pain. 2000;85(1–2):101–5.
9. Currin SS, Mirjalili SA, Meikle G, Stringer MD. Revisiting the surface anatomy of the sciatic nerve in the gluteal region. Clin Anat. 2015;28(1):144–9. https://doi.org/10.1002/ca.22449. Epub 2014 Aug 8. PMID: 25131147
10. Siqueira MG, Martins RS. Anatomia cirúrgica das vias de acesso aos nervos periféricos. (Portuguese version) Ed. Dilivros, Brasil 2005.
11. Beaton LE, Anson BJ. The relation of the sciatic nerve and of its subdivisions to the piriformis muscle. Anat Rec. 1937;70:1–5.
12. Atoni AD, Oyinbo CA, Francis DAU, Tabowei UL. Anatomic variation of the sciatic nerve: a study on the prevalence, and bifurcation loci in relation to the piriformis and popliteal fossa. Acta Med Acad. 2022;51(1):52–8. https://doi.org/10.5644/ama2006-124.370. PMID: 35695403; PMCID: PMC9982851
13. Kanawati AJ. Variations of the sciatic nerve anatomy and blood supply in the gluteal region: a review of the literature. ANZ J Surg. 2014;84(11):816–9. https://doi.org/10.1111/ans.12675. Epub 2014 May 20
14. Jankovic D, Peng P, van Zundert A. Brief review: piriformis syndrome: etiology, diagnosis, and management. Can J Anaesth. 2013;60(10):1003–12. https://doi.org/10.1007/s12630-013-0009-5.
15. Pokorny D, Jahoda D, Veigl D, Pinskerova V, Sosna A. Topographic variations of the relationship of the sciatic nerve and the piriformis muscle and its relevance to palsy after total hip arthroplasty. Surg Radiol Anat. 2006;28(1):88–91.
16. Singh AK, Sharma RC. Relationship between the sciatic nerve and piriformis muscle. Neurosci Res Lett. 2011;2(1):26–8.
17. Chiba S. Multiple positional relationships of nerves arising from the sacral plexus to the piriformis muscle in humans [in Japanese]. Kaibogaku Zasshi. 1992;67(6):691–724.
18. Uluutku MH, Kurtoglu Z. Variations of nerves located in deep gluteal region. Okajimas Folia Anat Jpn. 1999;76(5):273–6.
19. Berihu BA, Debeb YG. Anatomical variation in bifurcation and trifurcations of sciatic nerve and its clinical implications: in selected university in Ethiopia. BMC Res Notes. 2015;8:633. https://doi.org/10.1186/s13104-015-1626-6.
20. Georgakis E, Soames R. Arterial supply to the sciatic nerve in the gluteal region. Clin Anat. 2008;21:62–5.
21. Stolarczyk A, Papierski K, Adamczyk G, Sin'ski M, Sawionek L, Przybylski J. Functional studies on sciatic nerve blood flow in respect to its vascular supply and tonic neural activity. J Physiol Pharmacol. 2000;51:483–9.
22. Zamir M, Twynstra J, Vercnocke AJ, et al. Intrinsic microvasculature of the sciatic nerve in the rat. J Peripher Nerv Syst. 2012;17:377–84.
23. Pecina HI, Boric I, Smoljanovic T, Duvancic D, Pecina M. Surgical evaluation of magnetic resonance imaging findings in pririformis muscle syndrome. Skeletal Radiol. 2008;37:1019–23.
24. Russell JM, Kransdorf MJ, Bancroft LW, et al. Magnetic resonance imaging of the sacral plexus and piriformis muscles. Skeletal Radiol. 2008;37(8):709–13.
25. Guvencer M, Akyer P, Iyem C, Tetik S, Naderi S. Anatomic considerations and the relationship between the piriformis muscle and the sciatic nerve. Surg Radiol Anat. 2008;30(6):467–74.
26. Pecina M. Contribution to the etiological explanation of the piriformis syndrome. Acta Anat (Basel). 1979;105(2):181–7.
27. Boyajian-O'Neill LA, McClain RL, Coleman MK, Thomas PP. Diagnosis and management of piriformis syndrome: an osteopathic approach. J Am Osteopath Assoc. 2008;108(11):657–64.

28. Papadopoulos EC, Khan SN. Piriformis syndrome and low back pain: a new classification and review of the literature. Orthop Clin North Am. 2004;35(1):65–71.
29. Hopayian K, Song F, Riera R, Sambandan S. The clinical features of the piriformis syndrome: a systematic review. Eur Spine J. 2010;19(12):2095–109.
30. Byrd JW. Piriformis syndrome. Oper Tech Sports Med. 2005;13:71Y79.
31. Shane P, Cass DO. Piriformis syndrome: a cause of nondiscogenic sciatica. Curr Sports Med Rep. 2015;14(1):41–4.
32. Hallin RP. Sciatic pain and the piriformis muscle. Postgrad Med. 1983;74:69–72.
33. Durrani Z, Winnie AP. Piriformis muscle syndrome: an underdiagnosed cause of sciatica. J Pain Symptom Manage. 1991;6:374–9.
34. Reichel G. Treatment of piriformis syndrome with botulinum toxin. Pain Headache. 2003;14:140–58.
35. Huber HM. The piriformis syndrome – a possible cause of sciatica (German). Schweiz Rundsch Med Prax. 1990;79:235–6.
36. Pfeifer T, Fitz WF. The piriformis syndrome (German). Z Orthop Ihre Grenzgeb. 1989;127:691–4.
37. Fishman LM, Dombi GW, Michaelsen C, et al. Piriformis syndrome: diagnosis, treatment, and outcome – a 10-year study. Arch Phys Med Rehabil. 2002;83:295–301.
38. Fishman LM, Anderson C, Rosner B. Botox and physical therapy in the treatment of piriformis syndrome. Am J Phys Med Rehabil. 2002;81:936–42.
39. Benson ER, Schutzer SF. Posttraumatic piriformis syndrome: diagnosis and results of operative treatment. J Bone Joint Surg Am. 1999;81:941–9.
40. Parziale JR, Hudgins TH, Fischman LM. The piriformis syndrome. Am J Orthop (Belle Mead NJ). 1996;25:819–23.
41. Travell JG, Simons DG. Myofascial pain and dysfunction: the trigger point manual – the lower extremities, vol. 2. Baltimore: Lippincott Williams & Wilkins; 1992. p. 186–214.
42. Thiele GH. Coccygodynia and pain in the superior gluteal region and down the back of the thigh: causation by tonic spasm of the levator ani, coccygeus and piriformis muscles and relief by massage of these muscles. JAMA. 1937;109:1271–5.
43. Obach J, Aragones JM, Ruano D. The infrapiriformis foramen syndrome resulting from intragluteal injection. J Neurol Sci. 1983;58:135–42.
44. Pace JB. Commonly overlooked pain syndromes responsive to simple therapy. Postgrad Med. 1975;58:107–13.
45. Pace JB, Nagle D. Piriform syndrome. West J Med. 1976;124:435–9.
46. Benzon HT, Katz JA, Benzon HA, Iqbal MS. Piriformis syndrome: anatomic considerations, a new injection technique, and a review of the literature. Anesthesiology. 2003;98:1442–8.
47. Filler AG, Haynes BA, Jordan SE, et al. Sciatica of nondisc origin and piriformis syndrome: diagnosis by magnetic resonance neurography and interventional magnetic resonance imaging with outcome study of resulting treatment. J Neurosurg Spine. 2005;2:99–115.
48. Pace JB, Henning C. Episacroiliac lipoma. Am Fam Physician. 1972;6:70–3.
49. Peh WC, Reinus WR. Piriformis bursitis causing sciatic neuropathy. Skeletal Radiol. 1995;244:474–6.
50. Hockel M. Laterally extended endopelvic resection: surgical treatment of infrailiac pelvic wall recurrences of gynecologic malignancies. Am J Obstet Gynecol. 1999;180:306–12.
51. Arai Y, Kawakami T, Soga H, Okada Y. Psoas abscess associated with iliac vein thrombosis and piriformis and gluteal abscesses. Int J Urol. 1999;6:257–9.
52. Katati MJ, Vilchez R, Pinar L, et al. Haematoma of the piriformis muscle simulating a giant presacral tumour: unusual case of lumbosacral radiculopathy. Acta Neurochir. 1998;140:403–4.
53. Ku A, Kern H, Lachman E, Nagler W. Sciatic nerve impingement from piriformis hematoma due to prolonged labor. Muscle Nerve. 1995;18:789–90.
54. Cass SP. Piriformis syndrome: a cause of nondiscogenic sciatica. Curr Sports Med Rep. 2015;14(1):41–4.

55. Kulcu DG, Naderi S. Differential diagnosis of intraspinal and extraspinal nondiscogenic sciatica. J Clin Neurosci. 2008;15:124652.
56. Stewart JD. The piriformis syndrome is overdiagnosed. Muscle Nerve. 2003;28:644–6.
57. Fanucci E, Masala S, Sodani G, et al. CT-guided injection of botulinic toxin for percutaneous therapy of piriformis muscle syndrome with preliminary MRI results about denervative process. Eur Radiol. 2001;11:2543–8.
58. Childers MK. Use of botulinum toxin type A in pain management. Columbia/Austin: Academic Information Systems/Greenleaf Book Group; 2002.
59. Cassidy L, Walters A, Bubb K, Shoja MM, Tubbs RS, Loukas M. Piriformis syndrome: implications of anatomical variations, diagnostic techniques, and treatment options. Surg Radiol Anat. 2012;34:479–86.
60. Tillmann B. Variations in the pathway of the inferior gluteal nerve (author's transl) (German). Anat Anz. 1979;145:293–302.
61. Douglas S. Sciatic pain and piriformis syndrome. Nurse Pract. 1997;22:166–8.
62. Chen WS, Wan YL. Sciatica caused by piriformis muscle syndrome: report of two cases. J Formos Med Assoc. 1992;91:647–50.
63. Bendszus M, Rieckmann P, Perez J, Koltzenburg M, Reiners K, Solymosi L. Painful vascular compression syndrome of the sciatic nerve caused by gluteal varicosities. Neurology. 2003;61:985–7.
64. Sayson SC, Ducey JP, Maybrey JB, Wesley RL, Vermilion D. Sciatic entrapment neuropathy associated with an anomalous piriformis muscle. Pain. 1994;59:149–52.
65. Blaser-Sziede R. Piriformissyndrom — kritische beurteilung der literatur und diskussion der klinischen zusammenha¨nge (German). Man Ther. 2006;10:159–69.
66. Rodrigue T, Hardy RW. Diagnosis and treatment of piriformis syndrome. Neurosurg Clin N Am. 2001;12:311–9.
67. TePoorten BA. The piriformis muscle. J Am Osteopath Assoc. 1969;69:150–60.
68. Probst D, Stout A, Hunt D. Piriformis syndrome: a narrative review of the anatomy, diagnosis, and treatment. PM R. 2019;11(Suppl 1):S54–63. https://doi.org/10.1002/pmrj.12189. Epub 2019 Jul 22. PMID: 31102324
69. Solheim LF, Siewers P, Paus B. The piriformis muscle syndrome. Sciatic nerve entrapment treated with section of the piriformis muscle. Acta Orthop Scand. 1981;52(1):73–5.
70. Martin HD, Kivlan BR, Palmer IJ, Martin RL. Diagnostic accuracy of clinical tests for sciatic nerve entrapment in the gluteal region. Knee Surg Sports Traumatol Arthrosc. 2014;22(4):882–8.
71. Beatty RA. The piriformis muscle syndrome: a simple diagnostic maneuver. Neurosurgery. 1994;34(3):512–4. discussion 514
72. Pande A, et al. Piriformis syndrome and variants – a comprehensive review on diagnosis and treatment. J Spinal Surg. 2021;8(4):7–14.
73. Stark P, Hildebrandt-Stark HE. Calcific tendinitis of the piriform muscle. Rofo. 1983;138:111–2.
74. Ueno K, Matsuzawa H, Inoue A. 67 Ga imaging of gluteal muscle inflammation secondary to pyogenic sacroiliitis (PSI) (Japanese). Rinsho Hoshasen. 1985;30:319–22.
75. Fanucci E, Masala S, Squillaci E, et al. Piriformis muscle syndrome: CT/MR findings in the percutaneous therapy with botulinic toxin. Radiol Med. 2003;105:69–75.
76. Almanza MY, Poon-Chue A, Terk MR. Dual oblique MR method for imaging the sciatic nerve. J Comput Assist Tomogr. 1999;23:138–40.
77. Lee EY, Margherita AJ, Gierada DS, Narra VR. MRI of piriformis syndrome. AJR Am J Roentgenol. 2004;183(1):63–4.
78. Jankiewicz JJ, Hennrikus WL, Houkom JA. The appearance of the piriformis muscle syndrome in computed tomography and magnetic resonance imaging. A case report and review of the literature. Clin Orthop Relat Res. 1991;262:205–9.

79. Rossi P, Cardinali P, Serrao M, Parisi L, Bianco F, De Bac S. Magnetic resonance imaging findings in piriformis syndrome: a case report. Arch Phys Med Rehabil. 2001;82(4):519–21.
80. Russell JM, Kransdorf MJ, Bancroft LW, Peterson JJ, Berquist TH, Bridges MD. Magnetic resonance imaging of the sacral plexus and piriformis muscles. Skeletal Radiol. 2008;37(8):709–13.
81. Sikdar S, Shah JP, Gebreab T, et al. Novel applications of ultrasound technology to visualize and characterize myofascial trigger points and surrounding soft tissue. Arch Phys Med Rehabil. 2009;90(11):1829–38.
82. Kumbhare DA, Elzibak AH, Noseworthy MD. Assessment of myofascial trigger points using ultrasound. Am J Phys Med Rehabil. 2016;95(1):72–80.
83. Fusco P, Di Carlo S, Scimia P, Degan G, Petrucci E, Marinangeli F. Ultrasound-guided dry needling treatment of myofascial trigger points for piriformis syndrome management: a case series. J Chiropr Med. 2018;17(3):198–200.
84. McDonagh C, Alexander M, Kane D. The role of ultrasound in the diagnosis and management of carpal tunnel syndrome: a new paradigm. Rheumatology (Oxford). 2015;54(1):9–19.
85. Dumitru D, Nelson MR. Posterior femoral cutaneous nerve conduction. Arch Phys Med Rehabil. 1990;71:979–82.
86. Spinner RJ, Thomas NM, Kline DG. Failure of surgical decompression for a presumed case of piriformis syndrome. Case report. J Neurosurg. 2001;94:652–4.
87. Fishman LM, Zybert PA. Electrophysiologic evidence of piriformis syndrome. Arch Phys Med Rehabil. 1992;73:35964.
88. Dworkin RH, O'Connor AB, Bakonja M, et al. Pharmacologic management of neuropathic pain: evidence-based recommendations. Pain. 2007;132:237–51.
89. Lewit K, Simons DG. Myofascial pain: relief by post-isometric relaxation. Arch Phys Med Rehabil. 1984;65(8):452–6.
90. Retzlaff EW, Berry AH, Haight AS, et al. The piriformis muscle syndrome. J Am Osteopath Assoc. 1974;73(10):799–807.
91. Huerto AP, Yeo SN, Ho KY. Piriformis muscle injection using ultrasonography and motor stimulation–report of a technique. Pain Physician. 2007;10(5):687–90.
92. Lang AM. Botulinum toxin type B in piriformis syndrome. Am J Phys Med Rehabil. 2004;83(3):198–202.
93. Reus M, de Dios BJ, Vazquez V, Redondo MV, Alonso J. Piriformis syndrome: a simple technique for US-guided infiltration of the perisciatic nerve. Preliminary results. Eur Radiol. 2008;18(3):616–20.
94. Smith J, Hurdle MF, Locketz AJ, Wisniewski SJ. Ultrasoundguided piriformis injection: technique description and verification. Arch Phys Med Rehabil. 2006;87(12):1664–7.
95. Bennett JD, Miller TA, Richards RS. The use of Botox in interventional radiology. Tech Vasc Interv Radiol. 2006;9(1):36–9.
96. Betts A. Combined fluoroscopic and nerve stimulator technique for injection of the piriformis muscle. Pain Physician. 2004;7:279–81.
97. Fishman LM, Konnoth C, Rozner B. Botulinum neurotoxin type B and physical therapy in the treatment of piriformis syndrome: a dose-finding study. Am J Phys Med Rehabil. 2004;83(1):42–50.
98. Kirschner JS, Foye PM, Cole JL. Piriformis syndrome, diagnosis and treatment. Muscle Nerve. 2009;40:10–8.
99. Yoon SJ, Ho J, Kang HY, et al. Low-dose botulinum toxin type A for the treatment of refractory piriformis syndrome. Pharmacotherapy. 2007;27:657–65.
100. Michel F, Decavel P, Toussirot E, et al. Piriformis muscle syndrome: diagnostic criteria and treatment of a monocentric series of 250 patients. Ann Phys Rehab Med. 2013;56:371–83.
101. Rigaud M, Filip P, Lirk P, Fuchs A, Gemes G, Hogan Q. Guidance of block needle insertion by electrical nerve stimulation: a pilot study of the resulting distribution of injected solution in dogs. Anesthesiology. 2008;109:473–8.

102. Chan VW, Brull R, McCartney CJ, Xu D, Abbas S, Shannon P. An ultrasonographic and histological study of intraneural injection and electrical stimulation in pigs. Anesth Analg. 2007;104:1281–4.
103. Tsai TP, Vuckovic I, Dilberovic F, et al. Intensity of the stimulating current may not be a reliable indicator of intraneural needle placement. Reg Anesth Pain Med. 2008;33:207–10.
104. Altermatt FR, Cummings TJ, Auten KM, Baldwin MF, Belknap SW, Reynolds JD. Ultrasonographic appearance of intraneural injections in the porcine model. Reg Anesth Pain Med. 2010;35:203–6.
105. Finoff JT, Hurdle MF, Smith J. Accuracy of ultrasound-guided versus fluoroscopically guided contrast controlled piriformis injections. A cadaveric study. J Ultrasound Med. 2008;27:1157–63.

Chapter 13
Other Rare Entrapment Syndromes of Lower Limbs

13.1 Femoral Nerve Neuropathy

Femoral nerve neuropathy is a rare disease that can lead the patient to develop painful and motor symptoms. Because it is an uncommon neuropathy, its real incidence is unknown. Among the most commonly described causes in medical literature, iatrogenic causes stand out after surgical procedures and tumors [1].

13.1.1 Neuroanatomy of the Femoral Nerve

The femoral nerve (FN) is the largest branch originating from the lumbar plexus. It originates from the posterior division of the spinal nerves L2, L3, and L4. The FN has both motor and sensory functions in the lower limb (Fig. 13.1).

In the abdomen, the FN, after its formation, follows a path through the psoas major muscle, and more distally, it follows a path between the psoas major and iliacus muscles. Inside the pelvis, the FN is closely related to the external iliac artery, which is positioned anterior and medial to this nerve. More distally, the FN passes under the inguinal ligament, produces a branch for the pectineus muscle, and penetrates the femoral triangle [2, 3].

The femoral triangle is bounded laterally by the sartorius muscle, medially by the adductor longus muscle, and superiorly by the inguinal ligament. The floor of this triangle is made up of the iliopsoas, pectineus, and adductor longus muscles, and its roof is formed by the fasciae latae muscle [4, 5].

In its course, after leaving the inguinal ligament, about 4 cm from it, the FN branches into its anterior and posterior divisions [4].

M. J. S. Magalhães, *Lower Extremity Nerve Entrapments*,
https://doi.org/10.1007/978-3-031-90058-7_13

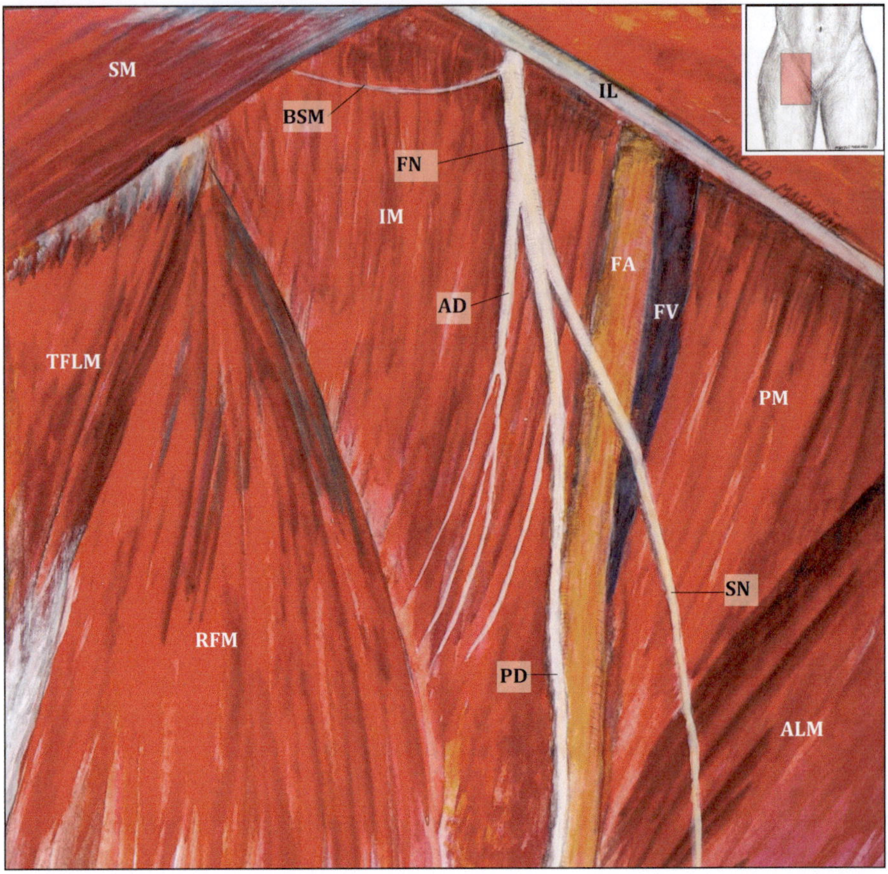

Fig. 13.1 Femoral nerve in right leg. Note that the sartorius muscle was detached and retracted laterally to better expose the femoral nerve and its branches. *AD* = anterior division of femoral nerve, *ALM* = adductor longus muscle, *BSM* = branch for sartorius muscle, *FA* = femoral artery, *FN* = femoral nerve, *FV* = femoral vein, *IL* = inguinal ligament, *IM* = iliacus muscle, *PD* = posterior division of femoral nerve, *PM* = pectineus muscle, *RFM* = rectus femoris muscle, *SM* = sartorius muscle, *SN* = saphenous nerve, *TFLM* = tensor fasciae latae muscle

The anterior division of the FN produces four branches: two motor branches for the sartorius muscle, the medial cutaneous nerve of the thigh, and the intermediate cutaneous nerve of the thigh. This muscle assists in the movement of hip flexion [5].

The posterior division produces the saphenous nerve, which is the longest branch of the FN. The saphenous nerve follows a medial course in the thigh and leg and is responsible for the sensitivity of the medial part of the knee, the medial part of the leg, the medial malleolus, and the medial arch of the foot, as well as the medial part of the big toe [5]. This division of the FN also produces the branch for the quadriceps femoris muscle (rectus femoris, vastus medialis, vastus intermedius, and vastus lateralis muscles). The quadriceps femoris muscle is responsible for knee extension. The branch that goes to the rectus femoris muscle also has a sensory innervation function of the hip joint. The other branches for the vastus medialis, vastus intermedius, and vastus lateralis muscles also have a sensory component for knee innervation [5]. The rectus femoris muscle in an anatomical study can receive between one and four motor branches, with the presence of two branches being the most common [6].

13.1.2 Signs and Symptoms of Femoral Nerve Neuropathy

A patient with FN neuropathy may present with clinical symptoms of pain, hypoesthesia, and paresthesias in the skin territory innervated by the sensory component of this nerve, especially in the area innervated by the saphenous branch. The patient may present these sensory changes in the inguinal region, anteromedial face of the leg, and medial part of the foot.

It is observed that the maneuver of hip extension may exacerbate the pain and can be evaluated during the patient's physical examination. The Tinel's sign should be evaluated along the course of the FN, especially near the inguinal ligament.

Regarding motor changes, trophic changes of the innervated musculature can be identified: pectineus, sartorius, and quadriceps. In patients with severe FN lesions, the hypotrophy of these muscles during inspection may be present. The patient should be asked about their gait, as weakness for knee extension can modify the patient's walk. Difficulty getting up from a chair may also be present in the patient's complaints.

The patellar reflex may be reduced or abolished, as the quadriceps can be compromised by the neuropathy. In the motor strength examination of the lower limbs, the patient may present paresis for hip flexion (psoas muscle involvement) and paresis for knee extension (quadriceps muscle involvement).

13.1.3 Classification of Femoral Nerve Neuropathy

The symptoms of FN neuropathy can present at least two well-defined patterns in terms of the speed of symptom manifestation: acute and chronic.

In the acute clinical picture, symptoms of pain and paresthesia develop quickly. In this group, the most commonly present etiologies are spontaneous hemorrhages. Iatrogenic and traumatic lesions also have immediate clinical manifestations. In the group with a chronic clinical picture, tumors, pregnancy, radiation, mononeuropathy, etc., are identified.

The etiology of FN neuropathy can also be classified into closed and open type lesions. Among the open lesions are those whose etiologies result from an event that violates the integrity of the skin, such as a penetrating traumatic injury (firearms, knives) and, surgical procedures of the hip and pelvis [7–11]. Among the lesions classified as closed type are tumors, radiation, pregnancy, hemorrhages, hypertrophic mononeuropathy, diabetic amyotrophy, and infections [12–15].

13.1.4 Differential Diagnoses of Femoral Neuropathy

Among the main differential diagnoses of FN neuropathy are high lumbar disc herniations (e.g., L2 and L3), avascular necrosis of the femoral head, rheumatic polymyalgia, lumbar plexopathy, and lumbar polyradiculopathy.

13.1.5 Additional Tests

For the diagnosis of femoral nerve neuropathy, different modalities of additional tests may be requested from patients. In the suspicion of hemorrhage as the cause of neuropathy, ultrasonography, computed tomography (CT), and magnetic resonance imaging (MRI) may be suitable tests. This same approach can assist in the diagnosis of tumor as the etiology of the disease [9, 10, 12, 16–18].

MRI and CT of the lumbosacral spine are useful tests for the exclusion of radiculopathy caused by disc hernias, especially those that occur at the most cranial levels of the lumbar spine. High-resolution MRI neurography can also be used as a complementary test for the investigation of patients with this neuropathy [19].

Among the additional tests for this group of patients, electroneuromyography (ENM) is considered the gold standard in the diagnosis of femoral nerve neuropathy. This test allows the evaluation of the motor and sensory conduction of the nerve. It is noted that a comparison between latency and amplitude can be performed between the affected side limb and the asymptomatic side. ENM also plays a relevant role in identifying the main differential diagnoses, such as lumbar spinal nerve radiculopathy, plexopathy, and polyradiculopathy. Another point of interest is the use of ENM for the evaluation of the recovery/progression process of the disease.

13.1.6 Treatment of Femoral Nerve Neuropathy: Overview

The first step after the complete investigation of the etiology of femoral nerve neuropathy is to define the best treatment. Patient management aims to control sensory symptoms which include pain and control of motor symptoms.

The patient with clinical symptoms resulting from hemorrhage, tumor, or masses to be clarified should opt for surgical treatment as the first option. On the other hand, those without tumoral or hemorrhagic etiology as the origin of their neuropathy should be candidates for conservative treatment.

In some patients, when a point of pinching of the femoral nerve along its path is identified, they are candidates for surgical decompression, especially in the absence of a satisfactory response after the implementation of conservative treatment [20].

13.1.7 Conservative Treatment of Patients with Femoral Nerve Neuropathy

Patients with acute symptoms of femoral nerve neuropathy may benefit from the use of ice, and patients with subacute symptoms may benefit from the use of local heat [1].

NSAID (non-steroidal anti-inflammatory) class medications may be useful for pain control, as well as, corticosteroid anti-inflammatory drugs. Another useful modality for pain control is the group of anticonvulsants such as carbamazepine, pregabalin, and gabapentin.

13.1.8 Surgical Treatment of Patients with Femoral Nerve Neuropathy

Patients with femoral nerve neuropathy in which tumoral lesions, hemorrhages [21], or compression points are identified may benefit from surgical treatment as a definitive treatment modality. When the integrity of the nerve is lost for some reason, such as, drainage of hematoma or tumor resection, nerve reconstruction should be performed with or without nerve graft.

It is interesting to recall that the literature describes the distal transfer of the motor branch of the obturator nerve to the femoral nerve with the aim of restoring the motor function of the quadriceps [6].

13.1.9 Surgical Approach to the Femoral Nerve

The patient is positioned in dorsal decubitus under general anesthesia, without the use of muscle blocker, and then undergoes asepsis of the lower limb, inguinal region, and lower abdomen. A cushion is placed under the knee of the limb to be operated on so that it is slightly flexed and abducted.

A marking of 1–2 cm is made on the longitudinal axis of the inguinal ligament, at a midpoint between the anterior superior iliac spine and the pubic branch. Another lateral line of approximately 10 cm is made from this midpoint in the direction of the longitudinal axis of the lower limb (Fig. 13.2).

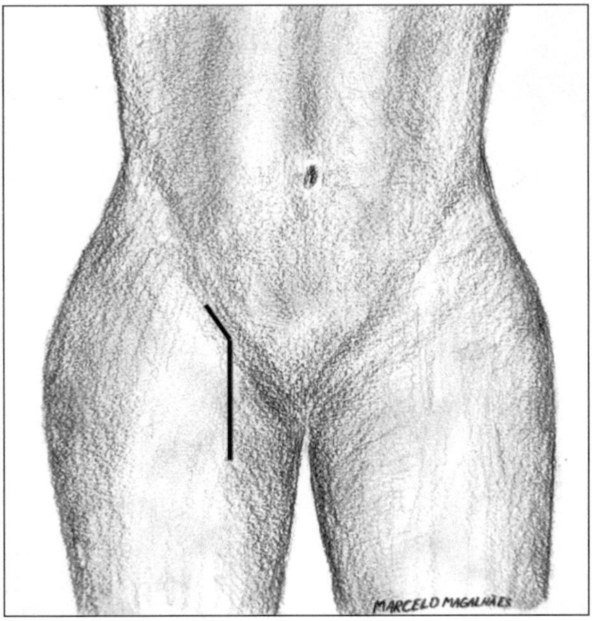

Fig. 13.2 Incision for surgical approach to the femoral nerve

After making the incision in the skin, the fascia of the thigh is identified under the areolar adipose tissue plane.

Preferably, the fascia of the thigh is incised parallel to the sartorius muscle. The sartorius muscle can then be pulled in the lateral direction and the femoral artery carefully pulled to the medial plane, with the aim to better identify the femoral nerve.

The dissection of the femoral nerve is performed proximally between the psoas major and iliacus muscles, under the inguinal ligament. The distal dissection is then performed to identify the distal branches, such as the saphenous (major branch) and anterior and posterior divisions [22].

13.1.10 Conclusion

Femoral nerve neuropathy is a rare clinical entity that should be investigated in patients with pain in the inner thigh, leg, as well as, patients with paresis for the performance of knee extension and hip flexion. The most commonly identified etiologies are spontaneous hemorrhages, surgical iatrogenies, traumas, tumors, pregnancy, radiation, and mononeuropathy. The conservative treatment is based on the use of local ice and heat, NSAIDs, steroid anti-inflammatory, and anticonvulsants. Patients with femoral nerve neuropathy, in which tumor lesions, hemorrhages, or compression points are identified, may benefit from surgical treatment.

13.2 Sural Nerve Neuropathy

13.2.1 Introduction

Sural nerve (SRN) neuropathy is a rare entity, even in large series of patients undergoing brachial plexus surgeries with the use of sural nerve grafts. The symptoms presented by patients are exclusively sensory, as the nerve only has sensory fibers in its constitution. Among the symptoms of this neuropathy, paresthesias, allodynia, pain in the lateral face of the leg, and lateral portion of the foot stand out [23].

13.2.2 Neuroanatomy of the Sural Nerve

The SRN is purely sensory located in the posterolateral part of the lower limb. Its relevance is due to the fact that the nerve is used as a graft in nerve reconstruction procedures. This nerve is responsible for the sensory innervation of a small portion of skin on the lateral part of the foot, including the lateral part of the ankle and fifth toe.

The SRN commonly originates from the union of a component from the tibial nerve (medial sural cutaneous nerve) and a component from the peroneal nerve which can be the lateral sural cutaneous nerve or fibers originated directly from the common peroneal nerve. However, it can be constituted by only the medial component from the tibial nerve or the lateral component from the common peroneal nerve (Fig. 13.3).

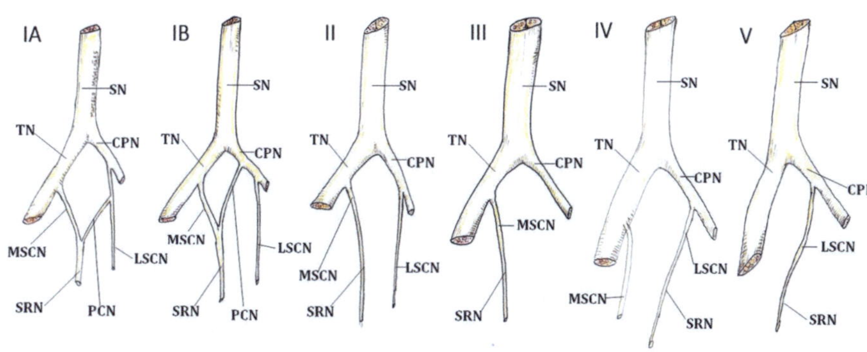

Fig. 13.3 Patterns of sural nerve formation from branches originating from the tibial and peroneal nerves. *CPN* = common peroneal nerve, *LSCN* = lateral sural cutaneous nerve, *MSCN* = medial sural cutaneous nerve, *PCN* = peroneal communicating nerve, *SRN* = sural nerve, *SN* = sciatic nerve, *TN* = tibial nerve

Thus, at least five patterns can be identified.

Pattern I = It is the most common pattern, with 63% of cases. The SRN is constituted by a medial component from the tibial nerve and a lateral component from the common peroneal nerve.

Pattern IA = SRN is constituted by fibers originating from the lateral sural cutaneous nerve.

Pattern IB = The lateral component originates directly from the common peroneal nerve through a peroneal communicating branch. In this pattern, the lateral sural cutaneous nerve may or may not be present.

Pattern II = Occurs in 27% of cases. The SRN is constituted only by the medial component from the tibial nerve and the lateral sural cutaneous nerve runs independently.

Pattern III = Occurs in 7% of cases. The SRN is constituted only by the medial component from the tibial nerve and the lateral sural nerve is absent.

Pattern IV = Occurs in 3% of cases. The SRN is constituted only by the lateral sural cutaneous nerve with the medial sural nerve running independently.

Pattern V = Very rare to be identified. The SRN is constituted only by the lateral sural cutaneous nerve and the medial sural cutaneous nerve is absent.

In the study by Riedl et al. (2013), it was shown that the medial sural cutaneous nerve was the nerve that was present in most of the specimens studied, with the exception of only one case. The medial sural cutaneous nerve almost always originates in the dorsal part of the circumference of the tibial nerve [24–31]. The medial sural cutaneous nerve originates outside the crural fascia, and its entry point to the subfascial space may contain a fibrous arcade positioned proximal to the musculotendinous junction of the gastrocnemius [24, 32–36].

As for the peroneal communicating branch, Huelke (1958) described that it originates from the common peroneal nerve in 42% of cases and that in 33% it originates from the lateral sural cutaneous nerve [23, 33]. Riedl et al. (2013) reveal that the lateral sural cutaneous nerve typically originates from the common peroneal nerve in its posteromedial quadrant [24].

The point of origin of the SRN is always in the proximal half of the leg. Regarding the disposition of the SRN in the fascial plane, it is noted that in 79% of cases, the origin of this nerve is positioned in the subfascial plane. More often, the pinching point of the SRN in the leg fascia is identified at the meeting of the second and third quarters of the leg [33, 37]. There are approximately 16 cm proximal to the lateral malleolus, the SRN perforates the crural fascia to reach a more lateral position in the leg, toward the lateral face of the calcaneus tendon. After perforating the fascia, the SRN follows a trajectory close to the small saphenous vein [22] (Fig. 13.4).

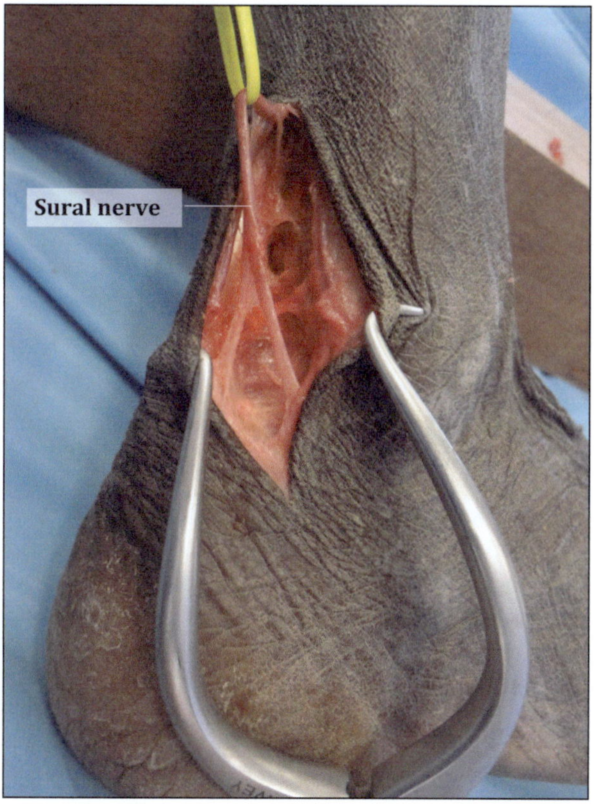

Fig. 13.4 Dissection of the sural nerve at its distal point on the lateral side of the right ankle

13.2.3 Etiology of Sural Nerve Neuropathy

The points of vulnerability of the SRN occur rarely in its proximal course. When they occur at this point, the causes include heterotopic calcification of the gastrocnemius muscle, injury to the gastrocnemius muscle, or a Baker's cyst. On the other hand, the distal involvement of the SRN can occur due to injury to the Achilles tendon, ankle fractures, or the fifth metatarsal [38]. Neuropathy can occur after biopsy and surgical treatments on the Achilles tendon and ankle, as well as, removal of the SRN for its use as a nerve graft.

13.2.4 Treatment of Sural Nerve Neuropathy

The conservative treatment of SRN neuropathy is usually directed at patients with idiopathic neuropathic etiology. In these cases, the patient should avoid the use of shoes and socks that can lead to nerve compression [39, 40].

Decompression of the sural nerve can be one of the treatment options, especially, in cases where the nerve undergoes a compressive process at its point of passage through the crural fascia.

Fabre et al. (2000) in their publication described the surgical treatment of eight athlete patients with compressive neuropathy of the SRN. In these described cases, the compressive process occurred due to thickening present in the crural fascia caused by a fibrotic band [41]. This is explained by the fact that the SRN originates at a point inside the fascia and that distally it needs to cross it, thus suffering compression [41, 42].

13.2.5 Surgical Approach to the Sural Nerve

13.2.5.1 Patient Position on the Surgical Table

The patient is positioned on the surgical table in two ways: prone or supine (Fig. 13.5a, b). The most ergonomic surgical approach for the surgeon is the one where the patient is positioned prone.

For the surgery of the patient in supine position, placing a cushion under the buttock area can assist in correct positioning. The patient's leg should be flexed at the hip and knee. For this, the patient's foot should be secured to the surgical table and the knee as well, to prevent it from being abducted during the procedure. This surgical position is the most used for cases of brachial plexus nerve reconstruction, as it allows the surgeon to approach the infra- and supraclavicular brachial plexus.

13.2.5.2 Type of Incision Used to Identify the Sural Nerve

Surgical approach to the sural nerve can be performed in several ways: a single longitudinal incision along its axis, endoscopic, and through three smaller incisions along its axis (Fig. 13.5a, b).

A. *Multiple Incisions*:

A 3 cm incision, lateral to the Achilles tendon, posterior to the lateral malleolus is made. A second 3 cm incision, at 19:00 h (left lower limb) or 17:00 h (right lower limb) on the clock, in the middle third of the calf and a third 3 cm incision, in the proximal third of the calf at 18:00 h on the clock is also made. In the supine position, it is advised that the surgeon perform the surgical approach seated, for better identification of the structures and greater ergonomics.

B. *Single Incision*

It is also possible to make a single and straight incision from the region lateral to the Achilles tendon to the proximal posterior third of the calf.

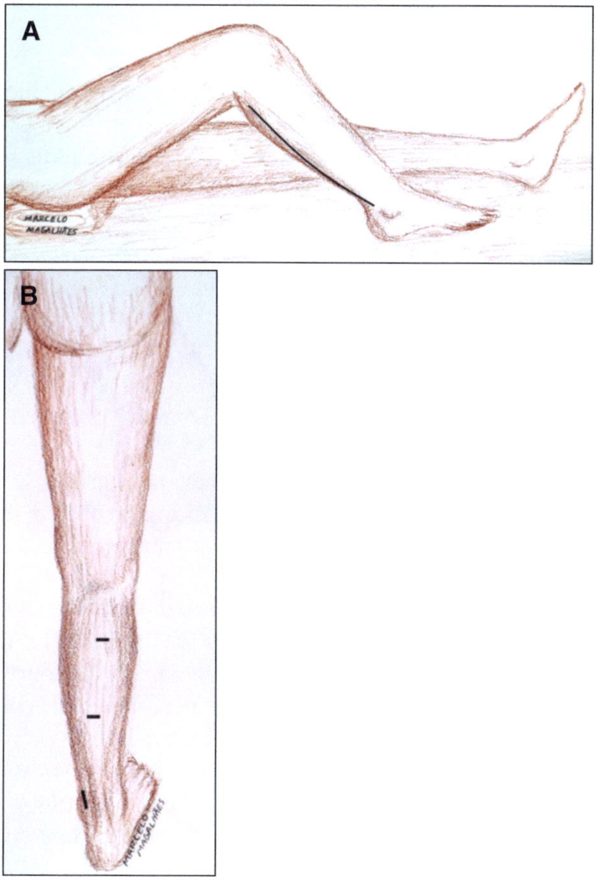

Fig. 13.5 (**a**) Patient position for surgical approach to the SRN in supine position. In this case, the illustration exemplifies how the incision is made in a single line. (**b**) Patient position for surgical approach in prone position. In this case, the illustration exemplifies the surgical approach to the sural nerve performed through 3 isolated incisions

C. *Dissection Details*

After making the incision in the skin, in the distal third of the leg, it is possible to identify the SRN in the subcutaneous plane. The small saphenous vein is positioned anterior to the nerve. The proximal dissection requires the opening of the leg fascia to expose the SRN. If the nerve is being dissected for its use as a graft in a nerve reconstruction surgery, it is first sectioned at its most distal point through the distal incision. Then, after applying slight traction, the SRN is sectioned proximally. The obtained graft should be kept inside saline solution until its use. Loose tissue adhered to the nerve should be resected before its use in nerve reconstruction [22].

13.2.6 Conclusion

Sural nerve neuropathy is a rare disease that should be investigated in patients with chronic pain in the region of its innervation territory, as well as in patients who have undergone surgeries or suffered some type of trauma where the nerve has a trajectory. Decompression can be one of the treatment options, especially, in cases where the nerve undergoes a compressive process.

13.3 Morton's Neuroma

13.3.1 Introduction

Morton's neuroma or intermetatarsal neuropathy is among the most common diseases that cause pain in the plantar region. The disease usually affects the third common plantar digital nerve, but it can also affect the second common plantar digital nerve [43].

In 1845, Lewis Durlacher described a painful syndrome that affected the plantar region, at the level of the metatarsals [44]. Only in 1876, Thomas Morton published a series of four cases of patients with pain in the fourth metatarsal joint. From this last publication, the term "Morton's neuroma" was coined [45]. Among the oldest anatomopathological descriptions of this painful syndrome in the medical literature is the publication by Civinini in 1935. In his cadaver study, this author identified the fusiform neuroma in the structure of the third digital common [46–49]. This pathological finding is identified in current imaging exams and aids in the diagnosis of this painful syndrome.

Despite the term "neuroma" referring to a tumor, it is believed that this neuropathy originates from a chronic inflammatory process [43].

13.3.2 Neuroanatomy of Digital Nerves

The plantar region has complex sensory innervation originating from several nerve branches: sural nerve (branch with a component of the tibial and peroneal nerves), saphenous nerve (branch of the femoral nerve), and medial and lateral plantar nerves (branches of the tibial nerve). The plantar surface of the toes is innervated by the terminal branches of the medial and lateral plantar nerves.

For a better understanding of the anatomy of the plantar digital nerves, knowledge of the complete anatomy of the tibial nerve is necessary.

The sciatic nerve is made up of nerve fibers originating from the spinal nerves L4-S3. The sciatic nerve, in turn, is responsible for the origin of the common peroneal and posterior tibial nerves, at the level of the distal third of the thigh [22].

The tibial nerve is a mixed type nerve that has motor, autonomic, and sensory fibers. In its constitution, there are nerve fibers from the spinal nerves L4-S3 [22]. The tibial nerve is responsible for the motility of the following lower limb muscles:

- Soleus muscle.
- Tibialis posterior muscle.
- Gastrocnemius muscle.
- Flexor hallucis longus muscle.
- Flexor digitorum longus muscle.
- Popliteus muscle.
- Quadratus plantae muscle.
- Adductor hallucis muscle.
- Flexor hallucis brevis muscle.
- Flexor digitorum brevis muscle.
- The first, second, third, and fourth lumbrical muscles of the foot.
- Abductor digiti minimi muscle.
- Flexor digiti quinti brevis muscle.
- Interosseous muscles of the foot.

After the tibial nerve passes through the popliteal fossa, it follows a trajectory over the popliteus muscle. It then reaches a deep trajectory in relation to the soleus muscle and a superficial trajectory in relation to the posterior tibial muscle. At the level of the medial malleolus, it penetrates the tarsal tunnel. Usually, the tibial nerve at the level of this osteofibrous tunnel emits the following branches: calcaneal, medial plantar, and lateral plantar [22].

The posterior tarsal tunnel (PTT) has as its roof, the flexor retinaculum that attaches to the medial malleolus and calcaneus. Inside the tunnel are the tendons of the tibialis posterior muscle, flexor digitorum longus, flexor hallucis longus, tibial nerve, tibial artery, and tibial veins [22]. The posterior limit of the PTT is the posterior process of the talus, the superior limit the medial malleolus, the lateral edge is constituted by the calcaneus, and the inferior edge the abductor hallucis longus muscle. The flexor retinaculum is also called the lancinate ligament or internal annular ligament.

The sensory fibers of the tibial nerve run through the medial sural cutaneous nerve, medial plantar branch, lateral plantar branch, and calcaneal branch.

It is noted that the sensory territory of the tibial nerve corresponds to the lateral portion of the foot, sole, and a small portion of skin located distally on the dorsum of the toes, excluding the skin located in the first interdigital space which is made by the deep peroneal nerve.

The medial plantar nerve commonly produces the first, second, and third common plantar digital nerve and the lateral plantar nerve produces the fourth common plantar digital nerve. Distally, each common plantar digital branch produces two proper digital branches that innervate the skin located between adjacent toes.

It is at the bifurcation of the common plantar digital nerve that Morton's neuroma is identified.

The existence of a communicating branch that makes anastomosis between the medial and lateral plantar nerves, at the level of the third common plantar digital nerve, is described in 51% of individuals [50–54] (Fig. 13.6).

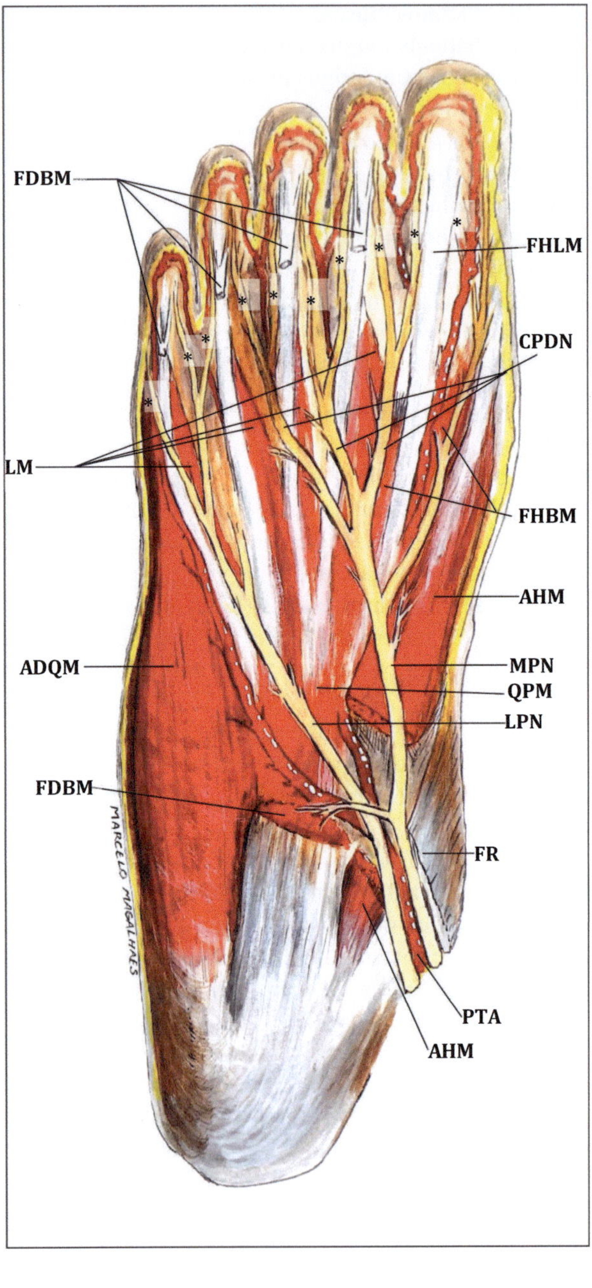

Fig. 13.6 Plantar nerves after resection of the flexor digitorum brevis and abductor hallucis muscles. * Proper plantar digital nerve. *ADQM* = abductor digiti quinti muscle, *AHM* = abductor hallucis muscle, *CPDN* = common plantar digital nerve, *FDBM* = flexor digitorum brevis muscle, *FDBM* = flexor digitorum brevis muscle (tendons), *FHBM* = flexor hallucis brevis muscle (tendon), *FHLM* = flexor hallucis longus muscle (tendon), *FR* = flexor retinaculum, *LM* = lumbrical muscles, *LPN* = lateral plantar nerve, *MPN* = medial plantar nerve, *PTA* = posterior tibial artery, *PTA* = posterior tibial artery, *QPM* = quadratus plantae muscle

13.3.3 Symptoms and Signs of Morton's Neuroma

According to Mak et al. (2020), this neuropathy is more common in middle-aged women. Among the identified risk factors is the use of high heels and pointed shoes. Among the symptoms most commonly described by patients is pain when walking. Usually, the pain is located in the metatarsal region which intensifies when wearing high heels or pointed shoes. The pain can have a character of radiation to the toes which the proper plantar digital branches innervate [43, 55, 56]. It is noted that manual palpation of the plantar region can also trigger symptoms and not infrequently, the patient reports the sensation of stepping on a stone, fold in the sock, or bump in the shoe floor [43, 56].

13.3.4 Differential Diagnoses of Morton's Neuroma

Among the most common differential diagnoses is fasciitis plantar and posterior tarsal tunnel neuropathy.

13.3.5 Additional Tests

The diagnosis is made through the patient's clinical history and physical examination; however, additional tests may assist in the diagnosis.

Foot radiography can assist in the diagnosis through indirect signs of the presence of the neuroma, such as the increase in the distal intermetatarsal space, which is called Sullivan's Sign [57].

Ultrasound (US) is the test of choice due to its low cost and the possibility of performing infiltration during its execution. Morton's neuroma presents as an ovoid hypoechoic aspect, at the level of the metatarsal heads, in the intermetastatic space. It can also be identified adjacent to the neuroma, the presence of tissue with a hyperechoic aspect, compatible with adipose tissue [43, 58, 59]. From the neuroma, continuity can be identified with the plantar digital nerve, which is around 1 to 2 mm [43, 59]. Sometimes, the presence of the bursa adjacent to the neuroma makes the image on the US larger than the actual size of the neuroma. Characteristically, the bursa can be filled with anesthetic/corticosteroid during US-guided puncture [43].

Magnetic resonance imaging (MRI) of the foot has similar sensitivity to US. It allows the examiner to identify cysts, tumors, tendinitis, fractures, and bursitis. Morton's neuroma on MRI appears hypointense or with intermediate intensity. In the T1W sequence, the neuroma appears isointense with skeletal muscle, with hyperintensity around it represented by adipose tissue [43].

13.3.6 Conservative Treatment of Morton's Neuroma

Among the conservative treatment options is infiltration with corticosteroid associated with local anesthetic. A relevant review on the subject showed clinical evidence that corticosteroid infiltration has a benefit in pain control in this group of patients. Another advantage of this treatment method is the confirmation of the diagnosis after immediate pain control after infiltration [43, 57, 60].

It is important to mention that the patient should be informed that the use of corticosteroids can trigger side effects, such as increased blood pressure and glycemic levels, skin depigmentation, and dermal and skin hypotrophy. Patients with an ongoing infectious process should not be candidates for corticosteroid treatment [61, 62].

The use of insoles and changing footwear is also described in the literature as treatment [63].

13.3.7 Surgical Treatment

Patients in whom conservative clinical treatment has failed may benefit from neurectomy of the neuroma. It is important to note that after surgery, the patient will present as a sequel, permanent hypoesthesia in the territory innervated by the common plantar digital nerve.

Surgical approach to the neuroma can be made through the plantar or dorsal route, and several techniques have already been described: isolated excision of the common plantar digital nerve, isolated division of the deep transverse metatarsal ligament, and a combination of these two techniques [64–66].

13.3.7.1 Dorsal Approach to Morton's Neuroma

The patient is positioned in dorsal decubitus, and after asepsis of the limb, local or regional anesthesia can be chosen. The use of a tourniquet at the level of the ankle or thigh to assist in hemostasis is optional [66].

A 3–4 cm incision is made longitudinally, starting at the head of the metatarsal and extending to the interdigital space. After the skin incision, the subcutaneous tissue is carefully retracted so as not to injure the dorsal digital nerves. After this maneuver, the deep fascia of the foot is opened through an incision parallel to that of the skin. Then, the deep transverse metatarsal ligament is identified and sectioned with the help of surgical instruments that allow the retraction of the metatarsals. Once the two proper plantar digital nerves, originating from the common plantar digital nerve, are identified, the former are sectioned.

Then, the common plantar digital nerve is pulled in the distal direction and sectioned at a proximal point, at the level of the metatarsal heads. After these maneuvers, the subcutaneous plane and skin are sutured. This technique has the advantage of the surgical wound not being located in the plantar region.

13.3.7.2 Plantar Approach to Morton's Neuroma

This technique is recommended for patients who have already undergone neurectomy for Morton's neuroma in a dorsal approach and who have evolved with recurrence of symptoms, due to the formation of a new neuroma [67–70].

The patient is positioned in dorsal decubitus, and after asepsis of the limb, local or regional anesthesia can be performed. The use of a tourniquet at the ankle or thigh is optional [66]. A plantar incision of approximately 4 cm is made longitudinally in the interdigital space, equidistant from the heads of the metatarsals. After opening the skin, the neuroma is already in the subcutaneous plane. Then, the common plantar digital nerve is identified and dissected, both proximally and distally. As soon as the neuroma is identified, it is resected, and the proximal stump of the common plantar digital nerve is introduced into the intrinsic musculature of the foot. After these maneuvers, the subcutaneous plane and skin are sutured [66].

13.3.7.3 Postoperative Care

Patients who undergo dorsal approach can, postoperatively, support the operated foot on the ground to walk. It is recommended that the surgical stitches be removed after 10–14 days. However, patients who undergo plantar surgical approach should remain for 2–3 weeks without supporting the operated foot on the ground. In this technique, it is recommended that the surgical stitches be removed only after this period [66].

13.3.8 Conclusion

Morton's neuroma is a disease that causes pain in the plantar region due to the usual involvement of the third common plantar digital nerve, and it can also affect the second common plantar digital nerve. Symptoms tend to intensify with the patient's gait. Its diagnosis is made through the patient's anamnesis, physical examination, and complementary exams. There are different modalities of conservative treatment, such as corticosteroid infiltration. In refractory cases, surgical treatment may be indicated.

13.4 Obturator Nerve Neuropathy

13.4.1 Introduction

Among the neuropathies described in the lower limbs, obturator nerve (ON) neuropathy is considered quite rare, especially when compared to other neuropathies, such as those affecting the peroneal nerve and tibial nerve at the level of the tarsal tunnel [71–73].

As identified in other compressive neuropathies, several risk factors have been described over time, such as pelvic/sacroiliac joint trauma, hematomas, tumors, hip positioning in full flexion during surgical procedures, and sports practices such as ice hockey, soccer, and rugby [74–80].

13.4.2 Neuroanatomy of the Obturator Nerve

The ON is a mixed nerve that carries both sensory and motor fibers. It is responsible for the innervation of the muscles located in the medial compartment of the thigh, as well as the sensitivity of the skin located on the medial face of the thigh and knee joint. It is constituted by the union of the fibers of the ventral branches of the spinal nerves L2, L3, and L4.

Regarding the formation of the ON, Tshabalala et al. (2022) described in a study with 181 limbs, that in 80% of the cases, the ON was constituted by the spinal nerves L2-L4 and in 20% by the spinal nerves L3-L4. These authors also mention that in 1.7% of the cases, the fusion of the fibers of the anterior branches of the spinal nerves occurred outside the psoas major muscle [81].

The formation of the ON trunk occurs inside the psoas major muscle and leaves it at its lateral edge. The ON penetrates the pelvic region approximately at the level of the sacroiliac joint. This nerve associated with the obturator vein and artery constitutes the neurovascular bundle that penetrates the obturator foramen. Still within the obturator canal, the ON divides into posterior, anterior, and muscular branches (Fig. 13.7).

It is important to mention that the point at the bifurcation of the ON is very variable and can occur both in the intrapelvic cavity, obturator canal, and on the medial face of the thigh [82–87].

Regarding the bifurcation of the ON into its branches, Tshabalala et al. (2022) showed that between 1% and 3% of the cases occurred still in the intrapelvic region, between 92% and 94% occurred inside the obturator canal, and finally, at an extrapelvic point, in 5% of the cases [81].

The anterior branch of the ON is responsible for the sensory innervation of the distal 2/3 of the medial face of the thigh. This branch is also responsible for the innervation of the muscles: adductor longus, adductor brevis, and gracilis [73, 81, 83, 85, 88].

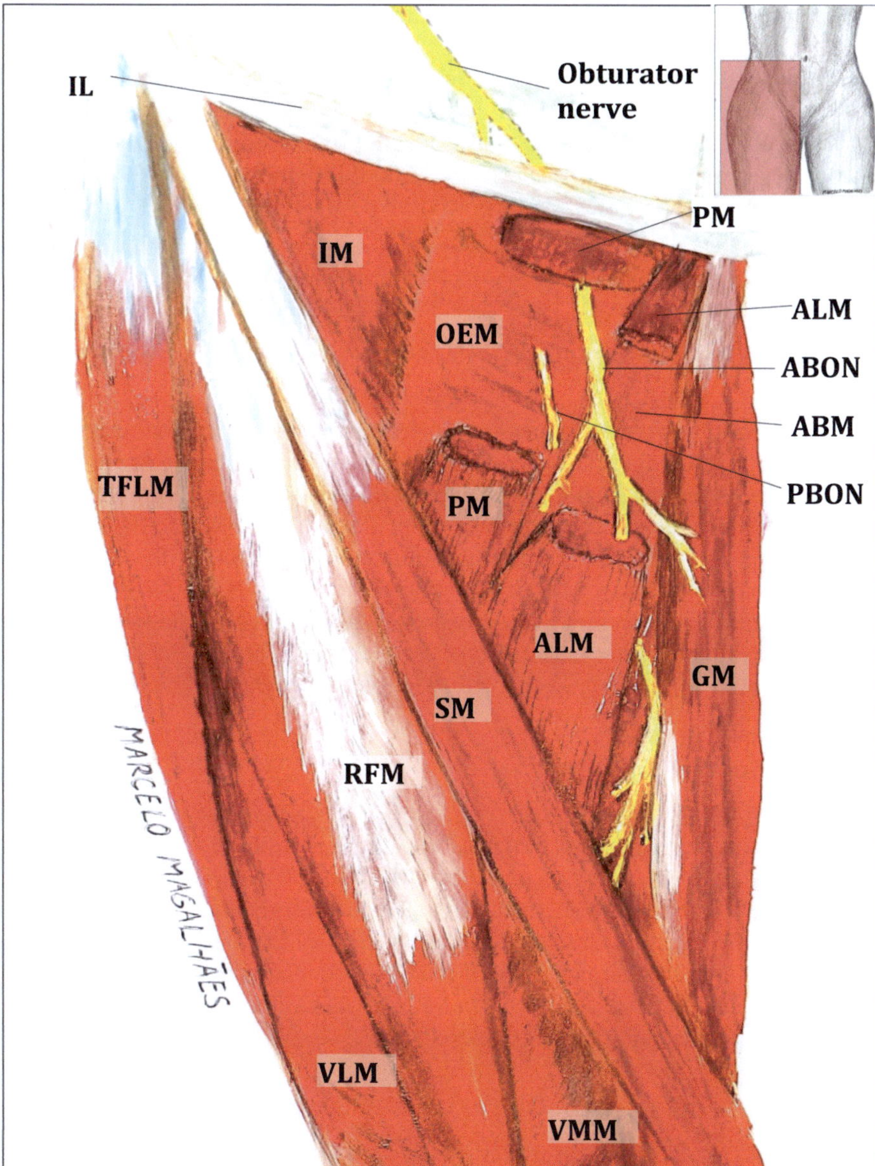

Fig. 13.7 Exposure of the obturator nerve after the resection of the pectineus and adductor longus muscles . *ABM* = adductor brevis muscle, *ABON* = anterior branch of obturator nerve, *ALM* = adductor longus muscle, *GM* = gracilis muscle, *IL* = inguinal ligament, *IM* = iliacus muscle, *OEM* = obturator externus muscle, *PBON* = posterior branch of obturator nerve, *PM* = pectineus muscle, *RFM* = rectus femoris muscle, *SM* = sartorius muscle, *TFLM* = tensor fasciae latae muscle, *VLM* = vastus lateralis muscle, *VMM* = vastus medialis muscle

The posterior branch of the ON produces motor fibers for a portion of the adductor magnus muscle.

Regarding the anatomical variation of this nerve, the presence of an accessory ON is described by some authors in anatomical studies. Tshabalala et al. (2022), Tubbs et al. (2005) [81, 89] did not identify the presence of an accessory ON. However, in the study by Akkaya et al. (2008) [90] the accessory ON was identified in 12.5% of the cases, and the study by Anloague and Huijbregts (2009) revealed a prevalence of 8.8% [91].

13.4.3 Signs and Symptoms of Obturator Nerve Neuropathy

Those suffering from this compressive syndrome may have pain and paresthesias located in the inguinal region, medial face of the thigh, and knee. Some patients may present symptoms such as the sensation of loss of power during their sports practices. Physical exertion can intensify complaints and rest can alleviate them. Rarely, there is paresis for adduction and internal rotation of the lower limb [92, 93].

Some patients may present in their neurological examination the loss of the hip adductor reflex on the affected side [71].

13.4.4 Pathophysiology

Regarding the pathophysiology of this neuropathy, it is believed that its origin could be associated with the compression of the ON when it crosses the obturator canal, which is an osteofibrous tunnel, or at a point located over the short brevis muscle, at the level of the thigh. The compressive process adjacent to the adductor brevis muscle would develop from an adhesion of the ON secondary to a local inflammatory process in the muscle fascia. Fibrosis in this anatomical location can be secondary to chronic tendinitis, adjacent to the nerve [71].

13.4.5 Differential Diagnosis of Obturator Nerve Neuropathy

Several diseases can lead to pain in the upper segment of the thigh: meralgia paresthesia, femoral nerve neuropathy, high lumbar radiculopathy resulting from disc herniation, and hip joint osteoarthritis.

Meralgia paresthesia causes pain in the lateral part of the thigh. Performing anesthetic block of the lateral femoral cutaneous nerve can be useful in confirming the diagnosis.

Lumbar disc herniation that causes an L4 radiculopathy can lead the patient to a clinical picture of paresis for knee extension, reduction or abolition of the patellar reflex, and in some more severe cases, hypotrophy of the quadriceps femoris muscle. The inverted Lasègue maneuver may be positive in patients with this L4 radiculopathy.

Hip osteoarthritis occurs more frequently in patients from the elderly group. Radiography and computed tomography of the hip joint can assist in the diagnosis.

Other differential diagnoses for ON neuropathy have already been cited in the literature: fractures of the femur neck, pubis, bursitis and iliopsoas synovitis, psoas muscle tendinopathy, enthesopathy of the inguinal ligament, and inguinal hernia [73].

13.4.6 Diagnosis of Obturator Nerve Neuropathy

The diagnosis of ON neuropathy is made through the patient's clinical history and physical examination.

Anesthetic block is an interesting option. The diagnosis is suggested when the patient presents control of symptoms after the anesthetic block [94–96]. After the nerve block, the presence of hypoesthesia in the medial face of the thigh and absence of pain in provocative tests suggests that the infiltration was performed in the correct place [71].

Electroneuromyography of the lower limbs may show signs of denervation of the adductor muscles [94, 95, 97].

Magnetic resonance imaging can assist in identifying inflammatory processes on the inner face of the thigh, as well as, pelvis. This exam can also display, in cases of severe ON neuropathy, the denervation of the pectineus and adductor muscles of the thigh [71].

13.4.7 Conservative Treatment

Tipton (2008) mentions that conservative treatment is based on physiotherapy, gradual return to physical activities, stretching, and corticosteroid infiltrations in the affected region with the help of imaging exams. This author also comments that, most of the time, pain control is temporary [73, 97, 98].

13.4.8 Surgical Treatment

The surgical approach of the ON, at the proximal level of the thigh, is described through decompression at the nerve pinching point.

Bradshaw et al. (1997) describe that decompression of the anterior branch of the obturator nerve is a treatment option for the symptoms of this neuropathy [71].

The surgical procedure is performed by opening the fascia, at its path point over the adductor brevis muscle, between the pectineus muscle and the adductor longus muscle [98].

Menderes et al. (2015) describe a case report in which a surgical approach was used as a treatment for iatrogenic injury of the ON. In this work, the nerve was reconstructed after being injured during pelvic lymphadenectomy for the treatment of endometrial carcinoma [99].

13.4.8.1 Approach to the Obturator Nerve via Intrapelvic and in the Thigh

The intrapelvic route is performed by a transabdominal extraperitoneal approach. With the patient in the dorsal decubitus position, a 6–7 cm oblique incision is made cranially to the inguinal ligament starting from the anterior superior iliac spine. The fibers that make up the abdominal oblique muscles are divulsed to identify the pre-peritoneal fat. The bladder and the peritoneum are retracted for better visualization of the ON in its intrapelvic trajectory [86, 100, 101].

13.4.8.2 Approach to the Obturator Nerve via Medial Face of the Thigh

With the patient in the dorsal decubitus position and with the thigh slightly extended and the knee slightly flexed, an oblique incision of 5–7.5 cm is made from the inguinal ligament.

The starting point of the incision is located halfway along a line that joins the femoral artery (located by palpation) and the pubic symphysis. Then the incision line extends from the lateral part of the adductor magnus muscle.

After the incision, the great saphenous vein should be identified, dissected, and is moved laterally. Thus, the fascia lata is identified and an incision is made along the lateral portion of the adductor longus muscle.

Through blunt dissection, the adductor longus muscle is separated from the pectineus. The anterior branch is positioned under a fascia that covers the short adductor muscle.

The fascia covering the adductor brevis muscle should then be incised and the ON dissected, from distal to proximal, where it will be possible to identify the posterior branch. By dissecting the branches of the ON proximally under the pectineus muscle, the obturator foramen is identified [102].

13.4.9 Conclusion

Obturator nerve neuropathy is considered quite rare. Some risk factors have been described over time: trauma to the pelvis/sacroiliac joint, hematomas, tumors, positioning of the hip in full flexion during surgical procedures, and sports practices. Among the most identified symptoms are pain/paresthesias located in the inguinal region and medial aspect of the thigh and knee. Conservative treatment provides transient results in symptom control. Surgical decompression of the nerve is an available option.

13.5 Ilioinguinal Nerve Neuropathy

13.5.1 Introduction

Ilioinguinal nerve neuropathy (IIN) is a neuropathy usually resulting from injury to this nerve after surgical procedures performed in the abdomen region. It is estimated that in the United States about 800,000 herniorrhaphies are performed annually, with 12% of patients developing chronic pain and 2% with IIN neuropathy [103–105].

Patients with this painful syndrome have pain in the genital region and upper part of the thigh. The diagnosis of this neuropathy is made through the patient's clinical history, physical examination, as well as complementary exams, such as ultrasound and electroneuromyography [106]. Initial treatment is conservative, with surgery reserved only for cases refractory to non-invasive measures [106].

13.5.2 Neuroanatomy of the Ilioinguinal Nerve

The ilioinguinal nerve (IIN) is a mixed type nerve that contains axonal fibers of both the motor and sensory types in its structure.

This nerve originates from fibers of the anterior branch of the spinal nerves T12 and L1 [103]. After its formation, the IIN emerges at the lateral edge of the psoas major muscle in a caudal direction, in the subperitoneal plane of the anterior abdominal wall, anterior to the quadratus lumborum muscle until it reaches the anterior superior iliac spine [103, 107] (Fig. 13.8).

From this point, the IIN crosses and innervates the transversus abdominis muscle and internal oblique muscle. As it follows a trajectory parallel to the inguinal ligament, this nerve takes a more superficial course to cross the superficial inguinal ring in men and the round ligament in women.

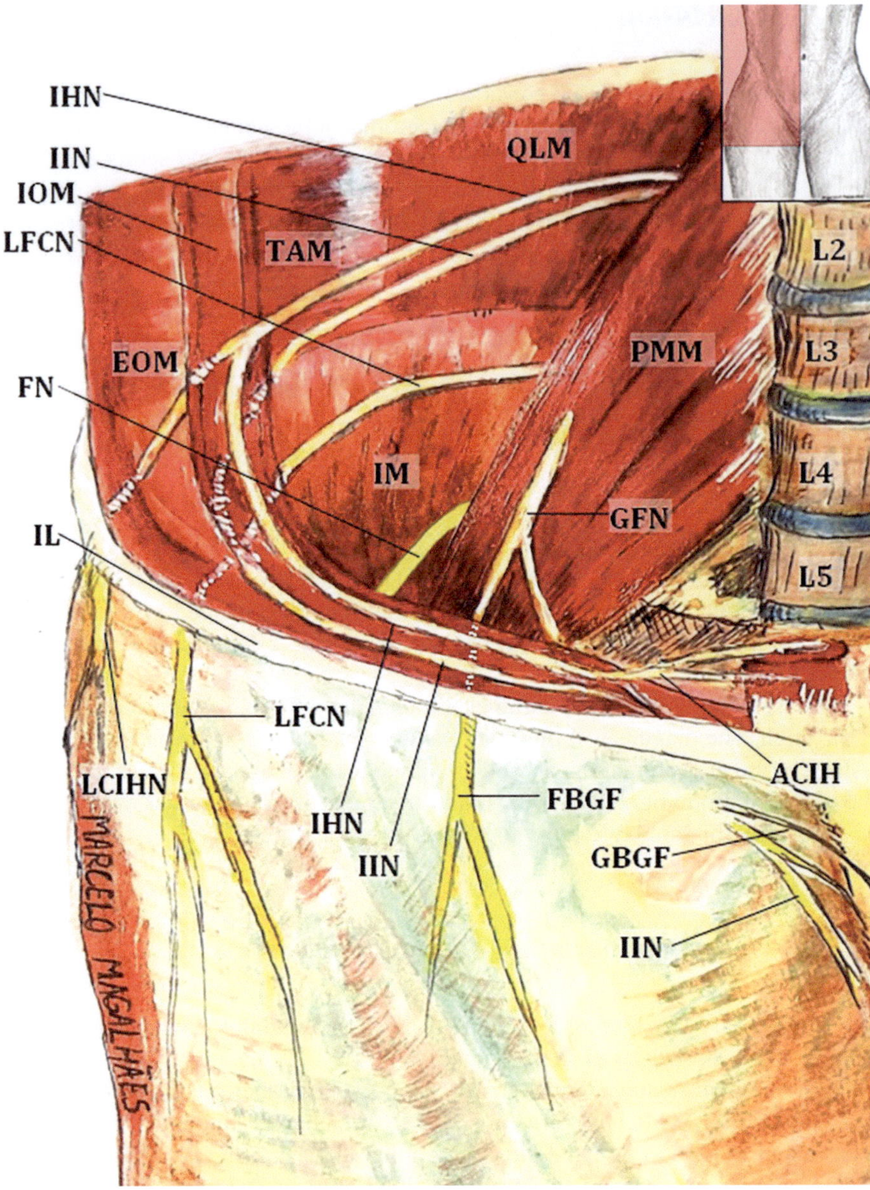

Fig. 13.8 Anatomy of the main nerves of the inguinal region and anterior region of the thigh. *ACIH* = anterior cutaneous branch of iliohypogastric nerve, *FBGF* = femoral branch of genitofemoral nerve, *FN* = femoral nerve, *GBGF* = genital branch of genitofemoral nerve, *GFN* = genitofemoral nerve, *IHN* = iliohypogastric nerve, *IIN* = ilioinguinal nerve, *IL* = inguinal ligament, *IM* = iliacus muscle, *LCIHN* = lateral cutaneous branch of iliohypogastric nerve, *LFCN* = lateral femoral cutaneous nerve, *LSCN* = lateral sural cutaneous nerve, *OEAM* = obliquus externus abdominis muscle, *OIAM* = obliquus internus abdominis muscle, *PMM* = psoas major muscle, *QLM* = quadratus lumborum muscle, *TAM* = transversus abdominis muscle

In women, the IIN is responsible for the sensory innervation of the pubic mound, large lips, and a small area of skin located in the anteromedial part of the thigh, and in men the skin of the anterior face of the scrotum, root of the penis, and a small part of the anteromedial region of the thigh [103, 107].

13.5.3 Etiology of Ilioinguinal Nerve Neuropathy

Among the most identified etiologies of IIN neuropathy are surgical procedures in the abdomen, such as appendectomy and hysterectomy. This neuropathy is also described in orchiectomy and testicular surgery, when the surgical approach is performed through the inguinal route [3, 106]. Other causes are described: tissue stretching occurred during childbirth and injury due to the use of a trocar during laparoscopic surgery [106].

However, some patients with this neuropathy do not have an identifiable cause, being classified as carriers of idiopathic IIN neuropathy [107–110].

13.5.4 Differential Diagnosis of Ilioinguinal Nerve Neuropathy

Diseases that affect nerves with a trajectory in the pelvic region and inguinal region can lead the patient to develop a painful clinical picture similar to those identified in IIN neuropathy.

In this group of diseases, we can mention lumbar radiculopathies, meralgia paresthetica, and femoral nerve neuropathy.

Lumbar disc herniation, at more cranial levels, can trigger pain in the anterior region of the thigh in the patient, in addition to changes in the patellar reflex and in some cases paresis for knee extension. The inverted Lasègue sign may be present. MRI of the lumbar spine and electroneuromyography of the lower limbs can assist in this diagnosis [112].

Femoral nerve neuropathy can also trigger pain in the anterior region of the thigh and the inner region of the leg. Some patients with this neuropathy may evolve with paresis for knee extension. Femoral nerve block, guided by ultrasound, can assist in confirming this diagnosis, as well as the examination of electroneuromyography of the lower limbs [113].

Meralgia paresthetica, which results from the involvement of the lateral femoral cutaneous nerve, is a potential differential diagnosis for IIN neuropathy. Patient may evolve with pain and paresthesias in the superolateral face of the thigh. In meralgia paresthetica, there is no motor impairment since the lateral femoral cutaneous nerve is purely sensory. The block test with local anesthetic guided by ultrasound can assist in the diagnosis [114].

13.5.5 Clinical and Complementary Diagnosis of Ilioinguinal Nerve Neuropathy

The diagnosis of IIN neuropathy can be suggested by the pattern of pain described by the patient in the sensory territory of the IIN and also by the history of surgeries that are known to be potential risk factors for the disease [106].

As in other neuropathies, a local anesthetic block can be used, in which symptom control after the test strengthens the diagnosis of IIN neuropathy. However, a negative test does not exclude this diagnosis [106, 115, 116].

Electroneuromyography of the lower limbs is not very useful for the diagnosis of this neuropathy. However, it is a complementary examination advantageous for the identification of other neurological diseases, such as radiculopathies, plexopathies, and polyneuropathies [6].

Ultrasound may be useful for performing the anesthetic block test. It is important to note that it is a low-cost and more accessible examination. It has become a useful tool in the investigation of compressive neuropathies. This examination modality allows for the identification the IIN from the anterior superior iliac spine to the external inguinal ring [20, 21].

Magnetic resonance imaging of the pelvis and lumbosacral spine can assist in identifying other potential differential diagnoses such as lumbar disc herniation. In patients with more severe IIN, the pelvic examination may show denervation of the internal oblique and transverse abdominal muscles. Patients who have undergone surgery in the inguinal region this examination can be especially useful [10].

13.5.6 Conservative Treatment of Ilioinguinal Nerve Neuropathy

As the pain in IIN neuropathy can be transient, the first step is to instruct the patient to avoid activities that require maintenance of the body with hip extension or long periods of walking. The resting position in bed with the hip and knees slightly flexed can provide relief from pain symptoms [106].

Oral medications are similar to those used in other compressive neuropathic syndromes: non-steroidal anti-inflammatory drugs (NSAIDs); tricyclic antidepressants such as amitriptyline; anticonvulsants such as gabapentin and pregabalin; and serotonin reuptake inhibitor antidepressants. Opioid analgesics can also be used [106].

Randomized studies on the use of capsaicin and lidocaine in skin patches for control of post-herniorrhaphy IIN neuropathy did not reveal satisfactory results [117, 118].

In addition to oral and topical medication, rehabilitation can assist in symptom control. Acupuncture, transcutaneous nerve electrical stimulation, and myofascial release are described in the literature for the treatment of these patients. It is emphasized that if pain symptoms persist for more than 6 months, other therapeutic measures should be indicated [119, 120].

Infiltration of the IIN with anesthetic, as a form of treatment for neuropathy, can be an option. Kastler et al. (2012) showed that symptoms were controlled by infiltration for an average period of only 1.6 months. Studies reveal that the control of IIN neuropathy symptoms through infiltration of anesthetics and corticosteroids guided by ultrasound is uncertain. Pain control rates remained between 55% and 75% [103, 121, 122].

13.5.7 Minimally Invasive Treatment of Ilioinguinal Nerve Neuralgia

Various procedures have been described in the literature for the treatment of patients with IIN neuropathy: cryoneurolysis, dorsal root ganglion stimulation, spinal cord stimulation, peripheral nerve stimulation, pulsed radiofrequency ablation, and selective spinal nerve block.

Cryoneurolysis is a treatment modality in which the nerve is cooled to the point of creating a structural lesion, typically guided by ultrasound. Studies show that control of pain symptoms can last for a period of 6 to 12 months [123–125].

A case report published by Elias (2000) explores the use of spinal cord stimulation (SCS) in the treatment of chronic post-herniorrhaphy pain. The patient in question had a pain condition that lasted for 2 years without adequate control. After the implantation of spinal stimulation, there was a 50% reduction in pain intensity, with persistence of the analgesic effect for at least 6 months after the procedure [126].

Stimulation of the sensory ganglion of the spinal nerve is an interesting procedure for the control of patients with IIN neuropathy. In the work of Schu et al. (2015) involving 10 patients, there was an average reduction of 70% in the pain of patients who used this treatment technique. The follow-up of the cases varied between 3 and 12 months. About 80% of patients were satisfied with the treatment [127].

Werner et al. (2012) conducted a systematic review on the use of pulsed radiofrequency for the treatment of post-inguinal herniorrhaphy pain. This review included five works. A success rate in pain control between 50% and 70% was identified. The patients in these studies were followed for a period from 3 to 12 months [128].

13.5.8 Surgical Treatment of Ilioinguinal Nerve Neuralgia

The patient is positioned in dorsal decubitus and asepsis is performed on the abdomen, root of the thigh, and inguinal region. A cushion is positioned under the gluteal region ipsilateral to the surgical approach.

The incision presents an inferomedial line, aligned with the longitudinal axis of the inguinal ligament. It is usually made medial and 2–3 cm cranial to the anterior superior iliac spine, with an extension of approximately 6 cm directed toward the midline. After identifying the subcutaneous tissue plane, this tissue is retracted to expose medially, the fibers of the rectus abdominis muscle and laterally, the fascia of the obliquus externus abdominis muscle. From this point, the fascia should be incised, as well as the fibers of the obliquus externus abdominis muscle.

The IIN can be identified on the obliquus internus abdominis muscle and below the fibers of the obliquus externus abdominis muscle. It is a nerve that has an approximate diameter of 1 mm and has a trajectory with direction to the inguinal region. It is noted that next to the IIN, in its trajectory, it is possible to identify a smaller caliber vein.

Usually, the dissection of the IIN should proceed medially to the point where the nerve penetrates the scar area secondary to previous surgery, if that is the clinical case in question. Then, the IIN is sectioned as proximally as possible from its exit point from the retroperitoneum. As this is a neurectomy, the patient will develop a permanent hypoesthesia in the skin area supplied by the IIN [122].

13.5.9 Complications of Ilioinguinal Nerve Neurectomy

Among the complications described after IIN neurectomy, is the sensory deficit in the innervated territory. Some patients may have some degree of hypersensitivity due to the deafferentation process that can occur.

There may also be flaccidity of the denervated abdominal muscles, especially when the neurectomy is performed at a proximal anatomical point, such as in the retroperitoneal space. As the IIN provides part of the sensory innervation of the genitals, the patient may present impairment of sexual activity [129].

Before neurectomy, an anesthetic block should always be performed so that the patient is aware of the permanent sensory effects that will be present after the neurectomy procedure.

13.5.10 Conclusion

IIN neuropathy usually results from injury to this nerve after surgical procedures in the abdominal region. Patients present with pain in the genital region and upper part of the thigh. The diagnosis is made through the patient's clinical history, physical examination, and complementary exams, such as ultrasound and electroneuromyography. Initial treatment is performed conservatively, with surgery reserved for cases refractory to non-invasive measures.

13.6 Iliohypogastric Nerve Neuropathy

13.6.1 Introduction

Iliohypogastric nerve (IHN) neuropathy is a disease usually associated with surgeries of the abdominal and inguinal region. More rarely, idiopathic IHN cases are identified. The most frequent cause of chronic pain after abdominal surgeries is due to injuries that occurred in the IIN and IHN or branches of the genitofemoral nerve [106, 130].

The pathophysiology of these nerve injuries usually reveals mechanical and/or thermal damage. The heat of the electric scalpel, surgical stitches, prostheses, and fibrosis in the path of the nerves may be involved in the genesis of the disease [106].

The manifestations of IHN neuropathy are already present in the immediate postoperative period of the patient. The most described symptom is neuropathic pain in the inguinal region [130].

The objective of this topic is to describe the anatomy of the IHN and the treatment of IHN neuropathy.

13.6.2 Anatomy of the Iliohypogastric Nerve

The IHN is a mixed type nerve that is responsible for the sensory innervation of the skin located in the hypogastrium, upper and lateral gluteal portion, and for supplying motor fibers to the lower part of the obliquus internus abdominis and transversus abdominis muscles.

It usually originates from the ventral branch of the spinal nerve L1; however, some or all of its fibers may originate from the spinal nerve T12.

The IHN is positioned more cranially than the ilioinguinal nerve. The IHN once formed crosses the psoas major muscle and leaves it at its superior lateral edge. It is a nerve that has an oblique trajectory behind the kidneys, passing on the anterior surface of the quadratus lumborum muscle at the level of the L1/L2 intervertebral disc.

After passing adjacent to the quadratus lumborum muscle, this nerve presents a trajectory in the lateral abdominal wall region until it pierces the aponeurosis of the transversus abdominis muscle at a cranial point, between the anterior superior iliac spine and the end of the 12th rib. From this point, the IHN follows a route under the aponeurosis of the obliquus internus abdominis muscle.

About 3 cm medial to the anterior superior iliac spine, the IHN can be identified in a plane, between the transversus abdominis and obliquus internus abdominis muscles. From this location, the nerve presents a course parallel to the inguinal ligament, under the aponeurosis of the obliquus externus abdominis muscle, but at a point cranial to the ilioinguinal nerve [130–136] (Fig. 13.8).

13.6.3 Iliohypogastric Neuralgia Diagnosis

IHN neuropathy can occur spontaneously due to congenital tendinous bands or as a result of complications from surgical procedures performed in the lower abdominal wall or inguinal region. Among the surgeries most often described as causing this neuropathy are inguinal herniorrhaphy, appendectomy, gynecological surgeries with Pfannenstiel incision, and retroperitoneal surgeries [130].

The pain resulting from IHN neuropathy is located in the region above the pubis, especially in a territory cranial to the inguinal ligament [130].

A test that can assist in the diagnosis is the performance of a block with local anesthetic at the point medial to the anterior superior iliac spine. Symptom relief after infiltration can strengthen the diagnosis of IHN neuropathy [130].

Imaging exams of the thoracolumbar spine can assist in identifying high lumbar disc herniations, which can cause similar symptoms.

Infiltration of spinal nerves T11, T12, L1, or L2 can assist in the diagnostic process [130].

13.6.4 Infiltration as Treatment for IHN Neuropathy

Cooke et al. (2019), in a retrospective study on infiltration for the treatment of IHN and IIN involving 131 patients, mention that 465 infiltration procedures with local anesthetic and/or triamcinolone were performed. In this study, among other data collected, the efficacy of the first infiltration was evaluated, which showed symptom control in 70% ($n = 69$) of 99 patients, whose data were available, 9% ($n = 9$) showed partial pain control, 18% ($n = 18$) without response, and 3% ($n = 3$) with pain exacerbation. In the group of non-responders, there was statistical significance for the factors' presence of vulvodynia and unilateral pain [137].

13.6.5 Surgical Treatment of IHN Neuropathy

Different modalities of surgical treatments are described for pain control in patients with IHN neuropathy: nerve decompression, neurectomy, and sensory root ganglionectomy [130].

13.6.5.1 Neurectomy for the Treatment of IHN Neuropathy

In this surgical technique, the nerve is severed at a point proximal to the pain region. It is an ablative procedure, in which the patient ends up with a permanent sequel of hypoesthesia in the skin territory innervated by the IHN.

It is indicated for the treatment of cases where nerve decompression failed or in cases where the iliohypogastric nerve is trapped in fibrosis. The success rates of this surgical technique for neuropathic pain control are around 60% [130].

13.6.5.2 Surgical Approach for the Neurectomy of the Iliohypogastric Nerve

The incision presents an inferomedial line that follows the direction of the longitudinal axis of the inguinal ligament. Usually, medial and 2–3 cm cranial to the anterior superior iliac spine, with an extension of approximately 6 cm directed toward the midline. After identifying the subcutaneous tissue plane, this tissue is retracted to expose medially the fibers of the rectus abdominis muscle and laterally, the sheath of the obliquus externus abdominis muscle. From this point, the sheath should be incised, as well as the fibers of the obliquus externus abdominis muscle, about 2 cm cranial to the line of the skin incision. About 3 cm medial to the anterosuperior iliac crest, the iliohypogastric nerve is identified in a plane between the transversus abdominis and obliquus internus abdominis muscles.

Distally, the iliohypogastric nerve perforates the obliquus internus abdominis muscle and continues cranial to the inguinal ligament. In some cases of IHN neuropathy, a fibrotic band may be present pinching the nerve when it leaves the obliquus internus abdominis muscle [130].

Usually, the dissection of the iliohypogastric nerve should proceed medially to the point where the nerve penetrates the scar area secondary to previous surgery, if that is the case in question. Then the nerve is severed as proximally as possible from its exit point from the retroperitoneum.

As this is a neurectomy, the patient will develop a permanent area of hypoesthesia in the hypogastrium [109, 111].

13.6.5.3 Dorsal Root Ganglionectomy

Dorsal root ganglionectomy (DRG) is an ablative treatment modality for patients with IHN who have already undergone nerve decompression/neurectomy without success. The procedure consists of severing the spinal nerve proximal to the sensory ganglion of T11, T12, and L1. It is important to note that this surgery results in a permanent sensory deficit in the inguinal region. The success rate in controlling neuropathic pain reported in the literature is around 50% [138].

13.6.6 Conclusion

IHN neuropathy is a disease usually associated with surgeries in the abdominal and inguinal region. More rarely, cases of idiopathic IHN are identified. Currently, there are different treatment modalities for such neuropathy, such as infiltration with anesthetics/corticosteroids, neurectomies, and ganglionectomies. However, the rates of control of painful symptoms in the literature do not exceed 60%.

References

1. Clinchot DM, Earl JC. Femoral neuropathy. In: Frontera WR, Silver JK, Rizzo TD, editors. Essentials of physical medicine and rehabilitation. 4th ed. Elsevier; 2020. p. 303–6.
2. Basinger H, Hogg JP. Anatomy, abdomen and pelvis: femoral triangle. StatPearls [Internet]. Treasure Island (FL): StatPearls Publishing; 2023.
3. Clar DT, Bordoni B. Anatomy, abdomen and pelvis: femoral region. StatPearls [Internet]. Treasure Island: StatPearls Publishing; 2022.
4. Orebaugh SL. The femoral nerve and its relationship to the lateral circumflex femoral artery. Anesth Analg. 2006;102(6):1859–62.
5. Refai NA, Black AC, Tadi P. Anatomy, bony pelvis and lower limb: thigh femoral nerve. In: StatPearls [Internet]. Treasure Island: StatPearls Publishing; 2024. Available from: https://www.ncbi.nlm.nih.gov/books/NBK556065/
6. Rastrelli M, Tocco-Tussardi I, Tropea S, Rossi CR, Rizzato S, Vindigni V. Transfer of the anterior branch of the obturator nerve for femoral nerve reconstruction and preservation of motor function: a case report. Int J Surg Case Rep. 2018;51:58–61. https://doi.org/10.1016/j.ijscr.2018.08.004. Epub 2018 Aug 9. PMID: 30144711; PMCID: PMC6107892.
7. Chhabra A, Faridian-Aragh N. High-resolution 3-T MR neurography of femoral neuropathy. AJR Am J Roentgenol. 2012;198:3–10.
8. Dumitru D, Amato A, Zwarts M. Electrodiagnostic medicine. Philadelphia: Hanley & Belfus; 2001.
9. Eaton RP, Qualls C, Bicknell J, et al. Structure-function relationships within peripheral nerves in diabetic neuropathy: the hydration hypothesis. Diabetologia. 1996;39:439–46.
10. Finnerup NB, Sindrup SH, Jensen TS. The evidence for pharmacological treatment of neuropathic pain. Pain. 2010;150:573–81.
11. Leung P, Kudrna J. Growth of an intrapelvic pseudotumor associated with a metal-on-metal total hip arthroplasty after revision arthroplasty causing femoral nerve neuropathy. Arthroplasty Today. 2016;2:105–9.
12. Geiger D, Mpinga E, Steves MA, Sugarbaker PH. Femoral neuropathy: unusual presentation for recurrent large-bowel cancer. Dis Colon Rectum. 1998;41:910–3.
13. Gruber H, Peer S, Kovacs P, et al. The ultrasonographic appearance of the femoral nerve and cases of iatrogenic impairment. J Ultrasound Med. 2003;22:163–72.
14. El-Ghanem M, Malik A, Azzam A, et al. Occurrence of femoral nerve injury among patients undergoing transfemoral percutaneous catheterization procedures in the United States. J Vasc Interv Neurol. 2017;9(4):54–8.
15. Kalita J, Misra U, Singh R, Bhoi S. Sports induced femoral neuropathy: review of the literature. Neurol India. 2016;64:1303–4.
16. Flack S, Anderson C. Ultrasound guided lower extremity blocks. Paediatr Anaesth. 2012;22:72–80.
17. Kim DH, Murovic JA, Tiel RL, Kline DG. Intrapelvic and thigh-level femoral nerve lesions: management and outcomes in 119 surgically treated cases. J Neurosurg. 2004;100:989–96.

18. Kimura J. Electrodiagnosis in diseases of nerve and muscle: principles and practice. 4th ed. New York: Oxford Press; 2013.
19. Oh SJ, Hatanaka Y, Ohira M, et al. Clinical utility of sensory nerve conduction of medial femoral cutaneous nerve. Muscle Nerve. 2012;45:195–9.
20. Ducic I, Dellon L, Larson EE. Treatment concepts for idiopathic and iatrogenic femoral nerve mononeuropathy. Ann Plast Surg. 2005;55(4):397–401. https://doi.org/10.1097/01.sap.0000181359.19366.4d.
21. Takao M, Fukuuchi Y, Koto A, et al. Localized hypertrophic mononeuropathy involving the femoral nerve. Neurology. 1999;52:389–92.
22. Siqueira MG, Martins RS. Anatomia cirúrgica das vias de acesso aos nervos periféricos. São Paulo: Dilivros; 2005.
23. Craig A. Nerve compression/entrapment sites of the lower limb. In: Tubbs RS, Rizk E, Shoja MM, Loukas M, Barbaro N, Spinner RJ, editors. Nerves and nerve injuries. Academic Press; 2015. p. 755–70.
24. Riedl O, Frey M. Anatomy of the sural nerve. Plast Reconstr Surg. 2013;131(4):802–10. https://doi.org/10.1097/prs.0b013e3182818cd4.
25. Riedl O, Koemuercue F, Marker M, Hoch D, Haas M, Deutinger M. Sural nerve harvesting beyond the popliteal region allows a significant gain of donor nerve graft length. Plast Reconstr Surg. 2008;122:798–805.
26. Coert JH, Dellon AL. Clinical implications of the surgical anatomy of the sural nerve. Plast Reconstr Surg. 1994;94:850–5.
27. Mahakkanukrauh P, Chomsung R. Anatomical variations of the sural nerve. Clin Anat. 2002;15:263–6.
28. Sokolow P. Zur Anatomie des Nervus suralis beim Menschen und Affen. Z Gesamte Anat. 1933;100:194–217.
29. Aktan Ikiz ZA, Uçerler H, Bilge O. The anatomic features of the sural nerve with an emphasis on its clinical importance. Foot Ankle Int. 2005;26:560–7.
30. Mestdagh H, Drizenko A, Maynou C, Demondion X, Monier R. Origin and make-up of the human sural nerve. Surg Radiol Anat. 2001;23:307–12.
31. Ortiguela ME, Wood MB, Cahill DR. Anatomy of the sural nerve complex. J Hand Surg Am. 1987;12:1119–23.
32. Romanes GJ. Cunningham's textbook of anatomy. 12th ed. Oxford, England: Oxford Medical Publications; 1981.
33. Huelke DF. A study of the formation of the sural nerve in adult man. Am J Phys Anthropol. 1957;15:137–47.
34. Sekiya S, Suzuki R, Miyawaki M, Chiba S, Kumaki K. Formation and distribution of the sural nerve based on nerve fascicle and nerve fiber analyses. Anat Sci Int. 2006;81:84–91.
35. Husson JL, Mathieu M, Briand B, Meadeb J, Barumbi O, Masse A. Syndrome of compression of the external saphenous nerve (or the sural nerve) (in French). Acta Orthop Belg. 1989;55:491–7.
36. Andreassi. Osservazioni intorno all'origine, comportamento e distribuzione dei nervi cutaneo mediale della sura, ramo anastomotico peoniero e cutaneo laterale della sural nell'uomo. Ricerche di Morfologia. 1931;11:83–100.
37. Lange JF, Wijsmuller AR, van Geldere D, Simons MP, Swart R, Oomen J, Kleinrensink GJ, Jeekel J, Lange JF. Feasibility study of three-nerve-recognizing Lichtenstein procedure for inguinal hernia. Br J Surg. 2009;96:1210–4.
38. Bryan BM 3rd, Lutz GE, O'Brien SJ. Sural nerve entrapment after injury to the gastrocnemius: a case report. Arch Phys Med Rehabil. 1999;80(5):604–6. https://doi.org/10.1016/s0003-9993(99)90206-x. PMID: 10326928.
39. Kim KH, Park BK, Kim DH. A case of lateral calcaneal neuropathy: lateral heel pain. Muscle Nerve. 2016;54(4):801–4.
40. Heaslet M, Patel D. Entrapment involving the lateral calcaneal branch of the sural nerve: a case study. J Am Podiatr Med Assoc. 2012;102(1):75–7.

41. Fabre T, Montero C, Gaujard E, Gervais-Dellion F, Durandeau A. Chronic calf pain in athletes due to sural nerve entrapment. A report of 18 cases. Am J Sports Med. 2000;28(5):679–82.
42. Bojovic M, Dimitrijevic S, Olory BCR, Eirale C, AlSeyrafi O, AlBaker AA, Krivokapic B, Jeremic D, DHooghe P. Overview of nerve entrapment syndromes in the foot and ankle. Int Orthop. 2025 Apr;49(4):853-862. https://doi.org/10.1007/s00264-025-06469-5.
43. Mak MS, Chowdhury R, Johnson R. Morton's neuroma: review of anatomy, pathomechanism, and imaging. Clin Radiol. 2021;76(3):235.e15–23. https://doi.org/10.1016/j.crad.2020.10.006.
44. Durlacher L. A treatise on corn, bunions, the diseases of nails and the general management of the feet. London: Simpkin, Marshall and Co; 1845.
45. Morton TG. A peculiar and painful affection of the fourth metatarso-phalangeal articulation. Am J Med Sci. 1876;71:37–45.
46. Murphey MD, Smith WS, Smith SE, et al. From the archives of the AFIP. Imaging of musculoskeletal neurogenic tumors: radiologic-pathologic correlation. Radiographics. 1999;19(5):1253–80.
47. Jain S, Mannan K. The diagnosis and management of Morton's neuroma: a literature review. Foot Ankle Spec. 2013;6(4):307–17.
48. Adelman KA, Wilson G, Wolf JA. Anterior tarsal tunnel syndrome. J Foot Surg. 1988;27(4):299–302.
49. Morscher E, Ulrich J, Dick W. Morton's intermetatarsal neuroma: morphology and histological substrate. Foot Ankle Int. 2000;21(7):558–62.
50. Sharma S, Bhardwaj S. Variation in the presence of the communicating branch of lateral plantar nerve. Sch J App Med Sci. 2015;3(2F):922–4.
51. Govsa F, Bilge O, Ozer MA. Anatomical study of the communicating branches between the medial and lateral plantar nerves. Surg Radiol Anat. 2005;27(5):377–81.
52. Frank PW, Bakkum BW, Darby SA. The communicating branch of the lateral plantar nerve: a descriptive anatomic study. Clin Anat. 1996;9(4):237–43.
53. Levitsky KA, Alman BA, Jevsevar DS, et al. Digital nerves of the foot: anatomic variations and implications regarding the pathogenesis of interdigital neuroma. Foot Ankle. 1993;14(4):208–14.
54. Jones JR, Klenerman L. A study of the communicating branch between the medial and lateral plantar nerves. Foot Ankle. 1984;4(6):313–5.
55. Hassouna H, Singh D. Morton's metatarsalgia: pathogenesis, aetiology and current management. Acta Orthop Belg. 2005;71(6):646–55.
56. Mulder JD. The causative mechanism in Morton's metatarsalgia. J Bone Joint Surg Br. 1951;33-B(1):94–5.
57. Sobiesk GA, Wertheimer SJ, Schulz R, et al. Sonographic evaluation of interdigital neuromas. J Foot Ankle Surg. 1997;36(5):364–6.
58. Maeseneer MD, Madani H, Lenchik L, et al. Normal anatomy and compression areas of nerves of the foot and ankle: US and MR imaging with anatomic correlation. Radiographics. 2015;35(5):1469–82.
59. Quinn TJ, Jacobson JA, Craig JG, et al. Sonography of Morton's neuromas. AJR Am J Radiol. 2000;174(6):1723–8.
60. Thomson CE, Beggs I, Martin DJ, et al. Methylprednisolone injections for the treatment of Morton neuroma: a patient-blinder randomized trial. J Bone Joint Surg Am. 2013;95(9):790–8.
61. Stepan JG, London DA, Boyer MI, et al. Blood glucose levels in diabetic patients following corticosteroid injections into the hand and wrist. J Hand Surg Am. 2014;39(4):706–12.
62. Shin WY, An MJ, Im NG, et al. Changes in blood glucose level after steroid injection for musculoskeletal pain in patients with diabetes. Ann Rehabil Med. 2020;44(2):117–24.
63. Saygi B, Yildirim Y, Saygi EK, et al. Morton neuroma: comparative results of two conservative methods. Foot Ankle Int. 2005;26(7):556–9.
64. McGlamry ED, Banks AS, Downey MS. Comprehensive textbook of foot surgery. Baltimore: Williams & Wilkins; 1992. p. 304–20.

65. Thomson CE, Gibson JN, Martin D. Interventions in the treatment of Morton's neuroma. Cochrane Database Syst Rev. 2004;2004(3):CD003118.
66. Singh SK, Ioli JP, Chiodo CP. The surgical treatment of Morton's neuroma. Curr Orthop. 2005;19(5):379–84.
67. Mann RA, Reynolds JC. Interdigital neuroma—a critical clinical analysis. Foot Ankle. 1983;3:238–43.
68. Coughlin MJ, Pinsonneault T. Operative treatment of interdigital neuroma: a long-term follow-up study. J Bone Joint Surg. 2001;83A:1321–8.
69. Johnson JE, Johnson KA, Unni KK. Persistent pain after excision of an interdigital neuroma: results of reoperation. J Bone Joint Surg Am. 1988;70:651–7.
70. Beskin JL, Baxter DE. Recurrent pain following interdigital neurectomy—a plantar approach. Foot Ankle. 1988;9:34–9.
71. Bradshaw C, McCrory P, Bell S, Brukner P. Obturator nerve entrapment: a cause of groin pain in athletes. Am J Sports Med. 1997;25:402–8.
72. Brukner P, Bradshaw C, McCrory P. Obturator neuropathy: a cause of exercise-related groin pain. Phys Sportsmed. 1999;27:62–73.
73. Tipton JS. Obturator neuropathy. Curr Rev Musculoskelet Med. 2008;1:234–7. https://doi.org/10.1007/s12178-008-9030-7.
74. Bowman AJ, Carpenter AA, Iovino J, Ward C. Intrapelvic complications of hip surgery: a case report of obturator nerve entrapment. Orthopedics. 1979;2:504–6.
75. Barrick EF. Entrapment of the obturator nerve in association with a fracture of the pelvic ring: a case report. J Bone Joint Surg Am. 1998;80:258–61.
76. Van Ba OL, Wagner L, de Tayrac R. Obturator neuropathy: an adverse outcome of a trans-obturator vaginal mesh to repair pelvic organ prolapse. Int Urogynecol J. 2014;25:145–6.
77. Hong BY, Ko YJ, Kim HW, Lim SH, Cho YR, Lee JI. Intrapartum obturator neuropathy diagnosed after cesarean delivery. Arch Gynecol Obstet. 2010;282:349–50.
78. Langebrekke A, Qvigstad E. Endometriosis entrapment of the obturator nerve after previous cervical cancer surgery. Fertil Steril. 2009;91:622–3.
79. Manny TB, Gorbachinsky I, Hemal AK. Lower extremity neuropathy after robot-assisted laparoscopic radical prostatectomy and radical cystectomy. Can J Urol. 2010;17:5390–3.
80. Holub Z. Obturator neuropathy after laparoscopic retroperitoneal surgery. Int J Gynaecol Obstet. 2006;95:165–6.
81. Tshabalala ZN, Human-Baron R, van der Walt S, Louw EM, van Schoor AN. The anatomy of the obturator nerve and its branches in a South African cadaver sample. Transl Res Anat. 2022;27:100201.
82. Wasse M. Interadductor approach to obturator nerve blockade for spastic conditions of adductor thigh muscles. Anesthesiol Pain Med. 1993;18(1):13–7.
83. Larson MR, Ryan W. Anatomy, abdomen and pelvis, obturator muscles. In: StatPearls [Internet]. Treasure Island: StatPearls Publishing; 2024. [cited 2023 Sep 29]. Available from: https://www.ncbi.nlm.nih.gov/books/NBK589636/
84. Vloka JD, Hadić A. Obturator and genitofemoral nerve blocks. Tech Reg Anesth Pain Manag. 1999;3(1):28–32.
85. Ricciardi E, Jakimovska M, Maniglio P, Schimberni M, Frega A, Kobal B, Moscarini M. Laparoscopic injury of the obturator nerve during fertility-sparing procedure for cervical cancer. World J Surg Oncol. 2012;10(1):1–3.
86. Moore KL, Dalley AF, Agur AM. Clinically oriented anatomy. 8th ed. Wolters Kluwer Health; 2013. p. 555–7.
87. Kumka M. Critical sites of entrapment of the posterior division of the obturator nerve: anatomical considerations. J Can Chiropr Assoc. 2010;54(1):33.
88. Anagnostopoulou S, Kostopanagiotou G, Paraskeuopoulos T, Chantzi C, Lolis E, Saranteas T. Anatomic variations of the obturator nerve in the inguinal region: implications in conventional and ultrasound regional anesthesia techniques. Anesthesiol Pain Med. 2009;34(1):33–9.
89. Tubbs RS, Salter EG, Wellons JC III, Blount JP, Oakes WJ. Anatomical landmarks for the lumbar plexus on the posterior abdominal wall. J Neurosurg Spine. 2005;2(3):335–8.

90. Akkaya T, Comert A, Kendir S, Acar H, Gumus H, Tekdemir I, Elhan A. Detailed anatomy of accessory obturator nerve blockade. Minerva Anestesiol. 2008;74(4):119–22.
91. Anloague PA, Huijbregts P. Anatomical variations of the lumbar plexus: a descriptive anatomy study with proposed clinical implications. J Man Manip Ther. 2009;17(4):107E–14E. https://doi.org/10.1179/106698109791352201.
92. Dawson DM, Hallet M, Wilbourn AJ. Miscellaneous uncommon syndromes of the lower extremity. In: Entrapment neuropathies. 3rd ed. Philadelphia: Lippincott-Raven; 1988. p. 369–79.
93. Mumenthaler M, Schliack H. Lesions of individual nerves of the lower limb plexus and the lower extremity. In: Peripheral nerve lesions: diagnosis and therapy. New York: Thieme Medical Publishers; 1991. p. 297–343.
94. Kendir S, Akkaya T, Comert A, Sayin M, Tatlisumak E, Elhan A, et al. The location of the obturator nerve: a three-dimensional description of the obturator canal. Surg Radiol Anat. 2008;30:495–501.
95. Locher S, Burmeister H, Bohlen T, Eichenberger U, Stoupis C, Moriggl B, et al. Obturator nerve block: a technique based on anatomical findings and MRI analysis. Pain Med. 2008;9:1012–5.
96. Yamamuchi M, Sato Y. Ultrasound-guided obturator nerve block. Masui. 2008;57:588–95.
97. Felsenthal G. Nerve blocks in the lower extremities: anatomical considerations. Arch Phys Med Rehabil. 1974;55:504–7.
98. Sorenson EJ, Chen JJ, Daube JR. Obturator neuropathy: causes and outcome. Muscle Nerve. 2002;25:605–7.
99. Menderes G, Vilardo N, Schwab CL, Azodi M. Incidental injury and repair of obturator nerve during laparoscopic pelvic lymphadenectomy. Gynecol Oncol. 2016;142(1):208. https://doi.org/10.1016/j.ygyno.2016.05.023.
100. Kitagawa P, Kim D, Reid N, Kline D. Surgical management of obturator nerve lesions. Neurosurgery. 2009;65:A24.
101. Fricker RM, Troeger H, Pfeiffer KM. Obturator nerve palsy due to fixation of an acetabular reinforcement ring with transacetabular screws: a case report. J Bone Joint Surg Am. 1997;79:444–6.
102. Bradshaw C, McCrory P. Obturator nerve entrapment. Clin J Sport Med. 1997;7:217–9.
103. Kastler A, Aubry S, Piccand V, Hadjidekov G, Tiberghien F, Kastler B. Radiofrequency neurolysis versus local nerve infiltration in 42 patients with refractory chronic inguinal neuralgia. Pain Physician. 2012 May–Jun;15(3):237-44. PMID: 22622908.
104. Loos MJ, Roumen RM, Scheltinga MR. Chronic sequelae of common elective groin hernia repair. Hernia. 2007;11(2):169–73. https://doi.org/10.1007/s10029-007-0185-x.
105. Hammoud M, Gerken J. Inguinal Hernia. In: StatPearls [Internet]. Treasure Island: StatPearls Publishing; 2023. [PubMed: 30020704]
106. Elsakka KM, Das JM, Leslie SW, et al. Ilioinguinal Neuralgia. [Updated 2024 Feb 18]. In: StatPearls [Internet]. Treasure Island: StatPearls Publishing; 2024. Available from: https://www.ncbi.nlm.nih.gov/books/NBK538256/
107. Whiteside JL, Barber MD, Walters MD, Falcone T. Anatomy of ilioinguinal and iliohypogastric nerves in relation to trocar placement and low transverse incisions. Am J Obstet Gynecol. 2003;189(6):1574–8. discussion 1578. [PubMed: 14710069]
108. Ndiaye A, Diop M, Ndoye JM, Konaté I, Ndiaye AI, Mané L, et al. Anatomical basis of neuropathies and damage to the ilioinguinal nerve during repairs of groin hernias (about 100 dissections). Surg Radiol Anat. 2007;29(8):675–81. [PubMed: 17985072]
109. Starling JR, Harms BA, Schroeder ME, Eichman PL. Diagnosis and treatment of genitofemoral and ilioinguinal entrapment neuralgia. Surgery. 1987;102(4):581–6. [PubMed: 3660235]
110. Cho HM, Park DS, Kim DH, Nam HS. Diagnosis of ilioinguinal nerve injury based on electromyography and ultrasonography: a case report. Ann Rehabil Med. 2017;41(4):705–8. [PMC free article: PMC5608680] [PubMed: 28971057]

111. Kim DH, Murovic JA, Tiel RL, Kline DG. Surgical management of 33 ilioinguinal and iliohypogastric neuralgias at Louisiana State University Health Sciences Center. Neurosurgery. 2005;56(5):1013–20. discussion 1013–20. [PubMed: 15854249]
112. Al Qaraghli MI, De Jesus O. Lumbar Disc Herniation. [Updated 2023 Aug 23]. In: StatPearls [Internet]. Treasure Island (FL): StatPearls Publishing; 2024. Available from: https://www.ncbi.nlm.nih.gov/books/NBK560878/
113. Santilli AR, Martinez-Thompson JM, Speelziek SJA, Staff NP, Laughlin RS. Femoral neuropathy: A clinical and electrodiagnostic review. Muscle Nerve. 2024;69(1):64–71. doi: https://doi.org/10.1002/mus.27994. Epub 2023 Nov 8. Erratum in: Muscle Nerve. 2024 Apr;69(4):505. https://doi.org/10.1002/mus.28055.
114. Gomez YC, Remotti E, Momah DU, Zhang E, Swanson DD, Kim R, et al. Meralgia Paresthetica review: update on presentation, pathophysiology, and treatment. Health Psychol Res. 2023;(11):71454. https://doi.org/10.52965/001c.71454. PMID: 36937080; PMCID: PMC10019995.
115. Lichtenstein IL, Shulman AG, Amid PK, Montllor MM. Cause and prevention of postherniorrhaphy neuralgia: a proposed protocol for treatment. Am J Surg. 1988;155(6):786–90. [PubMed: 3377120]
116. ter Meulen BC, Peters EW, Wijsmuller A, Kropman RF, Mosch A, Tavy DL. Acute scrotal pain from idiopathic ilioinguinal neuropathy: diagnosis and treatment with EMG-guided nerve block. Clin Neurol Neurosurg. 2007;109(6):535–7.
117. Bischoff JM, Petersen M, Uçeyler N, Sommer C, Kehlet H, Werner MU. Lidocaine patch (5%) in treatment of persistent inguinal postherniorrhaphy pain: a randomized, double-blind, placebo-controlled, crossover trial. Anesthesiology. 2013;119(6):1444–52. [PubMed: 23887198]
118. Bischoff JM, Ringsted TK, Petersen M, Sommer C, Uçeyler N, Werner MU. A capsaicin (8%) patch in the treatment of severe persistent inguinal postherniorrhaphy pain: a randomized, double-blind, placebo-controlled trial. PLoS One. 2014;9(10):e109144. [PMC free article: PMC4188585] [PubMed: 25290151]
119. Amid PK, Hiatt JR. New understanding of the causes and surgical treatment of postherniorrhaphy inguinodynia and orchalgia. J Am Coll Surg. 2007;205(2):381–5.
120. Sen H, Sizlan A, Yanarateş O, Senol MG, Inangil G, Sücüllü I, et al. The effects of gabapentin on acute and chronic pain after inguinal herniorrhaphy. Eur J Anaesthesiol. 2009;26(9):772–6.
121. Khan JS, Rai A, Sundara Rajan R, Jackson TD, Bhatia A. A scoping review of perineural steroids for the treatment of chronic postoperative inguinal pain. Hernia. 2016;20(3):367–76.
122. Bischoff JM, Koscielniak-Nielsen ZJ, Kehlet H, Werner MU. Ultrasound-guided ilioinguinal/iliohypogastric nerve blocks for persistent inguinal postherniorrhaphy pain: a randomized, double-blind, placebo-controlled, crossover trial. Anesth Analg. 2012;114(6):1323–9.
123. Campos NA, Chiles JH, Plunkett AR. Ultrasound-guided cryoablation of genitofemoral nerve for chronic inguinal pain. Pain Physician. 2009;12(6):997–1000. [PubMed]
124. Smiley A, McGuire J. Cryoneurolysis for the treatment of sensory nerve pain. AANA J. 2018;86(6):495–503. [PubMed]
125. Friedman T, Richman D, Adler R. Sonographically guided cryoneurolysis: preliminary experience and clinical outcomes. J Ultrasound Med. 2012;31(12):2025–34. [PubMed]
126. Elias M. Spinal cord stimulation for post-herniorrhaphy pain. Neuromodulation. 2000;3(3):155–7. [PubMed]
127. Schu S, Gulve A, ElDabe S, Baranidharan G, Wolf K, Demmel W, et al. Spinal cord stimulation of the dorsal root ganglion for groin pain-a retrospective review. Pain Pract. 2015;15(4):293–9.
128. Werner MU, Bischoff JM, Rathmell JP, Kehlet H. Pulsed radiofrequency in the treatment of persistent pain after inguinal herniotomy: a systematic review. Reg Anesth Pain Med. 2012;37(3):340–3.
129. Siqueira MG, Martins RS. Lesões traumáticas de nervos periféricos. 1st ed; 2022.

130. Melville K, Schultz EA, Dougherty JM. Ilionguinal-iliohypogastric nerve entrapment. Ann Emerg Med. 1990;19:925–9.
131. Eckmann. Ein Beitrag zur Kenntnis des terminalen Verlaufs des N. ilioinguinalis. Anat Anz. 1976;140:15–30.
132. Katkhouda N, Mavor E, Friedlander MH, et al. Use of fibrin sealant for prosthetic mesh fixation in laparoscopic extraperitoneal inguinal hernia repair. Ann Surg. 2001;233:18–25.
133. Köninger J, Redecke J, Butters M. Chronic pain after hernia repair: a randomized trial comparing Shouldice, Lichtenstein and TAPP Langenbecks. Arch Surg. 2004;389:361–5.
134. Pitman AG, Moss D, Stringer MD. Posterior abdominal wall and retroperitoneum. In: Standring S, editor. Gray's anatomy: anatomical basis of clinical practice. Amsterdam: Elsevier; 2016.
135. Poobalan AS, Bruce J, King PM, Chambers WA, Krukowski ZH, Smith WC. Chronic pain and quality of life following open inguinal hernia repair. Br J Surg. 2001;88(8):1122–6.
136. Rauchwerger JJ, Giordano J, Rozen D, Sehgal N. On the therapeutic viability of peripheral nerve stimulation for ilioinguinal neuralgia: putative mechanisms and possible utility. Pain Pract. 2008;8(2):138–43.
137. Cooke CM, Flaxman TE, Chen I, Singh SS. Safety and efficacy of ilioinguinal and iliohypogastric nerve blocks for treatment of pelvic pain. J Endometr Pelvic Pain Disord. 2019;11(1):37–44. https://doi.org/10.1177/2284026518823383.
138. Vanderlinden RG, Midha R, Vanderlinden L. Ilioinguinal/iliohypogastric neuropathy. In: Bendavid R, Abrahamson J, Arregui ME, Flament JB, Phillips EH, editors. Abdominal wall hernias. New York: Springer; 2001. p. 697–702. https://doi.org/10.1007/978-1-4419-8574-3_115.

Index

M. J. S. Magalhães, *Lower Extremity Nerve Entrapments*,
https://doi.org/10.1007/978-3-031-90058-7

MIX
Papier aus verantwortungsvollen Quellen
Paper from responsible sources
FSC® C105338

If you have any concerns about our products,
you can contact us on
ProductSafety@springernature.com

In case Publisher is established outside the EU,
the EU authorized representative is:
Springer Nature Customer Service Center GmbH
Europaplatz 3, 69115 Heidelberg, Germany

Printed by Libri Plureos GmbH
in Hamburg, Germany